The W
Hema
Subs

The Washington Manual™ Hematology and Oncology Subspecialty Consult

Faculty Advisor
Morey Blinder, M.D.
Associate Professor
Department of Medicine
Hematology Division
Department of Pathology and Immunology
Laboratory Medicine Division
Washington University School of Medicine
St. Louis, Missouri

The Washington Manual™ Hematology and Oncology Subspecialty Consult

Editors

Giancarlo Pillot, M.D.
Resident Physician
Department of Internal Medicine
Washington University School of Medicine
Barnes-Jewish Hospital
St. Louis, Missouri

Marcia L. Chantler, M.D.
Assistant Professor of Medicine
Director of Palliative Care and Pain Center
Department of Medical Oncology
Eastern Virginia Medical School of the
Medical College of Hampton Roads
Norfolk, Virginia

Holly M. Magiera, M.D.
Resident Physician
Department of Internal Medicine
Washington University School of Medicine
Barnes-Jewish Hospital
St. Louis, Missouri

Shachar Peles, M.D., M.B.B.C.H.
Resident Physician
Department of Internal Medicine
Washington University School of Medicine
Barnes-Jewish Hospital
St. Louis, Missouri

Geoffrey L. Uy, M.D.
Resident Physician
Department of Internal Medicine
Washington University School of Medicine
Barnes-Jewish Hospital
St. Louis, Missouri

Judah D. Friedman, M.D.
Resident Physician
Department of Internal Medicine
Washington University School of Medicine
Barnes-Jewish Hospital
St. Louis, Missouri

Matthew A. Ciorba, M.D.
Resident Physician
Department of Internal Medicine
Washington University School of Medicine
Barnes-Jewish Hospital
St. Louis, Missouri

Timothy J. Malins
Medical Student
University of Washington School
    of Medicine
Seattle, Washington

Series Editor
Tammy L. Lin, M.D.
Adjunct Assistant Professor of Medicine
Washington University School of Medicine
St. Louis, Missouri

Series Advisor
Daniel M. Goodenberger, M.D.
Professor of Medicine
Washington University School of Medicine
Chief, Division of Medical Education
Director, Internal Medicine Residency
Program
Barnes-Jewish Hospital
St. Louis, Missouri

 LIPPINCOTT WILLIAMS & WILKINS
A **Wolters Kluwer** Company
Philadelphia · Baltimore · New York · London
Buenos Aires · Hong Kong · Sydney · Tokyo

Acquisitions Editors: Danette Somers and James Ryan
Developmental Editors: Scott Marinaro and Keith Donnellan
Supervising Editor: Steven P. Martin
Production Editor: Brooke Begin, Silverchair Science + Communications
Manufacturing Manager: Colin Warnock
Cover Designer: QT Design
Compositor: Silverchair Science + Communications
Printer: RR Donnelley

Library of Congress Cataloging-in-Publication Data
The Washington manual hematology and oncology subspecialty consult / editors, Giancarlo Pillot ... [et al.].
   p. ; cm. -- (The Washington manual subspecialty consult series)
  Includes bibliographical references and index.
  ISBN 0-7817-4375-3
  1. Cancer--Handbooks, manuals, etc. 2. Oncology--Handbooks, manuals, etc. 3. Hematology--Handbooks, manuals, etc. 4. Blood--Diseases--Handbooks, manuals, etc. I. Title: Hematology and oncology subspecialty consult. II. Pillot, Giancarlo. III. Series.
  [DNLM: 1. Hematologic Diseases--Handbooks. 2. Neoplasms--Handbooks. 3. Diagnosis, Differential--Handbooks. 4. Drug Therapy--methods--Handbooks. WH 120 W319 2003]
  RC262.W265 2003
  616.99'4--dc21

                                           2003047747

The Washington Manual™ is an intent-to-use mark belonging to Washington University in St. Louis to which international legal protection applies. The mark is used in this publication by LWW under license from Washington University.

Care has been taken to confirm the accuracy of the information presented and to describe generally accepted practices. However, the authors, editors, and publisher are not responsible for errors or omissions or for any consequences from application of the information in this book and make no warranty, expressed or implied, with respect to the currency, completeness, or accuracy of the contents of the publication. Application of this information in a particular situation remains the professional responsibility of the practitioner.

The authors, editors, and publisher have exerted every effort to ensure that drug selection and dosage set forth in this text are in accordance with current recommendations and practice at the time of publication. However, in view of ongoing research, changes in government regulations, and the constant flow of information relating to drug therapy and drug reactions, the reader is urged to check the package insert for each drug for any change in indications and dosage and for added warnings and precautions. This is particularly important when the recommended agent is a new or infrequently employed drug.

Some drugs and medical devices presented in this publication have Food and Drug Administration (FDA) clearance for limited use in restricted research settings. It is the responsibility of health care providers to ascertain the FDA status of each drug or device planned for use in their clinical practice.

10 9 8 7 6 5 4 3 2 1

To the memory of
Matthew Arquette, M.D.

Contents

Contributing Authors

Leslie A. Andritsos, M.D.

Fellow
Department of Internal Medicine
Division of Hematology/Oncology
Washington University School of
Medicine
St. Louis, Missouri

Kristan Augustin, Pharm.D.

Clinical Pharmacist
Department of Pharmacy
Barnes-Jewish Hospital
St. Louis, Missouri

Ron Bose, M.D., Ph.D.

Resident Physician
Department of Internal Medicine
Washington University School of
Medicine
Barnes-Jewish Hospital
St. Louis, Missouri

Benjamin B. B. Brennan, M.D.

Resident Physician
Department of Neurology
Washington University School of
Medicine
Barnes-Jewish Hospital
St. Louis, Missouri

Amanda F. Cashen, M.D.

Resident Physician
Department of Internal Medicine
Washington University School of
Medicine
Barnes-Jewish Hospital
St. Louis, Missouri

Marcia L. Chantler, M.D.

Assistant Professor of Medicine
Director of Palliative Care and Pain
Center
Department of Medical Oncology
Eastern Virginia Medical School of the
Medical College of Hampton Roads
Norfolk, Virginia

Matthew A. Ciorba, M.D.

Resident Physician
Department of Internal Medicine
Washington University School of
Medicine
Barnes-Jewish Hospital
St. Louis, Missouri

Charles S. Eby, M.D.

Associate Professor of Pathology and
Medicine
Department of Pathology
Washington University School of
Medicine
St. Louis, Missouri

Judah D. Friedman, M.D.

Resident Physician
Department of Internal Medicine
Washington University School of
Medicine
Barnes-Jewish Hospital
St. Louis, Missouri

Neil S. Horowitz, M.D.

Instructor
Department of Obstetrics and
Gynecology
Division of Gynecologic Oncology
Washington University School of
Medicine
St. Louis, Missouri

Stacey K. Knox, M.D.

Resident Physician
Department of Internal Medicine
Washington University School of
Medicine
Barnes-Jewish Hospital
St. Louis, Missouri

Nicholas H. Laffely, M.D.

Resident Physician
Department of Medicine
Washington University School of
Medicine
Barnes-Jewish Hospital
St. Louis, Missouri

Tammy L. Lin, M.D.

Adjunct Assistant Professor of Medicine
Washington University School of
Medicine
St. Louis, Missouri

Lisa A. Mahnke, M.D., Ph.D.

Clinical and Research Fellow
Department of Internal Medicine
Division of Infectious Diseases
Washington University School of
Medicine
St. Louis, Missouri

Holly M. Magiera, M.D.

Resident Physician
Department of Internal Medicine
Washington University School of
Medicine
Barnes-Jewish Hospital
St. Louis, Missouri

Timothy J. Malins

Medical Student
University of Washington School of
Medicine
Seattle, Washington

Parag J. Parikh, M.D.

Resident Physician
Department of Radiation Oncology
Washington University School of
Medicine
Barnes-Jewish Hospital
St. Louis, Missouri

Shachar Peles, M.D., M.B.B.C.H.

Resident Physician
Department of Internal Medicine
Washington University School of
Medicine
Barnes-Jewish Hospital
St. Louis, Missouri

Giancarlo Pillot, M.D.

Resident Physician
Department of Internal Medicine
Washington University School of
Medicine
Barnes-Jewish Hospital
St. Louis, Missouri

Geoffrey L. Uy, M.D.

Resident Physician
Department of Internal Medicine
Washington University School of
Medicine
Barnes-Jewish Hospital
St. Louis, Missouri

Sarah Waheed, M.D., M.B.B.S.

Resident Physician
Department of Internal Medicine
Washington University School of
Medicine
Barnes-Jewish Hospital
St. Louis, Missouri

Stephen J. Wen, M.D.

Internal Medicine Hospitalist
St. John's Mercy Medical Center
St. Louis, Missouri

Jason D. Wright, M.D.

Fellow
Department of Obstetrics and
Gynecology
Division of Gynecologic Oncology
Washington University School of
Medicine
St. Louis, Missouri

Imran Zoberi, M.D.

Instructor of Radiation Oncology
Washington University School of
Medicine
St. Louis, Missouri

Chairman's Note

Medical knowledge is increasing at an exponential rate, and physicians are being bombarded with new facts at a pace that many find overwhelming. The Washington Manual™ Subspecialty Consult Series was developed in this context for interns, residents, medical students, and other practitioners in need of readily accessible practical clinical information. They therefore meet an important unmet need in an era of information overload.

I would like to acknowledge the authors who have contributed to these books. In particular, Tammy L. Lin, M.D., Series Editor, provided energetic and inspired leadership, and Daniel M. Goodenberger, M.D., Series Advisor, Chief of the Division of Medical Education in the Department of Medicine at Washington University, is a continual source of sage advice. The efforts and outstanding skill of the lead authors are evident in the quality of the final product. I am confident that this series will meet its desired goal of providing practical knowledge that can be directly applied to improving patient care.

Kenneth S. Polonsky, M.D.
Adolphus Busch Professor
Chairman, Department of Medicine
Washington University
School of Medicine
St. Louis, Missouri

Series Preface

The Washington Manual™ Subspecialty Consult Series is designed to provide quick access to the essential information needed to evaluate a patient on a subspecialty consult service. Each manual includes the most updated and useful information on commonly encountered symptoms or diseases and highlights the practical information you need to gather before formulating a plan. Special efforts have been made to organize the information so that these guides will be valuable and trusted companions for medical students, residents, and fellows. They cover everything from questions to ask during the initial consult to issues in subsequent management.

One of the strengths of this series is that it is written by residents and fellows who know how busy a consult service can be, who know what information will be most helpful, and can detail a practical approach to patient care. Each volume is written to provide enough information for you to evaluate a patient until more in-depth reading can be done on a particular topic. Throughout the series, key references are noted, difficult management situations are addressed, and appropriate practice guidelines are included. Another strength of this series is that it was written in concert. All of the guides were designed to work together.

The most important strength of this series is the collection of authors, faculty advisors, and especially lead authors assembled to write this series. In addition, we received incredible commitment and support from our chairman, Kenneth S. Polonsky, M.D. As a result, the extraordinary depth of talent and genuine interest in teaching others at Washington University is showcased in this series. Although there has always been house staff involvement in editing The Washington Manual™ series, it came to our attention that many of them also wanted to be involved in writing and making decisions about what to convey to fellow colleagues. Remarkably, many of the lead authors became junior subspecialty fellows while writing their guides. Their desire to pass on what they were learning, while trying to balance multiple responsibilities, is a testament to their dedication and skills as clinicians, teachers, and leaders.

We hope this series fulfills the need for essential and practical knowledge for those learning the art of consultation in a particular subspecialty and for those just passing through it.

Tammy L. Lin, M.D., Series Editor
Daniel M. Goodenberger, M.D., Series Advisor

Preface

The fields of hematology and oncology are rapidly changing, with a pace of discovery that likely will accelerate over the next several years. Emerging technologies in DNA expression analysis will likely allow for a greater understanding of the pathogenesis of hematologic and oncologic diseases and improved outcome in their treatment.

It is in this exciting and overwhelming time that we are proud to release *The Washington Manual™ Hematology and Oncology Subspecialty Consult*. We have attempted to create a reference for the internist, family practitioner, resident physician, and medical student that covers the basics of hematology and oncology. This volume does not attempt to be a chemotherapy manual nor does it attempt to be an exhaustive reference for the practicing hematologist or oncologist. Rather, its aim is to provide you with the general principles you need for an understanding of hematologic and oncologic disease in the "typical" patient. It provides you with the methods to evaluate common malignancies, including staging, an overview of the most common types of therapies, as well as the expected outcomes for these diseases. Given this information, the reader should be able to initiate an oncologic or hematologic evaluation, understand what information a consulted physician needs to see, and understand what is done with this information. It also gives the student or resident on a consult service the "basics" to aid with the evaluation of the patient.

A word of caution: Given the rapid changes in the field of hematology and oncology, one should be careful to access the most up-to-date sources regarding therapy. Chemotherapeutics can evolve rapidly, and a new chemotherapy manual is an invaluable reference. In addition, the staging of cancers is an evolving science. The newest American Joint Committee on Cancer staging manuals should be referred to for the newest staging systems. Although we have made every effort to ensure the accuracy and currency of this volume, errors in publication can occur. There is also considerable variation in management per local custom, as well as different interpretations of the currently available clinical evidence. As always, clinical judgment and experience are paramount in selecting the evaluation and therapy that are most appropriate for your individual patient, and this guide is not a substitute for these qualities.

We would like to express our gratitude for the reviewing attending physicians of the Washington University Medical Center and Barnes-Jewish Hospital in St. Louis, Missouri. Without their efforts, this manual could not have been written: Dr. Morey Blinder, Dr. Charles S. Eby, Dr. Philip Majerus, Dr. Douglas Tollefsen, Dr. Ramsaswamy Govindan, Dr. Joel Picus, Dr. Hanna Khouri, Dr. William Read III, Dr. William Clutter, Dr. Imran Zoberi, and Dr. J. Simpson.

G.P.
M.L.C.
H.M.M.
S.P.
G.L.U.
J.D.F.
M.A.C.

Key to Abbreviations

ACE	angiotensin-converting enzyme
ACTH	adrenocorticotropic hormone
AFP	alpha-fetoprotein
aPTT	activated partial thromboplastin time
ASA	acetylsalicylic acid
BP	blood pressure
CBC	complete blood count
CT	computed tomography
cDNA	complementary deoxyribonucleic acid
CMV	cytomegalovirus
CNS	central nervous system
DIC	disseminated intravascular coagulation
DNA	deoxyribonucleic acid
EBV	Epstein-Barr virus
ELISA	enzyme-linked immunosorbent assay
GI	gastrointestinal
GTP	guanosine triphosphate
hCG	human chorionic gonadotropin
Hct	hematocrit
HELLP	hemolysis, elevated liver enzymes, and low platelet (count)
Hgb	hemoglobin
HIV	human immunodeficiency virus
HLA	human leukocyte antigen
HTN	hypertension
ICU	intensive care unit
Ig	immunoglobulin
INR	international normalized ratio
LFT	liver function test
MAOIs	monoamine oxidase inhibitors
MESNA	2-mercaptopurine sulphonate sodium
MI	myocardial infarction
MRI	magnetic resonance imaging
NSAIDs	nonsteroidal antiinflammatory drugs
OR	operating room
PMNs	polymorphonuclear neutrophils
PT	prothrombin time
PTH	parathyroid hormone
PTT	partial thromboplastin time
RBC	red blood cell
RNA	ribonucleic acid
SIADH	syndrome of inappropriate secretion of antidiuretic hormone
SLE	systemic lupus erythematosus
TSH	thyroid-stimulating hormone
UA	urinalysis
U/S	ultrasound
VZV	varicella-zoster virus
WBC	white blood cell

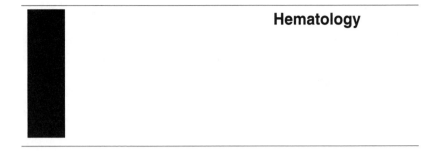

Hematology

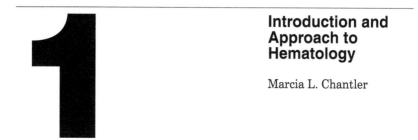

Introduction and Approach to Hematology

Marcia L. Chantler

INTRODUCTION

Primary hematologic diseases are uncommon, whereas secondary hematologic problems occur rather frequently. Therefore, a broad-based knowledge of medicine is important to the differential diagnosis of hematologic abnormalities. The use of the medical history and physical exam is fairly limited in the aid of diagnosing a primary hematologic disease. More information is often obtained from the lab tests. The goal of this handbook is to provide an understanding of the basic mechanisms for the hematologic disorders and the initial evaluation of them. The major clinical manifestations and the usual management options of these diseases are also discussed in each chapter.

APPROACH TO THE HEMATOLOGY PATIENT

Hematologic disorders can be approached by identifying the primary hematologic component that is affected: RBCs, WBCs, platelets, or the coagulation system. The major abnormalities in hematology are quantitative in nature, with either excessive or deficient production of one of the hematopoietic constituents.

History

The medical history is often limited in its usefulness in aiding in the diagnosis of primary hematologic disorders, except in the case of a strong family history for certain disorders, such as hemoglobinopathies or bleeding disorders. However, the medical history is still a key component to help establish a differential diagnosis in hematology. Table 1-1 offers some general questions for evaluation of a hematologic disorder.

Physical Exam

The physical exam is often nonspecific and also limited in its usefulness in the diagnosis of primary hematologic disorders. However, it should not be overlooked. Clues to aid in the differential diagnosis and in the guidance of lab testing are often found on exam. Table 1-2 offers some general physical exam findings that are useful in the hematology patient.

Lab Evaluation

The clinician should become comfortable using the CBC and peripheral smear (see Chap. 2, The Peripheral Smear) to evaluate patients for possible hematologic disorders. The role of the hematologist is to use the specialized lab testing, peripheral blood morphology, and basic pathophysiologic mechanisms to establish a differential diagnosis and to solve complex clinical problems in the field of hematology. Patients may be referred to a hematologist based on a lab abnormality that is drawn for an alternate reason other than the diagnosis of a primary hematologic disorder. The main question

TABLE 1-1. PERTINENT HISTORY IN THE HEMATOLOGY PATIENT

Pertinent medical history	Hematologic differential diagnosis
History of present illness:	
Recent infections:	
Fever, chills, rigors	Leukemias, lymphomas, multiple myeloma
Antibiotic use	Hemolysis
Bleeding:	
Hemorrhage, epistaxis, bleeding gums, petechiae, ecchymosis, menorrhagia	Thrombocytopenia, leukemias, coagulation disorder
Hemarthrosis	Clotting factor deficiency
Skin coloration:	
Pallor	Anemia
Jaundice	Hemolysis
Dyspnea, chest pain, orthostasis	Anemia
Pica	Iron deficiency
Abdominal fullness, early satiety	Splenomegaly
Alcoholism, poor nutrition, vegetarian	Megaloblastic anemia
Neurologic:	
Headache, neurologic deficits	Leukostasis, thrombocytopenia, thrombosis, Waldenström's macroglobulinemia
Pruritus	Polycythemia, Hodgkin's disease
Past medical history:	
Prior malignancies, chemotherapy	Secondary malignancies (leukemia), myelo-dysplasia
HIV risk factors	Anemia, thrombocytopenia
Previous hepatitis	Anemia, cryoglobulinemia
Pregnancy	Anemia, HELLP syndrome
Venous thrombosis	Thrombophilia
Family history:	
Bleeding disorders	Hemophilias, von Willebrand disease
Anemia (African-American, Mediterranean, Asian)	Hemoglobinopathies

HELLP, hemolysis, elevated liver enzymes, and low platelet count.

a practitioner faces is as follows: How abnormal must the test be to indicate a diagnostic or therapeutic action? There are certain limiting values in hematology that can help exclude or confirm the need for further testing or warn us of the possibility of potential physiologic consequences. Some of these limiting values are listed in Table 1-3.

TABLE 1-2. PHYSICAL EXAM IN THE HEMATOLOGY PATIENT

HEENT:	
Conjunctival or mucosal pallor	Anemia
Jaundice	Hemolysis, hyperbilirubinemia
Conjunctival or mucosal petechiae	Thrombocytopenia
Glossitis	Iron deficiency, vitamin B_{12} deficiency
Lymphadenopathy	Lymphoma
Skin/nails:	
Pallor	Anemia
Jaundice	Hyperbilirubinemia
Bronze appearance	Hemochromatosis
Spoon nails (koilonychia)	Iron deficiency
Ecchymosis, petechiae	Thrombocytopenia
Erythematous, indurated plaques	Mycosis fungoides
Cardiovascular:	
Tachycardia, S4, prominent PMI	Severe anemia with high-output cardiac failure
Abdominal:	
Splenomegaly	Hairy cell or other leukemias, polycythemia, lymphomas
Neurologic:	
Loss of vibratory sense and proprioception (dorsal and lateral columns)	Megaloblastic anemia
Musculoskeletal:	
Bone pain/tenderness	Multiple myeloma

HEENT, head, ears, eyes, nose, and throat.

KEY POINTS TO REMEMBER

- Hematologists are involved in the evaluation and treatment of bleeding and clotting disorders, blood cell count abnormalities, and abnormalities of blood cell morphology.
- The lab tests that often trigger referral to a hematologist are the CBC, PT, or PTT. There should be an appreciation of the degree and seriousness of the abnormality before any evaluation begins.
- The specific cell line or specific clotting pathway (i.e., intrinsic, extrinsic, or common) that is abnormal should be identified at the beginning of the workup: Is there a WBC, RBC, platelet, or multiple cell line abnormality? In bleeding or clotting, is the problem with platelets or the coagulation cascade (intrinsic, extrinsic, or common)?

TABLE 1-3. DECISION LIMITING VALUES FOR COMMON HEMATOLOGIC TESTS

Diagnostic test	Limiting value	Comments
Hgb	<5 g/dL	Transfusion indicated even in absence of symptoms
	<10 g/dL	Anemia workup indicated
Hct	>70%	Urgent phlebotomy indicated
Platelet count	<10,000/mm^3	Risk of spontaneous bleeding
	<50,000/mm^3	Risk of bleeding increased with surgery/trauma
	>2,000,000/mm^3	Risk for thrombosis
Neutrophil count	<500/mm^3	Greatest risk of infection
Blast count (acute myelo-blastic leukemia)	>100,000/mm^3	Risk of leukostasis, urgent treatment indicated
PT	<1.5 × control	No increased bleeding risk
	>2.5 × control	Risk for spontaneous bleeding
PTT	<1.5 × control	No increased bleeding risk
	>2.5 × control (>90 secs)	Risk for spontaneous bleeding
Bleeding time	>20 mins	Risk for spontaneous bleeding
Antithrombin III	<50% normal level	Risk for spontaneous thrombosis

REFERENCES AND SUGGESTED READINGS

Diggs LW, Sturm D, Bell A. *The morphology of human blood cells*. Abbott Park, IL: Abbott Laboratories, 1984:3–16.

Scnall SF, Berliner N, et al. Approach to the adult and child with anemia. In: Hoffman R, Silberstein LE, Benz EJ, et al., eds. *Hematology: basic principles and practice*. New York: Churchill Livingstone, 2000:367–382.

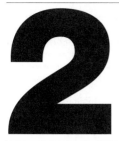

The Peripheral Smear

Shachar Peles

INTRODUCTION

Careful review of the peripheral smear should be included as part of the evaluation of every CBC. It represents an inexpensive yet powerful diagnostic test, and the information obtained, when combined with other clinical data, may allow determination of a definitive diagnosis. This chapter briefly reviews the elements of the peripheral smear and its evaluation. The reader should refer to a hematology atlas for visual representation of the cells referred to in the text. However, the best teacher of cell morphology is *frequent review of peripheral smears*. Automated hematology analyzers provide a large amount of data about blood counts and cell morphology and may even suggest a diagnosis. These machines, however, may not detect certain more subtle abnormalities. In addition, some diseases may have normal cell counts but abnormal cell morphology. In certain situations, such as suspected thrombotic thrombocytopenic purpura (TTP), hemolytic uremic syndrome (HUS) or RBC inclusion diseases such as malaria, review of the smear is mandatory.

PREPARATION

Slides for peripheral smear are typically prepared either by automated methods or by qualified technicians in a central laboratory and are rarely prepared by physicians today. Smears may be prepared on glass slides or coverslips. Ideally, blood smears should be prepared from uncoagulated blood and from a sample collected from a fingerstick. In practice, the vast majority of slides are prepared from blood samples containing anticoagulant and are thus prone to the introduction of morphologic artifacts. The general principle in making a slide or a coverslip involves placing a drop of blood on the slide and "smearing" it across the slide. The amount of blood placed on the coverslip or slide should not be too much or too little, as to avoid producing too thick or too thin a smear.

EXAM

Exam of the smear should proceed systematically and begin under low power to identify a portion of the slide with optimal cellular distribution and staining. RBCs in this part of the slide should be evenly spaced and should be almost touching one another but not overlapping. *Rouleaux formation* refers to RBCs that appear to stick together like stacked coins. This may represent artifact in thicker sections of the slide or may represent the presence of a myeloma paraprotein coating the red cells and resulting in loss of electrostatic repulsion between them. Under *low* power, one can also estimate the WBC count and determine the presence of abnormal populations of cells, such as blasts, by scanning over the entire smear. Under *high* power, each of the cell lineages is examined for any abnormalities in number of cells or morphology.

RBCs

- **Quantitative** assessment of RBCs is difficult on a peripheral smear. The diameter of the red cell should be approximately the same as a lymphocyte nucleus ($8\,\mu$m). Variation in red cell size is known as *anisocytosis*. Larger well-hemoglobinated cells are known as *macrocytes*, with smaller cells being known as *microcytes*. *Automated counters* measure RBC size as the mean cell volume. An erroneously normal mean cell volume may be reported if there are populations of both macrocytic and microcytic cells in the blood whose sizes "average each other out." This situation results in an elevation of the RBC distribution width, but exam of a smear would be required to appreciate these differing populations of cells.

- RBCs should be round with smooth cell membranes. Variation in shape of RBCs is known as *poikilocytosis*. Large oval cells are seen in megaloblastic anemia owing to vitamin B_{12} or folate deficiency. Schistocytes or red cell fragments and helmet cells are a feature of microangiopathic hemolytic anemia seen in TTP or DIC.
- RBCs should have a pale central area with a round rim of red hemoglobin. A very thin rim of hemoglobin and a larger pale area represent hypochromia. These red cells are often microcytic and are seen in iron deficiency—thalassemias and sideroblastic anemia. The reverse, termed *hyperchromia*, represents an increased hemoglobin concentration. Spherocytes are round, dense cells, lacking an area of central pallor and are found in autoimmune hemolytic anemia and hereditary spherocytosis. An increase in the ratio of cell membrane surface area to hemoglobin volume within the cell results in the formation of target cells. These have a central spot of hemoglobin surrounded by a ring of pallor, giving them a bull's eye appearance. The remnant RNA present in the cytoplasm of the less mature, macrocytic reticulocytes gives the cytoplasm a bluish tinge (polychromatophilia). In addition, the red cell cytoplasm may contain a variety of inclusions (detailed later).

RBC Abnormalities

- **Microcytosis:** (cells $<7\,\mu m$). Differential diagnosis includes iron-deficiency anemia, anemia of chronic disease, thalassemias, and sideroblastic anemia. These cells are usually hypochromic and have prominent central pallor.
- **Macrocytosis:** (cells $>8\,\mu m$). Seen in liver disease, alcoholism, aplastic anemia, and myelodysplasia. Megaloblastic anemias (B_{12} and folate deficiencies) have macroovalocytes—large oval cells. *Reticulocytes* are large immature red cells with polychromatophilia.
- **Schistocytes and helmet cells:** (fragmented cells). Caused by mechanical disruption of cells in the microvasculature by fibrin strands or by mechanical prosthetic heart valves. Differential diagnosis includes TTP/HUS; DIC; hemolysis, elevated liver enzymes, and low platelet count syndrome; and malignant HTN.
- **Acanthocyte/spur cell:** (spiculated cell with irregular projections of varying length). Seen in liver disease.
- **Burr cell/echinocyte/crenated cell:** (cell with short, evenly spaced cytoplasmic projections). May be an artifact of slide preparation or found in renal failure and uremia.
- **Bite cell:** (smooth semicircle extracted from cell). Due to spleen phagocytes that have removed Heinz bodies consisting of denatured hemoglobin. Found in hemolytic anemia due to glucose-6-phophate dehydrogenase deficiency.
- **Spherocyte:** (round, dense cell with absent central pallor). Seen in immune hemolytic anemia and hereditary spherocytosis.
- **Sickle cell:** (sickle-shaped cell). Due to polymerization of Hgb S. Found in sickle cell disease as well as SC disease but not in sickle cell trait.
- **Target cell:** (cell with extra Hgb in center surrounded by rim of pallor; bull's eye appearance). Due to redundancy of cell membrane. Found in liver disease, postsplenectomy, hemoglobinopathies, and thalassemia.
- **Teardrop cell/dacryocyte:** (teardrop-shaped cell). Found in myelofibrosis and myelophthisic states of marrow infiltration.
- **Ovalocyte:** (elliptical cell). Due to abnormal membrane cytoskeleton found in hereditary elliptocytosis.
- **Polychromatophilia:** (blue hue of cytoplasm). Due to presence of RNA and ribosomes in reticulocytes.
- **Howell-Jolly bodies:** (small, single purple cytoplasmic inclusions). Represent nuclear remnant DNA and are found after splenectomy or with functional asplenism.

- **Basophilic stippling:** (dark purple inclusions, usually multiple). Precipitated RNA found in lead poisoning and thalassemia.
- **Nucleated red cells:** Not normally found in peripheral blood. Found in hypoxemia and myelofibrosis or other myelophthisic condition, as well as with severe hemolysis.
- **Heinz bodies:** (inclusions seen only on staining with crystal violet). Represent denatured hemoglobin. Found in glucose-6-phosphate dehydrogenase after oxidative stress.
- **Parasites:** A variety of parasites, including malaria and babesiosis, may be seen within red cells.
- **Pappenheimer bodies:** (dark blue granules). Iron-containing granules found in sideroblastic anemia.
- **Rouleaux:** (red cell aggregates resembling a stack of coins). Loss of normal electrostatic charge repelling red cells due to coating by abnormal paraprotein such as in multiple myeloma.
- **Leukoerythroblastic smear:** (teardrop cells, nucleated red cells, and immature white cells). Found in marrow infiltration or fibrosis (myelophthisic conditions).

Platelets

- Platelets appear as small purplish cytoplasmic fragments, containing red/blue granules. They are 1–2 μm in diameter. Large platelets represent an accelerated marrow response, which may be associated with increased platelet destruction (e.g., in immune thrombocytopenic purpura).
- The platelet count can be estimated from the peripheral smear. The number of platelets per high-power field multiplied by 20,000 usually estimates the platelet count per μL. Alternatively, one should find one platelet for every 10–20 red cells. Pseudothrombocytopenia represents clumping of platelets in blood samples collected in ethylenediaminetetraacetic acid (EDTA), resulting in spuriously low platelet counts. These platelet clumps may be seen on the peripheral smear. This phenomenon can be avoided by using citrate to anticoagulate blood samples sent for blood counts.

WBCs

WBCs normally seen on the peripheral smear include neutrophils, lymphocytes, eosinophils, monocytes, and basophils. The presence of immature myeloid and lymphoid cells is abnormal. When performing a manual WBC differential, one should count at least 100 cells. When counting different populations of WBC counts, one should also be on the lookout for abnormal cellular morphology.

Neutrophils

- Neutrophils have nuclei containing 3–4 lobes and granular cytoplasm. Hypersegmented neutrophils contain >5 lobes and are found in megaloblastic anemias. Increased prominence of cytoplasmic granules is indicative of systemic infection or therapy with growth factors and is known as *toxic granulation*.
- Neutrophils develop from myeloblasts through promyelocyte, myelocyte, metamyelocyte, and band forms and progress on to mature neutrophils. Only mature neutrophils and bands may be normally found in peripheral blood. Metamyelocytes and myelocytes may be found in pregnancy, infections, and leukemoid reactions. The presence of less mature forms in the peripheral blood is indicative of hematologic malignancy.

Lymphocytes

Lymphocyte cells contain a clumped nucleus and scant rim of blue cytoplasm. Atypical (or reactive) lymphocytes seen in viral infections contain more extensive, malleable cytoplasm that may encompass surrounding red cells.

Eosinophils

Eosinophils are large cells containing prominent red/orange granules and a bilobed nucleus. Increased numbers are found in parasitic infections and allergic disorders.

Monocytes

Monocytes are the largest of the WBCs. They contain blue cytoplasm and a folded nucleus.

Basophils

Basophils comprise the smallest proportion of WBCs. Their cytoplasm contains dark blue granules. Increased numbers are seen in myeloproliferative disorders (e.g., chronic myeloid leukemia).

WBC Abnormalities

- **Pelger-Huet anomaly:** (neutrophils have a bilobed nucleus connected by a thin strand and decreased granulation). Seen in myelodysplastic syndromes.
- **Hypersegmented neutrophils:** (>5 nuclear lobes). Found in megaloblastic anemias (vitamin B_{12} and folate deficiency).
- **Blast cells:** (myeloblasts or lymphoblasts; large cells with large nuclei and prominent nucleoli). Seen in acute leukemia.
- **Auer rods:** (rod-like granules in blast cytoplasm). Pathognomonic for acute myelogenous leukemia.
- **Hairy cells:** (lymphoid cells with ragged cytoplasm). Seen in hairy cell leukemia.
- **Sézary cells:** (atypical lymphoid cells with cerebriform nuclei). Seen in cutaneous T-cell lymphoma.

KEY POINTS TO REMEMBER

- The peripheral slide should be manually reviewed by the physician in any case involving abnormalities of cell counts or coagulation.
- An area of the slide should be chosen in which RBCs are almost touching when reviewing a smear.
- The peripheral slide should be reviewed systematically every time, looking at every cell line. Failure to do so results in missed diagnoses.
- RBCs are usually monotonous, with one-third of their area demonstrating a central pallor.
- A quick estimation of platelet number is that one platelet per high-powered field equals 20,000 platelets per μL on an automated count.
- Thrombocytopenia discovered on an automatic blood count should first be assessed by review of the slide and resending the sample of blood in a citrate tube (rather than EDTA) to avoid clumping artifact.

REFERENCES AND SUGGESTED READINGS

Lee GR, Foerster J, Lukens J, et al. *Wintrobe's clinical hematology*, 10th ed. Philadelphia: Lippincott Williams & Wilkins, 1998.

Rosenthal DS, Mitus AJ, von Kapff C. Evaluation of the peripheral blood smear. In: Rose BD, ed. *UpToDate*. Wellesley, MA: UpToDate, 2002.

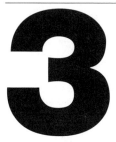

Bone Marrow Evaluation

Shachar Peles

INTRODUCTION

Diagnosis and staging of hematologic disease often requires an exam of the bone marrow. A bone marrow biopsy can be done at the bedside under local anesthesia, although some patients may require low doses of anxiolytics or opioids for the procedure. **Patient comfort** is paramount, especially during the patient's first bone marrow biopsy, as it "sets the stage" for the patient's expectations of subsequent biopsies. The exam of the bone marrow biopsy takes skill and experience and should be performed by those skilled in it. As with features of the peripheral smear, the reader should refer to a hematology atlas for visual examples of elements described herein.

Indications for bone marrow exam include further evaluation of hematologic abnormalities, workup of bone marrow malignancies, staging of marrow involvement by metastatic tumors, assessment of infectious diseases that may involve the bone marrow, and workup of metabolic storage diseases.

TECHNIQUE

The bone marrow biopsy involves aspiration of bone marrow cells as well as needle biopsy of the bone marrow. These are obtained from the posterior iliac crest, the anterior iliac crest, or the sternum, as hematopoiesis is largely limited to the axial skeleton in adults. Most often, the matierals needed to perform a bone marrow biopsy are in pre-packaged and sterilized kits. However, the proper specimen containers may need to be obtained separately. The **posterior iliac crest** is the preferred site, as it allows collection of both aspirate and biopsy specimens and is associated with minimal morbidity or complications. The procedure can be performed with little patient discomfort under local anesthesia, but anxious patients may be sedated. In most cases, a *Jamshidi* bone marrow aspiration and biopsy needle is used. Aspirate smears are often prepared at the bedside, the quality of which is assessed by observing for marrow spicules. Additional aspirate is often obtained for further studies such as flow cytometry, cytogenetics, and cultures. In some instances, marrow cannot be aspirated and only a biopsy is obtained (a "dry tap"). This could be due to technique or may signal myelofibrosis. In such cases, touch preparations of the biopsy can be made to allow for cytologic exam. The biopsy specimen is fixed in formalin before further histologic processing.

BONE MARROW EXAM

- The exam of bone marrow aspirates begins under **low power.** There should be gained an impression of overall cellularity, an initial scan for any abnormal populations of cells or clumps of cells, and an evaluation of the presence or absence of bone marrow spicules. Megakaryocytes are normally seen under low power as large multinucleated cells. Large clumps of cells often seen at the ends of the smear may be metastatic cancer cells or may represent a benign finding such as clumps of osteoblasts. The overall cellularity of the marrow should be estimated by observing the ratio of fat cells to hematopoietic cells. This is usually 30–60% but typically declines with advancing age and can only be reliably assessed on a bone marrow biopsy specimen, owing to possible peripheral blood dilution of aspirates. Increased cellularity may be seen in hematologic malignancies, whereas hypocellularity may be a feature of aplastic anemia or may be found after radiation therapy.

- The **myeloid to erythroid ratio** (M:E ratio) is also determined under low power and is normally 3–4:1. The ratio is increased in chronic myeloid leukemia due to an increase in granulocyte precursors and is increased in pure red cell aplasia due to a decrease of red cell precursors. The ratio is decreased in hemolytic disorders in which increased erythroid precursors are present or is decreased in agranulocytic conditions secondary to chemotherapeutic agents or other drugs.
- Under **high power,** the aspirate should contain a variety of cells representative of various stages in myeloid and erythroid maturation. Myeloid cells progress from myeloblasts to promyelocytes, myelocytes, metamyelocytes, band forms, and then mature neutrophils. As these cells mature, their nuclear chromatin condenses with a resultant decrease in the nuclear:cytoplasmic ratio. Their cytoplasm gradually develops granules seen in mature neutrophils.
- **Erythroid precursors** progress from proerythroblast through varying stages of normoblasts known as *basophilic, chromatophilic,* and *orthochromic.* Again, the nucleus gradually condenses, and the cytoplasm gradually takes on the pinkish hue of Hgb found in mature red cells.

ABNORMALITIES ON THE BONE MARROW SAMPLE

Listed below are some of the more common abnormal findings of the bone marrow. This list is by no means exhaustive, nor does it list all abnormalities noted on each condition.

- **Acute leukemia:** The presence of >20% blasts or immature cells in the bone marrow confirms the diagnosis of acute leukemia. The leukemias are classified as either myeloid or lymphoid. They are further classified on the basis of morphology according to the FAB classification. Acute lymphocytic leukemias consist of three types: L1–L3. Acute myeloid leukemia is classified into eight types: M0–M8.
- **Myelodysplastic syndrome:** This syndrome is characterized by immature erythroid precursors with loss of synchrony between nuclear and cytoplasmic maturation. Mature myeloid cells have decreased lobes (Pelger-Huet cells). Iron staining may reveal ring sideroblasts with iron granules surrounding the nucleus.
- **Chronic myeloid leukemia:** Findings include a hypercellular marrow with an increased M:E ratio. Myeloblasts represent <5% of cells with the marrow containing predominantly myelocytes, metamyelocytes, and mature neutrophils.
- **Chronic lymphocytic leukemia:** Hypercellular marrow with small, round, mature lymphocytes with a thin rim of blue cytoplasm.
- **Myelofibrosis:** This often is the cause of a "dry tap." Bone marrow biopsy will reveal marrow infiltration with collagen and fibrous tissue.
- **Essential thrombocytosis:** Megakaryocyte hyperplasia is a common finding.
- **Polycythemia vera:** This is characterized by a hypercellular marrow.
- **Multiple myeloma:** The marrow is replaced by large numbers of abnormal, often immature plasma cells with eccentric nuclei containing a cartwheel pattern of nuclear chromatin. Flame cells contain pink flame-like cytoplasm and are said to be associated with an IgA paraprotein.
- **Waldenström's macroglobulinemia:** Plasmacytic lymphocytes are seen infiltrating the marrow. These resemble smaller lymphocytes but have more cytoplasm and eccentrically placed nuclei.
- **Megaloblastic anemia:** Hypercellular marrow with abnormalities in myeloid and erythroid precursors. Megaloblasts are erythroid cells that are larger than normal with more nuclear chromatin. Giant megaloblasts and giant band forms are also found. There is loss of synchrony between nuclear and cytoplasmic maturation.
- **Hodgkin's disease:** One may find the characteristic Reed-Sternberg cells infiltrating the bone marrow in conjunction with lymphoid elements.
- **Storage diseases:** Macrophages with striated cytoplasm due to accumulation of cerebrosides may be seen in patients with Gaucher's disease. Individuals with Nie-

mann-Pick disease may have macrophages with a foamy cytoplasm secondary to contained sphingomyelin.

KEY POINTS TO REMEMBER

- Special care should be taken to ensure that a patient's first bone marrow biopsy is as comfortable as possible, as this will set the stage for subsequent biopsies.
- A bone marrow aspirate and biopsy should both be attempted in the bone marrow exam.
- Inability to aspirate bone marrow—a "dry tap"—may be due to technique or may signal myelofibrosis.

REFERENCES AND SUGGESTED READINGS

Lee GR, Foerster J, Lukens J, et al. *Wintrobe's clinical hematology*, 10th ed. Philadelphia: Lippincott Williams & Wilkins, 1998.

Rosenthal DS. Evaluation of bone marrow aspirate smears. In: Rose BD, ed. *UpToDate*. Wellesley, MA: UpToDate, 2002.

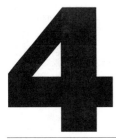

Disorders of Coagulation

Leslie A. Andritsos,
Charles S. Eby, and
Nicholas H. Laffely

INTRODUCTION

Normal coagulation is a complex sequence of reactions involving interactions between platelets, endothelium, and coagulation factors. Primary hemostasis, which is comprised of platelet activation and platelet plug formation, is followed by secondary hemostasis with activation of the coagulation cascade and formation of a stable fibrin complex. Fibrinolysis then limits the extent of thrombosis. Symptoms of mucosal bleeding, such as epistaxis, gum bleeding, hematochezia, melena, petechiae, or easy bruising, are often signs of defective primary hemostasis secondary to thrombocytopenia, platelet dysfunction, or abnormalities of von Willebrand factor (vWF). Hemarthroses, intramuscular hemorrhage, and bleeding into deeper structures are more commonly signs of secondary hemostasis disorders with coagulation factor deficiency or dysfunction. The evaluation of a patient with a coagulation disorder is performed in a systematic fashion and begins with a CBC, aPTT, and PT. Further workup depends on those results (Figs. 4-1, 4-2, and 4-3).

LAB TESTS IN THE WORKUP OF COAGULATION DISORDERS

The first lab tests that are obtained in the evaluation of a coagulation disorder are the CBC with peripheral slide, PT, aPTT, INR, and the thrombin time (TT). The aPTT, PT, and TT reflect the activity of the intrinsic, extrinsic, and common pathways of coagulation, respectively (Fig. 4-4). Mixing studies may also be performed to further evaluate abnormalities in the coagulation cascade. Bleeding times are less often performed, but evaluate problems with primary hemostasis.

CBC

The CBC is the first step in the evaluation of the bleeding patient. The CBC guides the clinician in determining the nature and urgency of the bleeding diathesis, reveals thrombocytopenia if present, and assesses whether the patient has developed clinically significant anemia. The finding of leukocytosis or leukopenia may implicate a hematologic malignancy as the cause of a patient's coagulopathy or thrombocytopenia. Examination of the peripheral smear yields information regarding the presence of microangiopathy, platelet clumping, and WBC morphology.

Coagulation Tests

Prothrombin Time

PT is a measure of the extrinsic (tissue factor) and common pathways. Prolongation of PT may be caused by antagonism of vitamin K owing to warfarin ingestion or deficiency owing to inadequate dietary intake, with subsequent decrease in the vitamin K–dependent factors (II, VII, IX, X). PT may also be prolonged by deficiency of factor V, direct thrombin inhibitors, or quantitative or qualitative disorders of fibrinogen. Historically, PT values have varied from institution to institution. As a result of institutional variation, the INR has evolved. This ratio standardizes all PT assays.

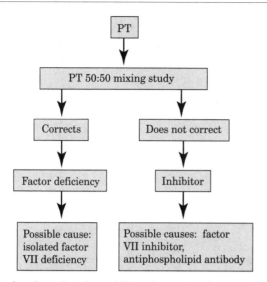

FIG. 4-1. General workup of an elevated PT in the setting of a normal aPTT.

Activated Partial Thromboplastin Time

The aPTT measures both the intrinsic and common pathways. Isolated factor deficiencies that prolong the aPTT and are associated with increased bleeding include factors IX, XI, and VIII. Total deficiencies of factor XII, prekallikrein, and high-molecular-weight kininogen markedly prolong the aPTT but are not associated with increased bleeding. Deficiencies or inhibitors of common pathway factors can also prolong the aPTT.

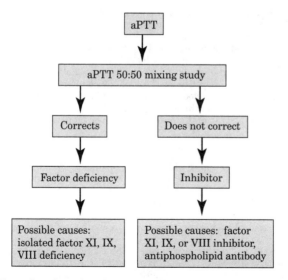

FIG. 4-2. General workup of an elevated aPTT in the setting of a normal PT.

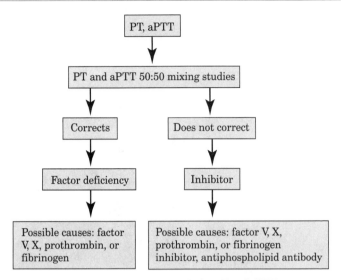

FIG. 4-3. General workup of an elevation of both the PT and aPTT.

Bleeding Time

To perform a bleeding time, a standardized incision is made in the patient's forearm, and the duration of time to cessation of bleeding is measured. Although it can be a useful test for identifying problems with primary hemostasis, many variables may artificially prolong the bleeding time, such as medications that interfere with platelet function, differences in operator procedure and interpretation, and SC edema or thinning of the skin.

Mixing Studies

Mixing studies are performed to determine whether a prolonged PT or aPTT is more likely due to factor deficiencies or inhibitors. In this test, a patient's plasma is mixed with normal plasma in a 1:1 ratio and the coagulation test in question, either the PT or the PTT, is performed immediately and after incubation at 37°C for 1 hr. Mixing studies are performed once, then routinely incubated for 1 hr and repeated. If a factor deficiency is the cause of the abnormal PT or PTT, it should correct completely or within a few seconds of the upper limit of the reference range when mixed with normal plasma. If the prolongation does not correct, if it is partial, or if the prolongation lengthens after incubation, an inhibitor is present. Further workup is then required to determine the nature of the inhibitor (i.e., nonspecific lupus anticoagulant vs factor specific).

Thrombin Time

The TT is performed by adding purified bovine or human thrombin to plasma and monitoring the time for fibrin clot formation. This measures the final common step in the coagulation cascade. The TT may be prolonged in a variety of coagulation disorders, including hypo- and dysfibrinogenemia, high levels of fibrinogen degradation products, monoclonal gammopathies, the presence of direct thrombin inhibitors such as lepirudin and argatroban, thrombin antibodies, and exposure to heparin or heparin-like inhibitors. When the TT is prolonged, a quantity of protamine sulfate is added to the patient's plasma, and the TT is repeated. If the TT corrects with protamine, then heparin or a heparin-like anticoagulant is present. If the TT does not correct, then one of the previously mentioned abnormalities may be the cause.

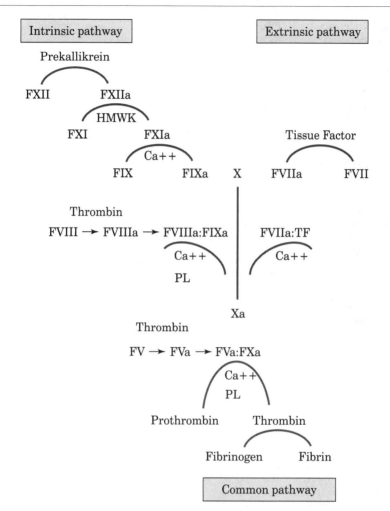

FIG. 4-4. General workup of elevated PT with normal aPTT: the normal coagulation cascade. It typically is split into the *intrinsic pathway* and the *extrinsic pathway*, either of which leads to activation of factor X to Xa. The factors after that point are referred to as the *common pathway*. Disorders of the intrinsic pathway are manifest as prolongation of the aPTT. Disorders of the extrinsic pathway are reflected by prolongation of the PT, whereas disorders of the common pathway will prolong both tests.

GENERAL WORKUP OF ELEVATED PROTHROMBIN TIME/ACTIVATED PARTIAL THROMBOPLASTIN TIME

The workup of an elevated PT or aPTT noted on lab evaluation involves first determining which (or both) pathway of the coagulation cascade is defective. A *mixing study* is then typically performed to determine whether the abnormality is due to an inhibitor present in the patient's serum or a deficiency of a factor in the coagulation cascade. This will provide the differential diagnosis for further testing (see condition-specific sections, later). Figures 4-2, 4-3, and 4-4 detail the workup and differential diagnoses based on the coagulation abnormality present.

INHERITED DISORDERS OF COAGULATION

Hemophilia A

Hemophilia A is an inherited coagulation disorder caused by point mutations, inversions, or deletions of the gene encoding factor VIII (FVIII). The incidence is approximately 1:5,000 live male births, and although affected males may inherit the abnormal gene from carrier females, approximately 30% of cases are the result of spontaneous mutations. The inheritance pattern is X-linked, and the gene that encodes FVIII is located on the long arm of the X chromosome (Xq28). Deficiencies or abnormalities of FVIII lead to impaired intrinsic pathway coagulation.

Clinical

Patients with hemophilia have normal primary hemostasis but experience delayed (hours to days) bleeding episodes after trauma or surgery, or spontaneous hemorrhage in cases of severe hemophilia. Hemophilia is classically characterized by hemorrhage into deep structures such as joint spaces or muscles. Over time, recurrent hemarthroses can lead to hemophilic arthropathy and joint destruction. The severity of the disease depends on the patient's FVIII level, with mild disease classified as a level 6–30% of normal, moderate as 2–5% of normal, and severe as ≤ 1% of normal. Both the severity of the disease and the type of hemorrhage determine the treatment of bleeding episodes.

Diagnosis

When hemophilia A is suspected, a FVIII activity assay is performed. This assay measures the activity of FVIII in the patient's plasma against a normal pooled plasma standard. The normal range is 50–150%. Prenatal diagnosis and carrier detection are now molecular-based procedures.

Treatment

- **DDAVP (desmopressin):** Patients with mild or moderate disease having minor bleeding episodes may be treated with DDAVP, which will increase FVIII levels by 3–5 times baseline. It may be given IV or SC at a dose of 0.3 μg/kg or intranasally at dose of 300 μg/kg. The half-life of FVIII after DDAVP administration is 5–8 hrs.
- **FVIII concentrates:** Patients with severe hemophilia require FVIII replacement for both mild and major bleeding challenges. It can consist of either purified FVIII concentrate from pooled plasma or recombinant FVIII. The choice of therapy is often determined by the availability of product, the patient's history of exposure to pooled plasma product, and patient preference. Patients who are HIV and hepatitis B or C negative usually receive recombinant FVIII, if available, to minimize the risk of viral transmission. In general, each unit/kg of body weight of FVIII replacement will raise the plasma level by 2%. The goal of therapy is determined by the clinical situation. For minor bleeding, plasma levels should reach 25–30% of normal. For more severe bleeding, the goal should be 50% of normal. For surgical procedures or life-threatening bleeding, levels should approach 75–100% of normal. The half-life of FVIII replacement is 8 hrs, and, therefore, the patient should receive a loading dose followed by redosing every 8–12 hrs, with 50% of the loading dose. Therapy should continue until there is resolution of bleeding or symptoms, and postop therapy is usually maintained for 10–14 days. Measuring peak and trough FVIII activities after the first dose and selected subsequent doses permits dose adjustments to ensure cost-effective therapy.
- **Recombinant factor VIIa (RFVIIa):** RFVIIa promotes hemostasis by activating the tissue factor/extrinsic pathway. It is currently approved for use in hemophilia A and B patients who have developed inhibitors to FVIII or factor IX (FIX) replacement therapy. RFVIIa is available in either 1.2- or 4.8-mg vials and is dosed at 90 μg/kg every 2 hrs until hemostasis is achieved.

- **Gene therapy:** Current studies in gene therapy involve use of either adenoviral or retroviral vectors to introduce the gene for FVIII into the genomes of somatic cells, or alternatively culturing a patient's dermal fibroblasts ex vivo and transfecting the cells with FIX cDNA. The cells are then reimplanted into the peritoneal fat. Although the adenovirus vector studies affected a small increase in FIX levels, the levels were not sufficient to eliminate dependence on factor replacement.

Hemophilia B

Hemophilia B (Christmas disease) results from abnormalities of the FIX gene, which is also located on the long arm of the X chromosome (Xq27). The incidence is approximately 1:30,000 in live male births. The clinical syndrome is indistinguishable from hemophilia A, but the distinction is important, as the treatment is different. FIX replacement consists of FIX concentrate or recombinant FIX, and each unit of concentrate/kg body weight results in a 1% increment in FIX levels. The half-life is approximately 24 hrs, and, therefore, the patient receives a loading dose followed by re-dosing every 18–24 hrs until hemostasis is achieved or 10–14 days postoperatively. Monitoring FIX activity should be done as described for FVIII replacement.

von Willebrand Disease

vWD is caused by quantitative or qualitative abnormalities of vWF, a glycoprotein that is involved in primary hemostasis—the initial step in platelet plug formation. The usual inheritance pattern of vWD is autosomal dominant, although incomplete penetrance may lead to mild vWD. There is an approximate incidence of 1:100–400. Clinically, a diagnosis of vWD is suspected when patients have mucocutaneous bleeding in the setting of a family history of a bleeding disorder and lab tests consistent with vWD. Although the majority of affected patients have mild vWD, patients with the most severe form may have life-threatening bleeding.

von Willebrand Factor

vWF is a protein synthesized by endothelial cells and platelets and is stored in the Weibel-Palade bodies of endothelial cells and the alpha granules of platelets. In addition to its role in primary hemostasis, vWF stabilizes and transports FVIII in the circulation. vWF is synthesized as a 300-kD subunit, which then assembles into multimers of a wide range of sizes. The largest multimers mediate platelet adhesion. Protein electrophoresis is used to identify whether a normal pattern of vWF multimers are present in the plasma. Several lab methods can be used to quantitate vWF antigen. Measurement of vWF platelet adhesion activity involves *in vitro* exposure of patient plasma, control platelets, and ristocetin—an antibiotic that stimulates vWF-platelet interaction.

Classification of von Willebrand Disease

vWD is not a single disease but a group of disorders caused by either qualitative or quantitative abnormalities of vWF. These have been subclassified into types 1, 2, and 3 (Table 4-1).

- **Type 1 vWD** is the most common form of vWD, accounting for 70–80% of diagnosed cases. The disease occurs as a result of a quantitative deficiency of vWF, with measured levels approximately 20–50% of normal. On protein electrophoresis, vWF multimers are present in smaller quantities but in normal proportions. The inheritance pattern is autosomal dominant.
- **Type 2 vWD** represents a group of vWF qualitative abnormalities. In these disorders, the plasma levels of vWF protein are mildly reduced or low normal, but the platelet adhesion is disproportionately lower. *Type 2a vWD* is the most common qualitative abnormality of vWF, which arises from either impaired intracellular assembly of vWF multimers or the increased susceptibility of vWF to proteolysis on release from storage granules. The net result is the loss of the high- and middle-molecular-weight multimers. DDAVP does not consistently have beneficial effects

TABLE 4-1. CLASSIFICATION OF VON WILLEBRAND DISEASE

Type 1: Partial quantitative deficiency of vWF (70% of cases)

Type 2: Qualitative abnormality/deficiency of vWF

   2A: Decreased vWF function associated with loss of large, or high molecular weight, vWF multimers

   2B: Defective vWF with increased affinity for platelets that leads to inappropriate binding and clearance

   2M: Normal multimer size/distribution but ineffective platelet binding

   2N: vWF with a defect in binding factor VIII

Type 3: Absence of vWF

vWF, von Willebrand factor.

in this disorder. In *Type 2b vWD*, the abnormal vWF has an increased affinity for the platelet receptor, Gp1b, leading to more avid binding of vWF to platelets. The bound vWF and platelet are cleared from plasma, resulting in both mild thrombocytopenia and diminished plasma levels of large multimers of vWF. Treatment with DDAVP may lead to worsening thrombocytopenia. Platelet counts may fall during pregnancy because of increased estrogen levels leading to increased vWF levels. *Type 2N vWD* (Normandy) is caused by mutations of the vWF FVIII binding region. This disorder is usually silent in heterozygotes but in homozygotes is clinically similar to mild or moderate hemophilia A. Female patients with unusually low FVIII levels may have type 2N vWD, as may males who appear to have an autosomally inherited hemophilia. *Type 2M vWD* is clinically similar to type 2A in that the defect involves a mutation that impairs binding of vWF to the Gp1b receptor; however, normal multimer patterns are obtained with protein electrophoresis. Pseudo-vWD results from an increased affinity of the Gp1b receptor for normal large vWF multimers and is clinically similar to type 2b.

- **Type 3 vWD** is a quantitative deficiency and is the most severe form of the disease. Patients have little or no detectible vWF and FVIII and a coagulation disorder similar to severe hemophilia. The inheritance pattern is autosomal recessive and usually arises as a result of a consanguineous relationship.

History and Physical Exam
The disease is associated with mild bleeding tendencies in many patients, but some have more significant bleeding episodes and may experience problems with surgery. A family history of bleeding problems is typically present and may be useful in suggesting the diagnosis. These patients will often seek medical advice for frequent bruising. They may give a history of epistaxis, bleeding gums, easy bruising, or menorrhagia. They may also develop hematomas. GI bleeding can be serious but is relatively rare. The mucosal bleeding can be a serious problem requiring transfusions.

Lab Evaluation
Initial tests include a **CBC** to evaluate platelet count (which may be mildly decreased in certain subtypes of vWF), and **PT/PTT** (PTT may be mildly prolonged as a result of decreased FVIII levels). These tests are most useful in suggesting alternate diagnoses. Diagnosis of vWD is often difficult and complex and requires the evaluation of the patient's vWF activity levels, antigen levels, multimer analysis, primary hemostasis as determined by a bleeding time, and a FVIII activity level. A family history of a bleeding disorder or known vWD is also important, as any or all of the previously mentioned tests may be normal or equivocal.

- **vWF antigen levels (vWF:Ag)** are used to quantify the total level of vWF in the patient's blood but will not measure the function of vWF and will not detect quali-

tative defects. The levels are measured against a normal reference sample and >50% activity is considered normal. It will detect all type 3, most type 1, and only some type 2 vWD. This test is inadequate alone.
- **Functional activity of FVIII** (**FVIII:C**) mixes plasma deficient in FVIII with the patient's plasma, which should give a quantitative corrected value of activity >50% if normal. Types 1, 3, 2A, and 2N are usually deficient, but other disorders, most notably hemophilia A, will give abnormal values. This test is not adequate alone to diagnose vWD.
- **Functional activity of vWF**, also known as **ristocetin cofactor assay** (**vWF:RCof**), is a test that will detect defects in vWF agglutination when normal vWF is present. The test uses comparison to a reference sample and >50% is considered normal. Patients with type 2A, 2B, 2M, and 3 will usually have abnormal values. Type 1 may also be abnormal. This test is useful when used with the vWF:Ag test in the Ag:RCof ratio.
- The **collagen binding assay** (**vWF:CBA**) uses ELISA and is especially useful for identifying the presence of high-molecular-weight forms of vWF. Because 2A and 2B are deficient in high-molecular-weight vWF, this test is useful in their diagnosis. As described earlier, reference comparison with >50% levels are considered normal. This test is used in comparison with the vWF:Ag test in the Ag:CBA ratio.
- The **vWF multimer assay** (**vWF:multimer assay**) is used only to clarify the subtype of vWD, if necessary, after the diagnosis is made and is frequently not readily available. It involves labor-intensive gel electrophoresis.
- The **ristocetin-induced platelet aggregation analysis** (**RIPA**) is used to assist in the diagnosis of type 2B and is used only after the diagnosis of vWD is made and further clarification of subtype is necessary.
- The **FVIII binding assay** (**vWF:FVIII binding assay**) is used to help diagnose type 2N.
- **Platelet function analyzers,** such as **PFA-100,** are automated tools that are sensitive to vWF problems but are not specific in the diagnosis of vWD. If available, they may be useful in urgent situations.

In general, a recommended initial panel would include PT/INR, PTT, platelet count, FVIII:C, vWF:Ag, and one of either vWF:RCof or vWF:CBA. When abnormal tests are found suggesting vWD, these tests should be repeated after 2 wks to confirm the diagnosis. If the two sets of tests do not agree, the test should be performed a third time. (For an excellent review of these tests, see Favaloro EJ. Laboratory assessment as a critical component of the appropriate diagnosis and sub-classification of von Willebrand's disease. *Blood Rev* 1999;13:185–204.)

Management

- **Treatment of bleeding episodes** and **prophylaxis for surgery** are the main indications for treatment of vWD. **DDAVP** is an analog of antidiuretic hormone, also known as *vasopressin*. It is the primary treatment for bleeding associated with type 1 vWD. It acts by releasing endothelial stores of vWF from Weibel-Palade bodies. This transiently increases the levels of FVIII and vWF in the plasma, providing for better hemostasis in bleeding type 1 vWD patents. Type 2 vWD does not respond as well to DDAVP as type 1, and it is contraindicated in type 2B patients in whom it may induce inappropriate agglutination and thrombocytopenia. Type 2A, 2M, and 2N bleeding patients may benefit from a trial of DDAVP, but it is not the definitive treatment for significant bleeding in these cases. It is entirely ineffective in type 3. The standard dose is 0.3–0.4 µg/kg in 50–100 mL of saline infused over 30 mins. DDAVP can also be administered SC and as a nasal spray. The spray may be useful for home therapy of menorrhagia and recurrent epistaxis.
- The use of blood products is the primary treatment when **significant bleeding** is involved, especially in non–type 1 disease. Because cryoprecipitate contains five- to tenfold higher concentrations of FVIII and vWF, it is more appropriate to use than fresh frozen plasma. Recently available are FVIII + vWF concentrates that are preferable (when available) to cryoprecipitate, owing to less chance of viral transmission. **Humate-P** is the concentrate of choice. Humate-P or similar concentrates should be used in all types of vWD but may be used in addition to DDAVP in cases in which DDAVP is effective. The recommended dose is 40–60 IU/kg in adults given

daily until adequate healing has occurred. Clinical judgment should guide repeated treatment schedules. Checking FVIII:C levels every 12 hrs the day of a surgical procedure, and daily after, appears warranted, but monitoring them for treatment of spontaneous bleeding is not standard practice.

- If an **operative procedure** is planned, patients with type 1 vWD usually receive DDAVP 1 hr before surgery and then daily for 2–3 days. For more invasive procedures, such as neurosurgery or cardiac surgery or in patients who are unable to achieve hemostasis postoperatively, plasma concentrates containing vWF/FVIII are indicated.

ACQUIRED DISORDERS OF COAGULATION

Vitamin K Deficiency

Vitamin K is a fat-soluble vitamin that is involved in the posttranslational modification of the vitamin K–dependent coagulation factors II, VII, IX, and X; protein C; and protein S. These reactions take place in the liver, where vitamin K serves as a cofactor for the conversion of glutamate to gamma-carboxyglutamic acid. This conversion enables the substrate to bind divalent cations and, therefore, to bind to phospholipid membranes, which is essential for normal coagulation. In the absence of vitamin K, glutamate is converted instead to des-gamma-carboxyl, and the net result is impaired coagulation. Vitamin K deficiency may occur secondary to inadequate dietary intake, which may deplete vitamin K stores in as little as 7 days. Antibiotic therapy can decrease the intestinal flora producing menaquinones, which are chemically similar to vitamin K. Malnourished patients receiving antibiotics are, therefore, most likely to develop vitamin K deficiency. The diagnosis is usually suspected when a prolonged PT that corrects after 50:50 mixing studies is encountered in such patients. Treatment may be PO, SC, or IV vitamin K. A recent study comparing PO vs SC vitamin K in patients requiring reversal of warfarin (Coumadin) anticoagulation suggests that PO replacement results in more rapid normalization of coagulation. Vitamin K absorption is variable when administered SC and may be impaired in edematous patients. IV vitamin K is effective but carries the risk of anaphylaxis. To minimize the risk of a vitamin K anaphylactoid infusion reaction, vitamin K may be diluted in 50 mL of 5% dextrose solution. Slow administration is recommended. With adequate replacement therapy, the PT should begin to normalize within 12 hrs and should normalize completely in 24–48 hrs.

Liver Disease

All coagulation factors with the exception of vWF, and possibly FVIII, are produced in the liver. Liver dysfunction leads to a number of coagulation abnormalities secondary to decreased factor synthesis, decreased clearance of activated clotting factors, production of abnormal fibrinogen (see Disorders of Fibrinogen), and circulating abnormal prothrombin, which results from impaired vitamin K–dependent carboxylation. The coagulopathy of liver disease is usually stable unless the liver synthetic function is rapidly worsening, such as in fulminant hepatic failure. Patients with liver synthetic dysfunction frequently also have thrombocytopenia secondary to portal HTN causing splenomegaly with splenic sequestration.

Disseminated Intravascular Coagulation

DIC is an acquired disorder of hemostasis that involves inappropriate small vessel thrombosis and thrombolysis. It leads to microangiopathic hemolytic anemia, thrombocytopenia, and coagulation abnormalities. See Chap. 8, Disorders of Platelets and Primary Hemostasis, for a complete discussion.

Acquired Inhibitors of Coagulation

- Acquired inhibitors of coagulation may arise *de novo* or may develop in patients with congenital coagulation disorders who are exposed to plasma products. These inhibitors, also known as *circulating anticoagulants*, either inhibit coagulation proteins directly or interfere with reactions affecting coagulation. Most are antibodies, specifically IgG, and can be directed against any of the clotting factors. Circulating anticoagulants usually arise *de novo* in patients with autoimmune diseases such as SLE. To assess for the presence of an inhibitor, a 50:50 mixing study of the plasma is performed. If the coagulation studies do not correct with mixing, specific factor levels are drawn depending on the likely affected factor. Treatment consists of immunosuppression, sometimes with IV Ig.

- Some inhibitors are molecules that directly or indirectly interfere with **anticoagulation.** Examples include amyloid, monoclonal antibodies, and heparin-like anticoagulants. Amyloid proteins are tissue-based inhibitors that classically bind to and inactivate factor X. Monoclonal antibodies may directly inhibit coagulation factors but more frequently interfere with fibrin polymerization. Heparin-like anticoagulants are not antibodies but glycosaminoglycans and usually develop in patients with malignancies or plasma cell dyscrasias. The characteristic lab findings are a prolonged aPTT that corrects with mixing studies, a prolonged TT that corrects with protamine sulfate, and a normal reptilase time. Treatment is directed at correction of the underlying cause.

Antiphospholipid Antibody Syndrome

Antiphospholipid antibodies are acquired antibodies that bind to anionic phospholipid-protein reagents. When they cause prolongation of aPTT or PT, or both, they are identified as lupus anticoagulants. This is not a true coagulopathy but a lab artifact resulting from antibody interference with phospholipid-dependent coagulation tests. The antibodies in fact may lead to a hypercoagulable disorder, discussed elsewhere in this manual (see Chap. 5, Thrombotic Disease).

Disorders of Fibrinogen

Fibrinogen is a precursor to fibrin that is produced in the liver and is an acute phase reactant. Disorders of fibrinogen may be either qualitative or quantitative and may be inherited or acquired. Congenital dysfibrinogenemias are rare and can be asymptomatic or associated with bleeding or thrombotic complications. Acquired dysfibrinogenemias are more common and are typically asymptomatic. Fibrinogen abnormalities leading to impaired coagulation include hypofibrinogenemia secondary to liver synthetic dysfunction and dysfibrinogenemia secondary to abnormal fibrinogen production. Abnormal fibrinogen production is usually seen in conditions that stimulate fibrinogen synthesis such as infiltration of the liver by metastatic disease, primary hepatocellular carcinoma, and occasionally paraneoplastic syndromes. The abnormal fibrinogen produced contains an increased sialic acid content that interferes with fibrin polymerization and causes delayed *in vitro* fibrin plug formation. Characteristic lab findings are prolonged thrombin and reptilase times and low fibrinogen blood levels based on rate of fibrin clot formation but normal fibrinogen antigen levels.

Factitious, Unsuspected, or Accidental Use of Anticoagulants

When abnormal coagulation tests results are present and an organic cause cannot be established, unsuspected exposure to an anticoagulant drug may be the culprit. For example, hospitalized patients frequently receive heparin during routine IV or central venous catheter flushes. Similarly, patients with central venous catheters may have had blood drawn from lines through which heparin is being infused. Patients with coagulation studies consistent with warfarin effect and an otherwise negative evaluation may be surreptitiously ingesting warfarin. A serum warfarin level can be drawn if this is suspected. Ingestion of anticoagulant rodenticides containing "superwarfarin" (i.e., brodifacoumarin) causes a prolonged elevation of the PT lasting up to 1 yr. Plasma products are indicated for patients with associated bleeding, along with high-dose (100–150 mg PO daily) vitamin K replacement, as standard doses of vitamin K do not usually correct the coagulopathy. Vitamin K should be continued until the PT normalizes.

KEY POINTS TO REMEMBER

* The initial step in evaluation of asymptomatic lab abnormalities in coagulation is to repeat the labs and evaluate for falsely abnormal studies (e.g., related to heparin in IV lines).
* The evaluation of the PT, PTT, and CBC is the first step in the determination of the step in the hemostatic process that is abnormal.
* Mixing studies helps distinguish between acquired factor inhibitor states and factor deficiencies when evaluating the elevated PT or PTT.
* Hemophilia A is a rare inherited disorder that involves decreased or absent activity of FVIII. Use of DDAVP or transfusion of plasma products is the mainstay of management.
* In general, a recommended initial panel would include PT/INR, PTT, platelet count, FVIII:C, vWF:Ag, and one of either vWF:RCof or vWF:CBA.

REFERENCES AND SUGGESTED READINGS

Bernard GR, Vincent JL, Laterre PF, et al. Efficacy and safety of recombinant human activated protein C for severe sepsis. *N Engl J Med* 2001;344:699–709.

Blanchard RA, Furie BC, Jorgensen M, et al. Acquired vitamin K-dependent carboxylation deficiency in liver disease. *N Engl J Med* 1981;305:242–248.

Budde U. Laboratory diagnosis of congenital von Willebrand disease. *Semin Thromb Hemost* 2002;28:173–190.

Butenas S, Brummel KE, Branda RF, et al. Mechanism of factor VIIa-dependent coagulation in hemophilia blood. *Blood* 2002;99:923–930.

Chua JD, Friedenberg WR. Superwarfarin poisoning. *Arch Intern Med* 1998;158:1929–1932.

Crowther MA, Douketis JD, Schnurr T, et al. Oral vitamin K lowers the international normalized ratio more rapidly than subcutaneous vitamin K in the treatment of warfarin-associated coagulopathy. *Ann Intern Med* 2002;137:251–254.

Dawson NA, Barr CF, Alving BM. Acquired dysfibrinogenemia. *Am J Med* 1985;78:682–686.

Favaloro EJ. Laboratory assessment as a critical component of the appropriate diagnosis and sub-classification of von Willebrand's disease. *Blood Rev* 1999;13:185–204.

Hoffman R, Furie B, Silberstein LE, et al. *Hematology: basic principles and practice,* 3rd ed. New York: Churchill Livingstone, 1999.

Hoyer L. Hemophilia A. *N Engl J Med* 1994;330:38–47.

Lackner H. Hemostatis abnormalities associated with dysproteinemias. *Semin Hematol* 1973;10:125–133.

Lechner K, Niessner H, Thaler E. Coagulation abnormalities in liver disease. *Semin Thromb Hemost* 1977;4:40–56.

Levi M, de Jonge E, van der Poll T, et al. Advances in the understanding of the pathogenetic pathways of disseminated intravascular coagulation result in more insight in the clinical picture and better management strategies. *Semin Thromb Hemost* 2001;27:569–575.

Levi M, Ten Cate H. Disseminated intravascular coagulation. *N Engl J Med* 1999;341:586–592.

Mannucci PM. Desmopressin (DDAVP) in the treatment of bleeding disorders: the first 20 years. *Blood* 1997;90:2515–2521.

Mannucci PM. How I treat patients with von Willebrand disease. *Blood* 2001;97:1915–1919.

Mannucci PM. The hemophilias—from royal genes to gene therapy. *N Engl J Med* 2001;344:1773–1779.

Nissen D. *Mosby's drug consult 2002.* Mosby–Year Book, 2002.

Sahud MA. Laboratory diagnosis of inhibitors. *Semin Thromb Hemost* 2000;26:195–203.

Schwaab R, Oldenburg J. Gene therapy of hemophilia. *Semin Thromb Hemost* 2001;27:417–424.

Thrombotic Disease

Shachar Peles and
Giancarlo Pillot

INTRODUCTION

Thrombotic disease involves the formation of a clot inappropriately in the venous or arterial circulation. Embolism of these clots can occur, causing pulmonary embolus (PE) when arising from the venous circulation or systemic emboli to vital organs when arising in the arterial circulation. The hematologist is often consulted to aid in the evaluation of these patients for a thrombophilia or hypercoagulable state, as well as decide on appropriate anticoagulant management and duration of therapy. However, it should be remembered that arterial and venous thrombi form in the presence of **Virchow's triad:** hypercoagulability, stasis, and endothelial damage.

DEEP VENOUS THROMBOSIS AND PULMONARY EMBOLUS

PE, the most feared complication of deep venous thrombosis (DVT), occurs in approximately 600,000 patients annually in the United States and contributes to as many as 100,000 annual deaths. Treatment of DVT is directed at preventing fatal PE and morbidity associated with the postphlebitic syndrome.

Diagnosis

- Clinical diagnosis of DVT and PE is highly unreliable and inaccurate, and definitive diagnosis should therefore be based on objective tests. Clinical findings suggestive of DVT include unilateral calf tenderness or swelling. Symptoms of acute PE include dyspnea, pleuritic chest pain, cough, anxiety, and hemoptysis. Physical exam may reveal tachypnea, tachycardia, and inspiratory crackles, but these findings are nonspecific.
- Doppler U/S is highly sensitive and specific for diagnosing DVT proximal to the calf. Venography has been the "gold standard" but is rarely done today. U/S is less invasive than venography and generally considered more accurate than impedance plethysmography and is thus the preferred method. If the Doppler study is positive, the patient should be treated for DVT. If negative, alternative diagnoses should be entertained. If the clinical suspicion is still high, repeating the Doppler study may be of benefit or venography may be pursued. CT venography may be comparable to U/S in this setting but at present remains experimental.
- Evaluation for acute PE should include ABG analysis, which may show hypoxemia and hypocapnia. $\dot{V}/\dot{Q}$ or CT scanning of the lung with a PE-specific protocol is usually used for diagnosis. The gold standard involves pulmonary angiography. The D-dimer is the result of fibrin breakdown and is generated under many circumstances. Measurements of D-dimer have been used for the diagnosis of venous thromboembolism but are most useful when negative, making the diagnosis much more unlikely. Patients with a positive D-dimer require further diagnostic evaluation. In cases of very high clinical suspicion, however, testing should be pursued despite a negative D-dimer.
- Diagnostic tests to identify individuals with thrombophilia and thus further guide decisions regarding the duration of anticoagulation should be pursued according to the guidelines outlined elsewhere in this chapter.

Treatment

- Treatment of diagnosed or highly suspicious DVT or PE should begin promptly with unfractionated heparin or low-molecular-weight heparin (LMWH). Thrombolytics may be considered in selected patients with hemodynamically significant PE. Individuals who are actively bleeding or at high risk for bleeding should be considered for inferior vena cava (IVC) filter placement.
- **Unfractionated heparin** involves an initial bolus followed by a continuous infusion. The dose is usually adjusted according to the aPTT, as heparin has a narrow therapeutic range and large variability with regard to patient response. The target aPTT should be 1.5–2.5 times the control value. Achieving therapeutic aPTT levels quickly is desirable, as persistently subtherapeutic levels almost certainly increase the risk of recurrence. Use of heparin nomograms assist in more rapid attainment and maintenance of therapeutic heparin levels. **LMWHs** have several advantages over standard unfractionated heparin in that they have longer half-lives and a more predictable dose response. Lab monitoring is therefore not necessary. It is also possible that they are associated with fewer bleeding complications, while having equivalent anticoagulant effect. Either form of heparin provides prompt protection from extension of DVT and progression to PE, as well as helps to avoid the postphlebitic syndrome. Treatment with heparin or LMWH should be continued for at least 5 days and until the patient has a therapeutic level of anticoagulation on an oral anticoagulant.
- Long-term anticoagulation is achieved with **oral coumarins.** These are vitamin K antagonists, warfarin being the most widely used. The dose is adjusted according to the INR, which is a form of the PT that is controlled for variations in testing reagents. Treatment should be started within 24 hrs of initiation of heparin, with a goal INR of 2–3.
    - **Duration of warfarin therapy** is variable and depends on a number of factors, including underlying thrombotic risk and on the risk of bleeding. One should include not only the risk of recurrence but also its effect (i.e., patients with cardiorespiratory disease might tolerate recurrent PE poorly).
    - Current data indicate that patients have lower rates of recurrence when treated with longer courses of warfarin, whereas those with idiopathic thrombosis have significantly higher rates of recurrence than those with an identifiable trigger (e.g., surgery, immobilization, trauma) that is subsequently resolved.
- **Anticoagulation failure** results in symptomatic recurrence of venous thromboembolism. Recurrence should be documented using objective studies, as the postphlebitic syndrome can be difficult to distinguish from recurrence. Early failure may be due to inadequate anticoagulant dosage or heparin-induced thrombocytopenia (HIT).
    - Management possibilities include intensifying therapy for inadequate dosage, substitution of heparin with another agent, or possibly the insertion of an IVC filter. Treatment failure may occur at any time in patients with overt or occult cancer or in those with the antiphospholipid syndrome.
    - **Trousseau syndrome** is a hypercoagulable state associated with malignancy and is characterized by DIC and recurrent arterial or venous thrombotic events. Treatment involves anticoagulation with heparin or LMWH.

Calf Vein Thrombosis
Only 20% of calf vein thrombi extend proximally and thus pose a significant risk for PE. It is generally considered safe to withhold anticoagulant therapy in patients with suspected venous thrombosis with normal results on serial exams with Doppler U/S, although some will have calf vein thrombi. Calf vein thrombi are not dangerous, provided they remain confined to the calf. An antiinflammatory agent may benefit many patients.

Venous Thrombosis during Pregnancy
Coumarin derivatives are able to cross the placenta and can cause fetal hemorrhage as well as being teratogenic (FDA pregnancy rating D). Pregnant women with documented thromboembolism should be given unfractionated heparin or LMWH until delivery. Calcium supplements should be given to avoid the complication of osteoporosis that heparins can cause. LMWHs have the advantage of causing less bleeding and osteoporosis; however, they are more expensive. Warfarin is appropriate to use for postpartum women and safe to use while breast-feeding.

Inferior Vena Cava Filters

The use of IVC filters represents an important alternative to anticoagulation to prevent PE in the short term. However, because filters are associated with an increased risk of DVT, IVC thrombosis, and postphlebitic limb and as long-term safety and efficacy remain uncertain, their use should be restricted to situations in which anticoagulation is clearly contraindicated. Absolute contraindications to anticoagulation include CNS hemorrhage or trauma, large cerebrovascular accident, cerebral metastases, retroperitoneal hemorrhage, GI hemorrhage, or severe thrombocytopenia. Filters may also be used under certain circumstances in which apparently adequate anticoagulation has failed and patients have recurrent venous thromboembolism. Those patients should continue anticoagulants if there are no contraindications. Temporary IVC filter devices are in development and may provide the benefits of permanent filters without the potential long-term side effects.

Thrombolytics

Thrombolytics provide several potential benefits in the management of PE. Rapid clot lysis results in improved pulmonary perfusion and overall hemodynamics, as well as reduces the incidence of recurrent PE by lysing peripheral venous thrombi. In practice, these benefits have no impact on overall morbidity and mortality, and the risks of thrombolytic therapy are, thus, not often warranted because there is a substantial risk of bleeding. Currently, the situation most often encountered in which the benefits of thrombolytics outweigh potential risks is in patients with shock secondary to massive PE. Further research is required to evaluate the effect on morbidity and mortality of thrombolytics in patients with other circumstances, such as large clot burden or right ventricular dysfunction, but without hemodynamic compromise. Thrombolytics should only be given by those experienced in their use.

THROMBOPHILIA

Virchow postulated three factors (Virchow's triad) predisposing for thrombosis, namely, alterations in the vessel wall, stasis of blood flow, and alterations in the composition of blood or so-called hypercoagulability. Hypercoagulability (i.e., thrombophilia) may be inherited or acquired. The presence of inherited thrombotic disorders has been appreciated for only a few decades, and clinicians can now determine major risk factors that were previously deemed idiopathic (Table 5-1).

TABLE 5-1. CAUSES OF HYPERCOAGULABILITY LEADING TO VENOUS THROMBOEMBOLISM

Acquired causes	Inherited causes
Surgery/trauma	Factor V Leiden mutation
Malignancy	Prothrombin G20210A mutation
Myeloproliferative disorders	Hyperhomocystinemia
Pregnancy	Protein C deficiency
Oral contraceptives	Protein S deficiency
Immobilization	Antithrombin deficiency
Congestive heart failure	Increased factor VIII activity
Nephrotic syndrome	
Obesity	
Antiphospholipid antibodies	
Lupus anticoagulant	
Anticardiolipin antibodies	
(Hyperhomocystinemia and antiphospholipid antibodies are considered risk factors for both venous and arterial thrombosis.)	

Activated Protein C Resistance/Factor V Leiden

Activated protein C resistance/factor V Leiden is the most common inherited thrombophilia. Using current assays, almost all cases are due to a substitution mutation
in the factor V gene, resulting in so-called factor V Leiden. This mutation slows
down the inactivation of active factor Va by activated protein C resulting in
increased generation of thrombin. It results in the failure of activated protein C to
prolong the PTT *in vitro* as detected in the activated protein C resistance assay. The
relative risk of thrombosis for carriers of the factor V Leiden mutation is thought to
be four- to fivefold for heterozygotes and 80-fold for homozygotes. The allele frequency among persons of European heritage is 4% but is much less common in other
populations. Factor V Leiden is detected in 20% of unselected patients with a first-
time venous thrombosis.

Prothrombin G20210A Mutation

Prothrombin G20210A mutation is a substitution mutation in the prothrombin gene
that results in increased levels of plasma prothrombin. It leads to increased generation of thrombin. The relative risk of thrombosis in heterozygotes is 2.8. The allele
frequency among persons of European heritage is 2% and, like factor V Leiden, is
extremely uncommon among the nonwhite population. It is detected in 4% of patients
with a first-time venous thrombosis. Patients who harbor both the factor V Leiden
and the prothrombin G20210A mutation are at increased risk compared with those
with a single abnormality.

Antithrombin Deficiency

Antithrombin deficiency defect involves impaired neutralization of thrombin. Deficiencies in antithrombin are identified in approximately 5% of patients with DVT. It is
a potent but uncommon risk factor for venous thrombosis. In addition to anticoagulation, treatment may involve infusion of antithrombin concentrate during high-risk
situations, such as during delivery or surgery.

Proteins C and S Deficiency

Proteins C and S are natural anticoagulants that are occasionally identified in
patients with venous thromboembolism. They pose a significant thrombotic risk and
should trigger a study of family members at risk.

Elevated Factor VIII Activity

Increased FVIII has been associated with an increased risk of thrombosis, and
increased levels have been the most common abnormality identified in individuals
with a first thrombotic episode. FVIII activity may increase as an acute-phase reactant during acute illness. At this point, it is unclear how elevated FVIII levels may
affect treatment of thromboembolism.

Workup of the Hypercoagulable State

Patients with hereditary thrombophilia most often present with DVT of the legs or
PE. Less commonly, they present with superficial venous thrombosis or thromboses
elsewhere in the vascular system. Acquired and genetic causes are often identified in
the majority of patients with hereditary thrombophilia, in which thrombosis is pro-
voked by an acquired event. The risk of recurrence after a thromboembolic event is
more common in patients with antithrombin deficiency, in patients with protein C or
protein S deficiency, in those with more than one inherited abnormality, and in those
homozygous for factor V Leiden or the prothrombin G20210A mutation. Current data
provide no clear indication whether the risk of a recurrent thromboembolic event is

greater among heterozygotes for factor V Leiden or the prothrombin G20210A mutation, as opposed to the "normal" population, so that altering treatment based on this finding is premature.

Screening symptomatic and asymptomatic individuals for the presence of these disorders has both benefits and drawbacks. Benefits include prevention of recurrence, a focus on attention for prophylaxis with anticoagulant therapy during further surgery/immobilization/pregnancy, an awareness of increased risk associated with oral contraceptive and hormone replacement therapy, and a benefit to other family members. Drawbacks may include difficulties in obtaining life-insurance coverage and possible overanticoagulation.

The optimal time for testing patients for hereditary defects is not well defined but conveniently done 6 mos after the thrombotic event. At this point, decisions need to be made regarding continuing anticoagulation. Performing the thrombophilic evaluation at the time of thrombosis can results in misleading test results. For example, acute thrombosis can cause low levels of antithrombin, protein C, and protein S. Therapy with heparin reduces antithrombin levels, and warfarin reduces proteins C and S levels. Table 5-2 lists the appropriate lab evaluation for a hypercoaguable state based on clinical characteristics.

Treatment Approach

The duration of anticoagulation in patients with hereditary thrombophilia should be tailored to the individual patient, but general guidelines available are shown in Table 5-3. Specific drug information regarding anticoagulation may be found in Chap. 13, Hematologic Drugs. In all patients with a history of a thromboembolic event, regardless of the presence or absence of hereditary thrombophilias, prophylaxis should be pursued with unfractionated heparin or LMWH during high-risk situations, including surgery, trauma, and immobilization. These individuals should also be advised to avoid oral contraceptives as well as hormone replacement therapy and warned of the increased risk of recurrent thrombotic events during pregnancy.

With the discovery of additional genetic abnormalities and further data regarding recurrence risks especially with recently identified abnormalities (e.g., increased FVIII levels), we will be better able to counsel patients and identify those at risk owing to the presence of multiple abnormalities.

ARTERIAL THROMBOEMBOLISM

Arterial thromboses are those that eventually lodge in the arterial side of the circulatory system. They may either occur *in situ* due to a damaged artery (e.g., by trauma, vasculitis, foreign body) or be the result of embolization from a proximal source (e.g., from the atria in atrial fibrillation, a ventricular or arterial aneurism, or proximal clot formed in an area of damaged artery). The symptoms are typically related to the acute ischemia of the organ in which the clot forms or lodges. Clots that form or embolize to the cerebral circulation manifest as acute stroke with neurologic deficits. Limb thromboses may present as cold, pulselss, pale, painful limbs or digits. Mesenteric thromboses may present with pain, ileus, hematochezia, and, in severe cases, hemodynamic instability.

The initial management of an arterial thrombus includes a search for its source as either an embolus from a distant site or its origin as a clot that formed *in situ*. As a general rule, emboli tend to be multiple; however, this can occur in the case of vasculitis as well. The ECG may reveal atrial fibrillation as a possible source. Echocardiography is often used to evaluate for a clot formed in one of the heart chambers. One possible source of embolus that should be considered is the case of a heart defect allowing a venous embolus to pass to the aterial circulation. Doppler ultrasonography may be used in certain arteries to evaluate blood flow, but typically angiography is required in the acute setting. The reader is referred to the *Washington Manual*™ *Cardiology Subspecialty Consult* for more information about atrial fibrillation and to the *Washington Manual*™ *Rheumatology Subspecialty Consult* regarding vaculitis.

TABLE 5-2. EVALUATION OF HYPERCOAGULABLE STATE BASED ON CLINICAL CONDITION

Clinical condition	Evaluation
Unprovoked thromboembolism in patient with one of the following characteristics: Age <45 yrs Family history of thromboembolic disease Recurrent events Cerebral or visceral vein thrombosis Recurrent spontaneous abortions	Complete evaluation Factor V Leiden mutation or activated protein C resistance clotting assay Prothrombin G20210A mutation Antithrombin functional assay Protein C functional assay Protein S functional assay, as well as free and total protein S levels Lupus anticoagulant Anticardiolipin antibodies Fasting total plasma homocysteine levels
First unprovoked thromboembolism with any of the following: Age >45 yrs Thromboembolism associated with pregnancy, oral contraceptive use, or hormone replacement therapy Provoked proximal vein thrombosis or pulmonary embolism	Factor V Leiden/activated protein C resistance Anticardiolipin antibodies Lupus anticoagulant Hyperhomocystinemia Prothrombin G20210A mutation Omit the protein C, protein S, and antithrombin tests, as these have a low yield in this population
First provoked thromboembolism in distal vein (i.e., associated with surgery, trauma, immobilization)	No screening necessary
Asymptomatic patients (no thromboembolic event) with a family history of thromboembolic events	Thorough counseling regarding both the benefits and drawbacks of screening Should also be informed of symptoms that require immediate attention
Asymptomatic patients without a family history but before or during exposure to thrombotic risk factors such as pregnancy, oral contraception, major surgery, or immobilization	No firm recommendations available; screening of healthy woman is generally not recommended because it would deny contraceptives to 5–10% of white women with the factor V Leiden or the prothrombin G20210A mutation while preventing very few fatal venous thromboemboli
Arterial thrombus	Fasting homocysteine levels Anticardiolipin antibodies Lupus anticoagulant

TABLE 5-3. GENERAL GUIDELINES FOR ANTICOAGULATION IN PATIENTS WITH HEREDITARY THROMBOPHILIA

Patient	Duration of anticoagulation
First event and an identifiable transient triggering factor	Between 3 and 6 mos, provided that trigger factor is removed
First event and no evidence of a triggering factor, including those with either the factor V Leiden mutation or the prothrombin G20210A mutation	6 mos
Active cancer, continued immobilization, venous insufficiency, deficiencies of protein C or protein S	12–24 mos
Single thromboembolic episode but more than just one allelic abnormality (e.g., those who are homozygous for factor V Leiden or those who are heterozygous for both factor V Leiden and the prothrombin G20210A mutation)	Lifelong anticoagulation
Life-threatening thrombosis such as massive pulmonary embolism, cerebral, mesenteric, portal, or hepatic thrombosis	Lifelong anticoagulation
≥ 2 thromboembolic events	Lifelong anticoagulation
Antiphospholipid antibodies	Lifelong anticoagulation
Antithrombin deficiency	Lifelong anticoagulation

After evaluation for an embolic source of thrombus and management of the acute ischemic event, the hematologist is often asked to evaluate for the possibility of a hypercoaguable state as an etiology of the arterial thrombus. Arterial thromboses may be associated with hyperhomocysteinemia and antiphospholipid syndrome.

Hyperhomocystinemia

Homocysteine is an amino acid formed in the metabolism of methionine. Elevated levels are present in vitamins B_{12} and B_6 and folate deficiencies; chronic renal failure; hypothyroidism; malignant neoplasms; and the use of methotrexate, phenytoin, and theophylline. Elevated levels of homocysteine are associated with higher rates of recurrent thrombosis. Fasting homocysteine plasma levels are a sensitive indicator for the diagnosis. Patients deficient in folate, vitamin B_6, or vitamin B_{12} should be supplemented with these vitamins in sufficient doses to achieve normal levels. In the absence of specific deficiencies, plasma homocysteine levels can be reduced up to 50% by administering folate at doses of 1–2 mg/day, although it is uncertain whether this ultimately leads to a decreased frequency of adverse events.

Antiphospholipid Syndrome

The diagnosis of this syndrome should be considered in patients with thrombosis (venous and/or arterial) or recurrent fetal loss and antiphospholipid antibodies (anticardiolipin antibodies and/or lupus anticoagulant). The syndrome is considered primary if there is no accompanying autoimmune disease and secondary if the patient has SLE. Other features occasionally seen include thrombocytopenia and livedo reticularis. Lupus anticoagulants are IgG or IgM antibodies that react with negatively charged phospholipids. Thus, in vitro they act as anticoagulants and interfere with membrane surfaces in clotting assays, resulting in false prolongation of the aPTT and occasionally the PT. The presence of the lupus anticoagulant may be confirmed with the dilute Russell's viper venom assay or phospholipid neutralization assay. A higher risk of recurrent thrombosis seems to occur when the "normal" intensity anticoagulation is used, so that increasing the goal INR to 2.5–3.5 or the addition of ASA has been used.

KEY POINTS TO REMEMBER

- Keep in mind all components of Virchow's triad (endothelial damage, stasis, hypercoagulability) as possible sources of thrombi.
- The clinical diagnosis of DVT is highly unreliable. Use Doppler U/S to exclude it when the diagnosis is entertained.
- PE and DVT may be treated with unfractionated heparins or LMWH. They should be continued at least 5 days and until therapeutic PO anticoagulation is achieved.
- Calf vein thromboses may be followed safely in most patients using serial U/S.
- IVC filters are an important alternative to treatment of DVT/PE with anticoagulation but are clinically inferior and should be used only when absolutely needed.

REFERENCES AND SUGGESTED READINGS

Harris JM, Abramson N. Evaluation of recurrent thrombosis and hypercoagulability. *Am Fam Phys* 1997;56:1591–1596.
Hirsch JH, Lee AY. How we treat deep vein thrombosis. *Blood* 2002;99:3102–3110.
Hoffman R, ed. *Hematology: basic principles and practice*, 3rd ed. New York: Churchill-Livingstone, 2000.
Levine S. The antiphospholipid syndrome. *N Engl J Med* 2002;346:752–763.
Seligsohn U, Lubetsky A. Genetic susceptibility to venous thrombosis. *N Engl J Med* 2001;334:1222–1229.
Streiff MB. Vena caval filters: a comprehensive review. *Blood* 2002;95:3669–3677.

Evaluation of Complete Blood Count Abnormalities

Geoffrey L. Uy

INTRODUCTION

With the routine use of automated analyzers for measuring the CBC, CBC abnormalities are often detected in all settings whether through the routine preop testing of an asymptomatic individual or as part of the initial workup of a hospitalized patient. The abnormalities may be an incidental finding or may reflect the underlying disease for which the patient has come to seek medical attention.

ANEMIA AND POLYCYTHEMIA

Anemia is broadly defined as a decrease in the red cell mass characterized by a Hgb below the normal range, whereas *polycythemia* is defined as a red cell mass above the normal range. See Chap. 7, Anemia, and Chap. 10, Myeloproliferative Disorders, for further information.

THROMBOCYTOPENIA

Thrombocytopenia is defined as a platelet count less than a "normal" range, usually approximately $150,000/\mu L$. Surgical bleeding due solely to a reduction in the number of platelets does not generally occur until the platelet count is $<50,000/\mu L$, whereas spontaneous bleeding does not occur until the platelet count is $<10,000-20,000/\mu L$.

Pathophysiology and Differential Diagnosis

Thrombocytopenia generally occurs as the result of one of three mechanisms either alone or in combination.

Decreased Platelet Production

- Infection: HIV, hepatitis C, parvovirus, varicella, rubella, mumps
- Chemotherapy
- Radiation
- Congenital or acquired primary bone marrow failure: Fanconi anemia, megakaryocytic thrombocytopenia, paroxysmal nocturnal hemoglobinuria (PNH)
- Vitamin deficiencies: folate, B12
- Alcohol

Increased Platelet Destruction

- Drugs: heparin, valproic acid, quinine
- Autoimmune platelet destruction: ITP, TTP-HUS
- HELLP syndrome
- DIC

Pseudothrombocytopenia

- Splenic sequestration
- Platelet clumping

TABLE 6-1. DRUGS COMMONLY IMPLICATED IN THROMBOCYTOPENIA

Quinidine	Danazol	Amphotericin B	Ethambutol
Quinine	Ethanol	Vancomycin	NSAIDs
Rifampin	Heparin	Amiodarone	Acetaminophen
TMP-SMX	Digoxin	H_2-blockers	

History and Physical Exam

- The **initial evaluation** should include a careful bleeding history and the chronicity of events. Bleeding caused by thrombocytopenia commonly presents as bleeding either in mucosal membranes or in the skin. Patients may describe epistaxis, bleeding gums, or menorrhagia. The presence of petechiae or ecchymoses suggests severe thrombocytopenia and is caused by the rupture and small hemorrhages in the capillary system.
- A careful **medication history** is essential, as drugs are a frequent cause of thrombocytopenia or platelet dysfunction. The social history should inquire about alcohol use and HIV risk factors. Alcohol leads to thrombocytopenia either through direct toxic effects on the marrow or through cirrhosis of the liver leading to portal HTN and hypersplenism. HIV is associated with thrombocytopenia due to a direct effect of the virus on the bone marrow, immune-mediated increased platelet destruction, or through antiretroviral medications that affect platelet production (Table 6-1).
- **Systemic symptoms** such as weight loss, fevers, night sweats, and fatigue may indicate an underlying malignancy or infection. Hepatosplenomegaly and/or ascites suggest the presence of portal HTN and splenic sequestration as a cause of thrombocytopenia.

Evaluation

- The **initial lab evaluation** of thrombocytopenia generally includes a CBC, peripheral smear, PT, and PTT. Results of any prior tests will help establish the chronicity of the problem. The PT and PTT are important screening tests in a patient with a suspected bleeding problem to rule out abnormalities of coagulation. Additionally, in patients with suspected TTP-HUS, LDH, and creatinine are usually increased, but PT/PTT is commonly normal. The elevated LDH in this situation results from RBC destruction and tissue ischemia and is useful in monitoring disease response to therapy.
- The **platelet count** may be roughly estimated from a peripheral smear with the platelet count being approximately 20,000 × the number seen per high-power field. Exam of the peripheral smear may also reveal *pseudothrombocytopenia* from platelet clumping. Clumping often occurs from EDTA in the sample tube and may be avoided by redrawing the sample in either a heparinized or citrated tube. However, in patients with clinical manifestations of bleeding, one should not assume that clumping is the cause of the thrombocytopenia. Exam of the smear may also reveal **schistocytes**, which may be indicative of a *microangiopathic hemolytic anemia* found in DIC or TTP.
- **Heparin-dependent antiplatelet antibodies** may occur in patients who have experienced a platelet drop while on heparin. A serotonin release assay is a highly sensitive and specific test for *heparin-induced thrombocytopenia* for patients who experience thrombocytopenia while on heparin (see Chap. 8, Disorders of Platelets and Primary Hemostasis, for a detailed discussion of this disorder).
- A **DIC panel**, including measurement of fibrinogen and fibrin degradation products, may be appropriate when the coagulation profile is abnormal.
- **Bone marrow biopsy** to evaluate for the presence of megakaryocytes may be useful to establish whether thrombocytopenia results from accelerated destruction or decreased production.
- **Abdominal U/S or CT scan** can quantify the size of the spleen where hypersplenism is suspected.

Management

Current medications should be reviewed carefully, and when drugs that may interfere with platelet function, such as NSAIDs, are identified, they should be discontinued. Platelet transfusion therapy is indicated in thrombocytopenia associated with major bleeding. Prophylactic platelet transfusions for individuals with chronic thrombocytopenia may be indicated when the platelet count is $>10,000/\mu L$ to reduce the risk of spontaneous intracranial bleeding. A threshold of $10,000/\mu L$ is also appropriate for nonbleeding patients who are not producing platelets due to marrow suppression from chemotherapy. When treated as outpatients, a more appropriate threshold in these patients may be $20,000/\mu L$, as they are less closely monitored. For most minor procedures, including central line placement, lumbar puncture, skin biopsy, and many surgeries in stable patients without active consumption of platelets, a threshold of $50,000/\mu L$ may be appropriate. In cases of neurosurgical procedures or other procedures in which bleeding would be devastating, a threshold of $100,000/\mu L$ may be wise. Platelet transfusions generally are not indicated in individuals with immune-mediated thrombocytopenia.

THROMBOCYTOSIS

Thrombocytosis is defined as a platelet count of the "normal" range, often $>450,000/$ μL, although further evaluation is often not indicated unless the platelet count is $>600,000/\mu L$. Depending on the etiology, either thrombosis or bleeding may be present. See Chap. 10, Myeloproliferative Disorders, for further details.

PANCYTOPENIA

Pancytopenia is described as a reduction in all blood cell lines: RBCs, WBCs, and platelets. Patients usually present with pancytopenia as a consequence of bone marrow failure with symptoms of anemia, bleeding secondary to thrombocytopenia, or recurrent infections as a result of leukopenia.

Pathophysiology

Pancytopenias may be the result of processes that either directly affect bone marrow or the result of processes outside of it. The bone marrow evaluation is often diagnostic in the workup of pancytopenia. *Nonmarrow* causes include hypersplenism, consumption, vitamin deficiencies (B_{12} and folate), autoimmune disease, or overwhelming infection. Those that occur as a result of an insult to the marrow itself may be characterized by a decrease in hematopoietic elements (aplasia) or from ineffective hematopoiesis or infiltration of the bone marrow.

Aplastic States

Aplastic anemia is that which occurs when there is a failure of marrow to produce any cells. Aplastic anemia is characterized by a hypoplastic marrow with morphologically normal cells. An acquired aplastic anemia can be caused by an autoimmune mechanism, infection (including HIV, parvovirus, certain types of viral hepatitis, EBV), radiation injury, or cytotoxic drugs. Of the congenital anemias, Fanconi anemia is the most common. It is an autosomal recessive disease that, in addition to hematologic findings, patients manifest varying degrees of physical anomalies and mental delay. *Paroxysmal nocturnal hemoglobinuria* (PNH) is a rare disorder characterized by a defect in glycosyl-phosphatidylinositol–anchored GPI-linked proteins, particularly CD59 and CD55, which help protect cells from complement-mediated lysis and can sometimes cause pancytopenia. It may be diagnosed by flow cytometry for these proteins (CD59 and CD55); their absence confirms this diagnosis.

Ineffective and Infiltrative Processes

Other marrow causes are those that are related to a dysplastic marrow or infiltration by abnormal tissue. That is, there is cellularity of the bone marrow, but it fails to produce hematologic cells. These typically are processes that infiltrate the bone marrow, such as malignancy (whether hematopoietic or solid tumor) or myelodysplastic syndromes. Nonmalignant processes such as infection or granulomatous disease is also possible.

Diagnostic Evaluation

History and Physical Exam

A search for concomitant illnesses or infections, which may be responsible for pancytopenia, should be undertaken. Patients have increased susceptibility to infections with increasing severity proportional to the degree of neutropenia. Symptoms and signs of inflammation, such as erythema or pus production, may be minimal or absent. Lymphadenopathy may indicate infection or malignancy, whereas splenomegaly may indicate liver disease and/or pseudothrombocytopenia.

Lab Evaluation

- The diagnosis of a pancytopenia often requires **bone marrow biopsy.** Aplastic anemia is characterized by a hypoplastic marrow with morphologically normal cells, whereas those related to abnormal infiltration will be evident on bone marrow biopsy. Metastatic tumors or involvement by leukemia or lymphoma will be apparent on bone marrow exam. Myelodysplastic syndromes can be more challenging to diagnose but typically show disordered maturation in a cellular bone marrow. Cytogenetics and flow cytometry of the bone marrow aspirate are useful when a hematologic malignancy or leukemia is suspected. See Chap. 9, Myelodysplasia, and Chap. 30, The Leukemias, for further details. In an aplastic anemia, it is often difficult to determine the cause based on bone marrow biopsy results alone.
- Initial lab evaluation should involve a peripheral smear and reticulocyte count. HIV status, folate and B_{12} levels, and viral hepatitis studies should be obtained. PNH may be suspected in the presence of an elevated reticulocyte count or hemolysis, as well as recurrent venous thrombosis. If infection is suspected, the aspirate should be sent for culture with fungal isolators. Other viral studies (EBV, CMV, parvovirus) may be appropriate in the setting of a patient with decreased marrow reserve. When no other cause is obviously apparent, the medication list of the patient should be studied. Medications can be the culprit in a number of cases, and the removal of the offending agent may be therapeutic. Acute leukemias or myelodysplastic disorders are characterized by impaired maturation. See Chap. 9, Myelodysplasia, and Chap. 30, The Leukemias, for further details.

Management

Treatment is directed at preventing complications, and any underlying illnesses should be identified and treated. When possible, drugs that may be responsible for cytopenias should be discontinued. A response to withdrawal of the offending agent is usually seen within 5–7 days. Patients with aplastic anemia often require support with red cell and platelet transfusions. Antibiotics and antifungal agents are often required to fight recurrent infections caused by impaired host defenses. Individuals with an absolute neutrophil count <500/μL should be placed on neutropenic precautions. Fever >38.1°C for 1 hr or 38.3°C should be treated with empiric broad-spectrum antibiotics and a search for infectious etiologies undertaken. The use of granulocyte-stimulating factors may be indicated in select applications, but data are lacking for routine use in asymptomatic leukopenic patients.

KEY POINTS TO REMEMBER

- The evaluation of CBC abnormalities should always include evaluation of the peripheral smear.
- Immune-mediated thrombocytopenias are associated with a normal spleen size. An enlarged spleen suggests an alternate diagnosis.

- PNH should be suspected in patients with pancytopenia and either reticulocytosis or unexplained thrombosis.
- Bone marrow biopsy is typically indicated in the workup of pancytopenia.
- Platelet clumping is a possible artifactual reason for thrombocytopenia but should not be the assumed reason in a bleeding patient.
- Fanconi anemia is the most common congenital anemia. This autosomal recessive disease is manifested by anemia and varying degrees of physical anomalies and mental delay.

REFERENCES AND SUGGESTED READINGS

Davenport J. Macrocytic anemia. *Am Fam Physician* 1996;53:155.

George JN, Raskob GE, Berkowitz SD. Platelets: acute thrombocytopenia. *Hematology* 1998:371–383.

George JN, Raskob GE, Shah SR, et al. Drug induced thrombocytopenia: a systematic review of published case reports. *Ann Intern Med* 1998;129:886.

Hillman RS, Ault KA. Clinical approach to anemia. In: Hillman RS, Ault KA, eds. *Hematology in clinical practice*. New York: McGraw-Hill, 2001:29.

Young NS, Abkowitz JL, Luzzatto L. New insights into the pathophysiology of acquired cytopenias. *Hematology* 2000:18–38.

Anemia

Stephen J. Wen

Low RBC counts are a common problem in consultative hematology. The workup of anemia is best served by a systematic approach to quickly narrow down the diagnosis and help guide the subsequent diagnostic workup. This chapter briefly discusses key points about RBCs and anemia and then describes the approach to diagnosis. This chapter assumes that the other blood cell lines—the WBCs and platelets—are normal; the workup of pancytopenia is discussed in Chap. 6, Evaluation of Complete Blood Count Abnormalities.

HISTORY AND PHYSICAL EXAM

Clinical manifestations will vary according to degree of anemia, underlying etiology, and whether onset is acute or chronic. *Anemia* is defined as a decrease in the circulating RBC mass; the usual criteria are Hgb <12 g/dL (Hct <36%) in women and <14 g/dL (Hct <41%) in men. Patients can be asymptomatic, but those patients with a Hgb <7 g/dL will usually have symptoms. Acute symptoms will include those typical of hypovolemia (pallor, visual impairment, syncope, and tachycardia) and require immediate attention. Chronic symptoms will reflect tissue hypoxia (fatigue, headache, dyspnea, lightheadedness, angina). Potential sources of blood loss, family history, and medication history must be evaluated carefully. On exam, one can note pallor, alopecia, atrophic glossitis, angular cheilosis, congestive heart failure (with severe anemia), koilonychias (spoon nails), and brittle nails.

LAB TESTS

- The **CBC** contains not only the measurements of WBCs, Hgb, and platelets, but also measurements of the *red cell indices*. The most useful are the mean cell volume (MCV), red cell distribution width (RDW), and mean cell Hgb concentration. **MCV** is the mean size of the red cells, **RDW** is a measure of variability in the size of the red cells, and *mean cell Hgb concentration* describes the concentration of Hgb in each cell. The **Hgb** is a measurement of g/dL of Hgb in blood, whereas the **hematocrit** is the physical amount of space as a percentage of the whole that the red cells occupy. Remember that the Hgb and Hct are unreliable indicators of red cell volume in the setting of rapid shifts of intravascular volume (i.e., an acute bleed).
- Other values include the **reticulocyte count,** which measures the immature red cells in the blood as a percentage of the whole and reflects the bone marrow's (BM) response to anemia (i.e., a normal BM response is to increase the production of red cells in anemia so that the observed reticulocyte count goes up).
- The **absolute reticulocyte count** is calculated as

$$\text{\% reticulocytes} \times \text{total RBC count}$$

- The **peripheral smear** is a required part of the initial hematologic evaluation. Key points to look for are shape of the RBCs and presence or absence of abnormal forms, such as schistocytes, spherocytes, or teardrop cells. The other cell lines should also be noted, especially the presence or absence of platelets.
- A **BM biopsy** may be indicated in normocytic anemias with a low reticulocyte count in the absence of an identifiable cause. It is also indicated when anemia is associated with

other cytopenias, leading to suspicion of myelophthisic process (i.e., presence of tear-drop or fragmented cells, normoblasts, or immature WBCs on peripheral blood smear).

APPROACH TO THE WORKUP OF ANEMIA

While there can be some overlap, anemia can be divided into three broad categories: **blood loss (acute or chronic), increased destruction of RBCs (hemolysis), and decreased production of RBCs.** Blood loss can be evaluated by a careful evaluation of the patient, including volume status. The *reticulocyte count* will usually help differentiate between states with decreased production (reticulocyte count <2%) and those associated with increased destruction (implied when reticulocyte count is >2%).

ANEMIAS ASSOCIATED WITH DECREASED PRODUCTION

The approach to an anemia associated with decreased production of red cells is to divide them into categories based on red cell size with the MCV, described earlier. Normal size range is typically 80–100 fL. Cells of this volume are called *normocytic*, with smaller cells being described as *microcytic* and larger being described as *macrocytic*.

Microcytic Anemias
Causes

CAUSES OF MICROCYTIC ANEMIAS BY MCV

MCV 70–80	MCV <70
Iron deficiency	Thalassemia
Anemia of chronic disease	Iron deficiency
Thalassemia	
Sideroblastic anemia	

The degree of microcytosis may give a clue to the possible underlying diagnoses. Very low MCV typically do not represent anemia of chronic disease of sideroblastic anemia.

Iron-Deficiency Anemia
ETIOLOGIES

- **Dietary deficiency** is usually seen in infants who are milk fed. In early childhood it can be seen in meat-deficient diets. It can also occur in the setting of increased requirements, such as pregnancy or early childhood.
- **Malabsorption** can occur in the setting of partial gastrectomy (hypochlorhydria/achlorhydria impairs Fe absorption; decreased transit time through duodenum in which Fe is most actively absorbed); celiac sprue (refractory to PO Fe therapy); chronic diarrhea and other malabsorption syndromes; and inhibition of Fe absorption by tannates (tea), carbonates, and phosphates.
- **Chronic blood loss** is the most common cause of Fe deficiency in adults. It is usually lost via the GI tract by ulcerative disease, gastritis, cancer, hemorrhoids, or arteriovenous malformation, with ulcers and colon malignancies being the most common. Can also occur owing to menorrhagia/menstruation, hematuria due to genitourinary cancer, frequent blood donation, and frequent phlebotomy in hospitalized patients.
- In addition to the usual symptoms of anemia, Fe deficiency is often associated with **pica** (consumption of nonfood substances such as corn starch or ice).
- *It should be noted that the diagnosis of Fe deficiency in an adult mandates investigation of its cause to rule out malignancy.*

DIAGNOSIS

- Diagnosis involves serum testing of **Fe**. The serum **ferritin** can be checked and, when low, almost always signifies Fe deficiency. However, it is an acute phase reactant and can be falsely elevated in inflammatory states. The **transferrin saturation percent** is another measure of Fe in the serum but can be less reliable. The gold standard diagnosis is a BM biopsy with Fe staining.
- **Patients can have microcytic normochromic anemia that eventually progresses to microcytic hypochromic as the anemia progresses. With worsening Fe-deficient anemia, there is a gradual increase in anisocytosis and poikilocytosis (abnormally shaped cells).**

TREATMENT

- In addition to diagnosing the Fe deficiency, it is important to discover and treat the underlying disorder.
- **Fe replacement** may be given by PO Fe salts, which should be given between meals because food or antacids may decrease absorption. Ascorbic acid given with Fe sulfate may increase absorption. One replacement regimen is ferrous sulfate, 325 mg PO tid (equivalent of 65 mg elemental Fe tid). Enteric-coated forms are not well absorbed and should not be used.
- **Parenteral Fe** is given with indications including intolerance or failure to take PO Fe, Fe losses that exceed the capacity to replete PO, or malabsorption. There is a ≈ 1/300 risk of a serious reaction (including anaphylaxis), however, with IV Fe dextran. This is treated by stopping the infusion and giving epinephrine.
- The amount of Fe needed can be calculated as the amount of Fe needed to replace the missing Hgb added to the amount necessary to replete the total body Fe stores (usually estimated at approximately 1000 mg) from the formula below [1]:

$$\text{Total dose (in mg)} = ([\text{normal Hgb (g/dL)} - \text{patient Hgb (g/dL)}] \times \text{body weight [kg]} \times 2.2) + 1000 \text{ mg}$$

However, in practice, Fe is often infused at a dose of 1–1.2 g without formally calculating iron repletion.

FOLLOW-UP. One can expect an increase in the reticulocyte count within 7–10 days, and correction of anemia usually occurs within 6–8 wks if ongoing blood loss is stopped. Treatment should continue for approximately 6 mos (on PO Fe) to fully restore tissue stores.

Thalassemias

These patients are transfusion dependent and require chelation therapy to avoid Fe overload, usually at ferritin concentrations above 1000 ng/mL. Deferoxamine is the only effective long-term iron chelator currently approved for use in the United States. In general, thalassemia results from complete lack of or decreased synthesis of alpha or beta globin chains. *Beta-thalassemia* is more common in Mediterranean, African, and Southeast Asian populations and is thought to offer resistance to falciparum malaria. Beta-thalassemia major results from a total lack of production of beta-globin chain. It causes lack of adequate Hgb A formation, leading to microcytic, hypochromic cells. Complications of severe beta-thalassemia include skeletal deformities resulting from erythropoietin-stimulated expansion of BM, hepatosplenomegaly from extramedullary hematopoiesis, and secondary hemochromatosis from repeat blood transfusions and increased dietary absorption of Fe. Thalassemia minor is loss of only one of the two alleles coding for the beta-globulin gene. It is usually an asymptomatic condition manifest by microcytosis and a normal red cell distribution width. It is accompanied by a mild anemia (if any). *Alpha-thalassemia* results from decreased production of alpha-globin chains, of which there are four total. The severity of anemia depends on the number of defective alpha genes. Diagnosis is by Hgb electrophoresis for beta-thalassemia and severe alpha-thalassemia. Mild alpha-thalassemia may be detected by alpha:beta ratio or by molecular testing, although neither is widely available.

The treatment of thalassemias usually depends on the severity of the genetic defect and resultant clinical sequelae. The minor thalassemias are commonly asymptomatic and require no therapy while the major thalassemias may be treated by chronic transfusions, chelation therapy to avoid Fe overload (due to transfusions), and splenectomy.

Sideroblastic Anemias

Sideroblastic anemias are characterized by ineffective erythropoiesis and the presence of ringed sideroblasts in the BM. The term *ringed* refers to the accumulation of Fe in the mitochondria that surround the periphery of the nucleus. There are hereditary and idiopathic forms, as well as forms associated with drugs or toxins such as alcohol, lead, isoniazid (INH), and chloramphenicol. One final diagnosis to consider in cases of microcytic, hypochromic anemias is **lead poisoning.** It is a rare but treatable form of microcytic anemia in adults and usually results from a work or an environmental exposure. The diagnosis is suggested by finding basophilic stippling on the peripheral smear.

There is no cure for hereditary sideroblastic anemia, and treatment is aimed at preventing end-organ damage from Fe overload (chelation therapy). Drug-induced sideroblastic anemias are commonly reversible when the offending agent is discontinued. For sideroblastic anemia caused by isoniazid treatment, high-dose pyridoxine supplementation (up to 200 mg/day PO) often reverses the anemia and allows for continuation of the drug.

Normocytic Anemias

Normocytic anemias can be associated with an elevated reticulocyte count, which represents a hemolytic anemia or bleeding (see following sections), whereas a decreased reticulocyte count typically represents hypoproliferative disorder (Table 7-1). Normocytic anemia may be an early finding in BM failure. Aplastic anemia is actually a pancytopenia and is discussed in Chap. 6, Evaluation of Complete Blood Count Abnormalities. Pure RBC aplasia involves a selective destruction of RBC precursors and can be congenital or acquired. It is often associated with viral infections (e.g., parvovirus). Symptoms are related to the anemia. Diagnosis is via BM biopsy showing absence of erythroid elements but with preservation of other cell lines. Treatment includes supportive measures with transfusions as needed.

Anemia of Chronic Disease

This condition is often associated with malignancy, infection, and inflammatory states. It may occur in patients with chronic infections (e.g., osteomyelitis), HIV, or inflammatory diseases (e.g., lupus or rheumatoid arthritis). These disorders will have in common the

TABLE 7-1. CAUSES OF NORMOCYTIC ANEMIA ASSOCIATED WITH DECREASED RETICULOCYTE COUNT

Malignancies and other marrow infiltrative diseases
  Leukemia and lymphoma
  Metastatic cancer
  Plasma cell disorders
  Granulomatous disease
Stem cell disorders
  Myelofibrosis
  Aplastic anemia
  Pure red cell plasma
  Myelodysplasia
Due to other medical conditions
  Anemia of renal disease
  Anemia of chronic disease
  Endocrine disorders

inhibition of normal RBC synthesis due to the underlying disorder. They may act by inadequate release or insensitivity to erythropoietin. Other etiologies include deficiency in mobilization of Fe from the reticuloendothelial system. The anemia is most often a normocytic, normochromic anemia with a decreased reticulocyte count but may also present as a mild microcytic anemia. The serum Fe concentration and total Fe-binding capacity are usually both low, often giving a normal transferrin saturation (although this may be low or low-normal range). Serum ferritin is an acute phase reactant, often elevated in inflammatory diseases and infections. BM exam, if done, typically shows present Fe stores. Symptoms and physical exam of the anemia of chronic disease patient are dependent on the patient's underlying condition. The anemia is typically mild and does not require blood transfusion. The more appropriate treatment is to treat the underlying condition.

Myelophthisic Anemias

Myelophthisic anemias refer to those with evidence of hematopoiesis outside the BM or infiltration of the BM by nonhematologic cells. The most common cause is metastatic carcinoma to the BM (e.g., breast, lung, prostate, kidney). Other causes include myeloproliferative disorders, multiple myeloma, leukemias, and lymphoma. These are often suspected by a typical appearance of the peripheral smear (nucleated RBC, teardrop-shaped RBCs, and immature WBCs) and a "dry" tap on BM aspiration. BM biopsy results are dependent on the underlying disease. Treatment is based on the underlying disorder.

Myelodysplastic Syndromes

See Chap. 9, Myelodysplasia.

Anemia of Chronic Renal Failure

Anemia of chronic renal failure is due to erythropoietin deficiency. The anemia generally starts when CrCl <45 mL/min and worsens with increasing renal failure. When possible, treatment involves first treating the underlying renal dysfunction. Erythropoietin can be given at 50–100 U/kg IV or SC 3×/wk with readjustments based on response. In follow-up, expect an increase in Hct in 8–12 wks.

Endocrine Disorders

Anemia due to endocrine disorders is seen in hypothyroidism, adrenal insufficiency, and gonadal dysfunction. Estrogens tend to inhibit red cell synthesis, and testosterone tends to stimulate it. Correction of the underlying endocrine disorder may improve the anemia.

Macrocytic Anemias

The anemias that have a MCV of more than approximately 100 fL are the macrocytic anemias. These may be separated into two categories based on features seen on peripheral smear: megaloblastic and nonmegaloblastic. *Megaloblastic* features include the presence of oval macrocytes and hypersegmentation of the PMNs. They are a consequence of abnormal maturation of these cells and nuclear/cellular asynchrony in terms of maturation. *Nonmegaloblastic* features include the presence of round macrocytes without hypersegmentation of the PMNs.

Causes

- Megaloblastic anemia: oval macrocytes and hypersegmentation of PMNs on smear
  - Vitamin B_{12} deficiency
  - Folate deficiency
  - Drug-induced
- Nonmegaloblastic anemia: round macrocytes and no hypersegmentation of PMNs on smear
  - Liver disease
  - Hypothyroidism
  - Alcohol-induced
  - Reticulocytosis secondary to hemolytic anemia

Vitamin B$_{12}$ Deficiency

The daily requirement of vitamin B$_{12}$ is 2 μg/day, and a typical diet provides 5–15 μg/day, with the liver capable of storing approximately 2000–5000 μg. Thus, it takes up to 3–6 yrs for deficiency to develop once absorption completely ceases.

ETIOLOGIES. Etiologies include pernicious anemia (the most common cause), gastrectomy or gastric bypass surgery, ileal disorders (sprue, inflammatory bowel disease, lymphoma), bacterial overgrowth in the small intestine, fish tapeworms, and inadequate intake (this is very rare and only occurs in the strict vegetarian).

HISTORY AND PHYSICAL EXAM. Symptoms include burning sensation of the tongue, vague abdominal pain, diarrhea, numbness, paresthesia, and mental clouding. On exam, one can note glossitis, smooth tongue, dorsal column finding (decreased vibration and proprioception), and corticospinal tract findings (motor weakness, spasticity, Babinski sign). *Patients can present with neurologic signs without overt anemia.*

DIAGNOSIS. In cases of borderline low B$_{12}$ values, one can measure serum methylmalonic acid and homocysteine levels that are elevated in vitamin B$_{12}$ deficiency. Once deficiency is established, an attempt should be made to identify the etiology. The presence of antiintrinsic factor antibodies or antiparietal cell antibodies lends support to the diagnosis of pernicious anemia. Surgical history can reveal postsurgical etiologies. Suspicion of ileal disorder can be evaluated by endoscopy with or without biopsy. Stool ova and parasites should be performed if suspicious for parasitic infection or a therapeutic trial of antibiotics if bacterial overgrowth is suspected. The Schilling test is rarely used today but may delineate the underlying pathology.

TREATMENT. Treatment usually includes vitamin B$_{12}$, 1 mg IM or SC daily for 7 days, then weekly for 1 mo, followed by monthly doses thereafter. Failure to correct or identify the underlying mechanism of deficiency should result in lifetime therapy.

FOLLOW-UP. Reticulocytosis should occur in 5–7 days, with resolution of hematologic abnormalities in approximately 2 mos. Resolution of neurologic abnormalities depends on their duration before treatment and may take up to 18 mos but can also be permanent.

Folate Deficiency

The daily requirement of folate is 50–100 μg/day, with body stores approximately 5–10 mg. Depletion can occur after approximately 2–4 mos of persistent negative balance. Etiologies include inadequate intake (e.g., alcoholics), decreased absorption (e.g., sprue, bacterial overgrowth, certain drugs such as dilantin and oral contraceptives), or states of increased requirements (hemolytic anemia, pregnancy, chronic dialysis, exfoliative dermatitis). It can be iatrogenic during treatment with folic acid antagonists (e.g., methotrexate, trimethoprim). Symptoms and physical exam are similar to vitamin B$_{12}$ deficiency with the exception that neurologic features are **not** present. Make sure to measure both serum and RBC folate levels. Serum folate is more labile and subject to acute rise after a folate-rich meal; RBC folate is a better indicator of tissue stores. It is important to **rule out vitamin B$_{12}$ deficiency** before repletion with folate, because folate may improve the hematologic abnormalities in vitamin B$_{12}$ deficiency but will not correct the neurologic manifestations. Treatment is with PO folate (1 mg/day) with resolution of hematologic abnormalities in approximately 2 mos.

Drug-Induced Disorders

Several drugs can cause a macrocytic anemia by affecting DNA synthesis. Offenders include purine analogs (e.g., 6-mercaptopurine, azathioprine), pyrimidine analogs (5-fluorouracil, Ara-C), hydroxyurea, and anticonvulsants (dilantin, phenobarbital). Reverse transcriptase inhibitors (AZT, etc.) may cause macrocytosis without anemia. Therapy is cessation of the offending agent or tolerating a mild anemia if the drug is therapeutically needed.

Nonmegaloblastic Anemia

Nonmegaloblastic anemias typically have round macrocytes without hypersegmentation of PMNs on peripheral smear. MCV of nonmegaloblastic anemias is rarely >110–115. A value higher than this would tend to support a megaloblastic etiology. When the reticulocyte count is elevated, it suggests an etiology such as alcohol, hypothyroidism, or liver disease, and evaluation should seek to investigate these possible causes. Hemolytic

TABLE 7-2. CAUSES OF INCREASED RBC DESTRUCTION

Hereditary	Acquired
RBC membrane disorders	Immune related
Spherocytosis	Warm antibody
Elliptocytosis	Cold agglutinin
RBC enzyme disorders	Transfusion reaction
Pyruvate kinase deficiency	Nonimmune
Hexokinase deficiency	Microangiopathic hemolytic anemia
G-6-PD deficiency	Infection
Disordered Hgb synthesis	Hypersplenism
Hemoglobinopathy (i.e., sickle cell)	Paroxysmal nocturnal hemoglobinuria
Thalassemias	

anemia can produce a macrocytosis via increased production of reticulocytes. Nonmegaloblastic anemias are usually treated by identifying and treating the underlying etiology, such as discontinuation of alcohol use and thyroid hormone replacement.

ANEMIAS ASSOCIATED WITH INCREASED DESTRUCTION

Table 7-2 lists causes of anemia associated with increased RBC destruction. The following discussion is based on the acquired vs. hereditary classification.

Classification of Hemolytic Anemias

- **Extravascular** implies hemolysis occurring in the reticuloendothelial system, usually in the spleen, whereas **intravascular** is occurring within the circulation.
- **Intrinsic** implies a defect in the RBC membrane or contents, whereas **extrinsic** implies serum antibody, trauma within circulation, infection, etc.
- **In general, most intrinsic causes are hereditary, and most extrinsic causes are acquired.**

Hemolytic Anemias (HA)

Acute hemolysis may be accompanied by fever, chills, back and abdominal pain, and even shock. Also noted are jaundice, occasionally splenomegaly, and, in some cases, voiding brown or red urine. Signs of hemolysis on peripheral blood smear are often identified and include spherocytes (in autoimmune hemolytic anemia, hereditary spherocytosis), helmet cells or schistocytes (microangiopathic hemolytic anemia), sickle cells and Howell-Jolly bodies (sickle cell anemia), spur cells (liver disease), bite cells or Heinz bodies [G-6-PD (glucose-6-phosphate dehydrogenase)], and agglutination (cold agglutinin). Lab tests suggestive of hemolysis include increased lactate dehydrogenase, decreased haptoglobin, and increased unconjugated bilirubin. Typically associated are lab signs of increased RBC production via an increased reticulocyte count. **Positive direct Coombs test** is a direct antiglobulin test. The direct Coombs test detects antibodies (usually IgG) or complement (usually C3) bound to the surface of circulating RBCs by mixing *patient RBCs* with *anti-IgG*. Positive results may occur in cases of allo- or autoantibodies to RBC antigens or in cases of nonspecific adherence of other Ig or immune complexes to RBC surface. In the **indirect Coombs** test, the patient's **serum** is mixed with **normal** RBCs to detect antibody.

Sickle Cell Anemia

Sickle cell anemia is caused by a defect in the beta-globin chain, resulting in sickle cells. See Chap. 12, Sickle Cell Disease, for further details.

TABLE 7-3. PRECIPITANTS OF HEMOLYSIS IN GLUCOSE-6-PHOSPHATE DEHYDROGENASE DEFICIENCY

Infection (*E. coli*, salmonella, *S. pneumoniae*, viral hepatitis)

Drug-induced

    Antimalarials: primaquine and chloroquine

    Antibiotics: sulfonamides, dapsone (Dapsone USP, DDS), nitrofurantoin (Macrodantin)

    Phenazopyridine (Pyridium)

    Analgesics: in some cases, salicylates

Fava beans (in the Mediterranean variant only)

Naphthalene

Glucose-6-Phosphate Deficiency

G-6-PD is an X-linked disorder fully expressed in males and homozygous females and variably expressed in heterozygous females. The mechanism of hemolysis is that, in the presence of oxidative stress, G-6-PD deficiency results in an inability to maintain Hgb in a reduced state. This, in turn, leads to Hgb precipitation within RBCs (Heinz body formation) and intravascular hemolysis (Table 7-3). There are two main variants that lead to clinically significant hemolysis: *G-6-PD A–* and *G-6-PD Mediterranean*. G-6-PD A– occurs in 10% of black individuals, has normal enzyme activity in young RBCs, but older cells have marked deficiency of enzyme activity. When challenged, only the older cells lyse. This form is typically milder and self-limited. The G-6-PD Mediterranean variant occurs in people of Middle Eastern and Mediterranean descent. It is characterized by a nearly complete lack of G-6-PD. Hemolysis tends to be more severe compared to the A– variant. Diagnosis is suspected when hemolysis occurs after starting a drug known to precipitate hemolysis in a G-6-PD patient—Heinz bodies and "bite" cells may be seen on the smear. "Bite" cells result from the attempts by macrophages in the spleen to remove the Heinz bodies from the RBCs. Definitive diagnosis is made by measuring enzyme activity level. **In the A– variant, do not measure enzyme levels in the presence of acute hemolysis,** as you will be measuring the activity in reticulocytes and younger RBCs, which will be normal. It is advisable to **wait 3–4 wks after the acute episode** to get a true representation of the enzyme activity level. The same does not apply to the Mediterranean variant, as both younger and older red cells are affected. Treatment is supportive with transfusions as needed and documentation of oxidative precipitant and avoidance in the future.

Hereditary Spherocytosis (Membrane Defect)

Hereditary spherocytosis is an autosomal dominant disorder, most common in patients of Northern European descent, owing to a defect in a membrane cytoskeletal protein resulting in the formation of spherocytes. Symptoms are those of anemia; some patients may have symptoms of cholelithiasis. On physical exam, one finds splenomegaly secondary to extravascular hemolysis. Diagnosis is suspected when spherocytes are seen on the blood smear. The *osmotic fragility test* will note increased red cell lysis with incubation in hypotonic saline. Treatment may include splenectomy, which corrects the anemia but not the underlying defect, and supportive transfusions.

Acquired Immune Hemolytic Anemia

WARM ANTIBODY. Warm antibody is the most common form. Most are IgG and active at 37°C. 60% are *idiopathic* (or *primary*), whereas 40% are *secondary*. Secondary forms can be from chronic lymphocytic leukemia, non-Hodgkin's lymphoma, Hodgkin's lymphoma, autoimmune disorders (such as SLE), and drugs. **Drug-related antibodies** can occur by three main mechanisms:

- **Autoantibody:** production of antibody against Rhesus (e.g., methyldopa)
- **Hapten:** drug binds to RBC membrane; antibody directed against this complex; occurs 1–2 wks after treatment (e.g., penicillin, cephalosporins)

- **Immune complex:** drug binds to plasma protein, evoking an antibody response; drug-protein-antibody complex nonspecifically coats RBCs, resulting in complement-mediated lysis (e.g., quinidine, INH, sulfonamides)

Warm antibodies usually cause extravascular hemolysis by the spleen, leading to splenomegaly. Almost all are pan-agglutinins (i.e., reacts with most donor RBCs), making crossmatching difficult. Treatment consists of drug withdrawal when applicable (hemolysis will stop when the drug is cleared from the plasma) and steroids (prednisone) may be used, 1 mg/kg/day for severe hemolysis in idiopathic forms, continued until Hgb reaches normal levels over a few weeks, and then tapered. Splenectomy is an option for patients who relapse after steroid taper or who do not respond to steroids. If both steroids and splenectomy fail, then other immunosuppressives can be tried [e.g., cyclosporin (Sandimmune), azathioprine (Imuran)]. Attempts should be made to avoid transfusions, if possible, as this may result in more hemolysis.

COLD ANTIBODY. Most cold antibodies are IgM and active at <30°C. Acute onset is associated with mycoplasma pneumonia or infectious mononucleosis, whereas chronic forms occur with lymphoproliferative disorders or are idiopathic. The two main manifestations are acrocyanosis (ears, nose, distal extremities) and hemolysis (complement mediated). Symptoms mainly occur in distal body parts where temperature may be <30°C. In these cold temperatures, IgM will bind to the RBCs and cause complement fixation and hemolysis. The antibody dissociates from the RBC when the temperature rises above 30°C. Treatment involves avoidance of cold exposure and treatment of the underlying disorder, if possible. Immunosuppressive agents may be effective, but splenectomy and steroids are of limited value.

Nonimmune Hemolytic Anemia
TYPES. See Table 7-4.

TABLE 7-4. TYPES OF ACQUIRED NONIMMUNE HEMOLYTIC ANEMIAS

1. Microangiopathic hemolytic anemia
   a. TTP
   b. Disseminated intravascular coagulation
   c. HUS
   d. Eclampsia
   e. Malignant HTN
   f. Metastatic adenocarcinoma
2. Macroangiopathic hemolytic anemia
   a. Prosthetic valve
   b. Severe aortic stenosis
3. Physical and chemical
   a. Snake and spider venom
   b. Osmotic hemolysis from freshwater drowning
   c. Damage to RBC membranes from third-degree burns
4. Infection
   a. Malaria
   b. *Clostridium difficile*
   c. Babesiosis
5. Hypersplenism
6. Paroxysmal nocturnal hemoglobinuria

DISSEMINATED INTRAVASCULAR COAGULATION. DIC is an acquired disorder in which a microangiopathic hemolytic anemia occurs. It is usually secondary to another cause. It is diagnosed by demonstration of microangiopathic hemolytic anemia on a smear, with elevated fibrin split products and decreased fibrinogen in the appropriate clinical setting. Treatment is largely supportive and aimed at correcting the underlying deficit. Fresh frozen plasma can be given, as well as cryoprecipitate. Please see Chap. 8, Disorders of Platelets and Primary Hemostasis.

PAROXYSMAL NOCTURNAL HEMOGLOBINURIA. PNH is a rare defect in which all cell lines lack specific glycosylphosphotidylinositol-linked plasma membrane proteins, which are responsible for regulating activation of complement. Thus, the cells become sensitive to complement-mediated lysis. Complications include acute leukemia, aplastic anemia, and venous thrombosis (hepatic, portal, cerebral). It is diagnosed by the sucrose hemolysis, acid hemolysis (Ham), and flow cytometry (to evaluate for absence of various CD antigens) tests.

KEY POINTS TO REMEMBER

- Always consider active bleeding as a source of anemia.
- The initial workup of anemia always includes a thorough history and physical, assessment of cell counts and red cell indices, tests of the coagulation system, and viewing of the peripheral slide.
- The Hgb and Hct are often inaccurate in the setting of acute bleeding.
- Patients with Fe deficiency can have microcytic normochromic indices (early) that eventually progress to microcytic hypochromic. With worsening Fe deficiency anemia, there is a gradual increase in anisocytosis and poikilocytosis (abnormally shaped cells).
- In vitamin B_{12} deficiency, patients can present with neurologic signs without overt anemia.
- It is important to rule out vitamin B_{12} deficiency before repletion with folate, because folate can improve the hematologic abnormalities in vitamin B_{12} deficiency but will do nothing for the neurologic manifestations.
- In G6PD-A, do not measure enzyme levels during an acute hemolytic attack. It is best to wait 3–4 wks, because it is the older RBCs that have the marked deficiency in enzyme activity, which are the cells that have been lysed. Testing during an acute attack can render false-negative results.

SUGGESTED READING

Adams RJ. Stroke prevention and treatment in sickle cell disease. *Arch Neurol* 2001;58(4):565–568.

Berkow R, ed. Anemias. In: *The Merck manual*, 16th ed. Rahway, NJ: Merck Research Laboratories, 1992:1136–1174.

Blinder M. Anemia and transfusion therapy. In: Ahya, Flood, Paranjothi, eds. *The Washington Manual of medical therapeutics*, 30th ed. Philadelphia: Lippincott Williams & Wilkins, 2001:413–428.

Burd R. Hematology/oncology. In: Ferri FF, ed. *Practical guide to the care of the medical patient*, 3rd ed. St. Louis: Mosby, 1995:376–387.

Davenport J. Macrocytic anemia. *Am Fam Physician* 1996;53(1):155–162.

Division of Blood Diseases and Resources. *Management and therapy of sickle cell disease*, 3rd ed. Bethesda, MD: National Heart, Lung, and Blood Institutes, December 1995. (NIH publication no. 96-2117.)

Eckman JR. Orderly approach to the evaluation and treatment of anemia. *Emory Univ J Med* 1991;5(2):80–90.

Goroll AH. Evaluation of anemia. In: Goroll, AH, May LA, Mulley AG. *Primary care medicine: office evaluation and management of the adult patient*, 3rd ed. Philadelphia: J.B. Lippincott Company, 1995:447–455.

Robbins SL, Cotran RS, Kumar V. Diseases of red cells and bleeding disorders. In: Cotran RS, Robbins SL, Kumar V, et al. *Pathologic basis of disease*, 5th ed. Philadelphia: W.B. Saunders, 1994:583–616.

Rosse W, Bunn HF. Hemolytic anemias. In: Isselbacher KJ, Braunwald E, Wilson JD, et al., eds. *Harrison's principles of internal medicine*, 13th ed. New York: McGraw-Hill, 1994:1743–1754.

Sandstad J, McKenna RW, Keffer JH, ed. Erythrocyte disorders. In: Keffer JH, ed. *Handbook of clinical pathology*. Chicago: ASCP Press, 1992:193–211.

Steensma DP, Hoyer JD, Fairbanks VF. Hereditary red blood cell disorders in Middle Eastern patients. *Mayo Clin Proc* 2001;76(3):285–293.

Steinberg MH. Management of sickle cell disease. *N Engl J Med* 1999;340(13):1021–1030.

Vichinsky E, Styles L. Pulmonary complications. *Hematol Oncol Clin North Am* 1996;10(6):1275–1287.

Vichinsky EP, Haberkern CM, Neumayr L, et al. A comparison of conservative and aggressive transfusion regimens in the perioperative management of sickle cell disease. *N Engl J Med* 1995;333(4):206–213.

Wayne AS, Kevy SV, Nathan DG. Transfusion management of sickle cell disease. *Blood* 1993;81(5):1109–1123.

REFERENCE

1. Massey A. Microcytic anemia, differential diagnosis and management of iron deficiency anemia. *Med Clin North Am* 1992;76(3):549–566.

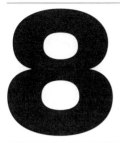

Disorders of Platelets and Primary Hemostasis

Nicholas H. Laffely,
Leslie A. Andritsos,
and Charles S. Eby

INTRODUCTION

Platelets are essential for primary hemostasis—the process in which a platelet plug forms to initiate clotting. When the platelet number is too low or the platelets are not functioning properly, bleeding may result. The general approach to thrombocytopenia is addressed in Chap. 6, Evaluation of Complete Blood Count Abnormalities. This chapter expands on disorders that cause thrombocytopenia, as well as those that are associated with problems of primary hemostasis. Disorders of the coagulation pathways, including von Willebrand disease (vWD), are discussed in Chap. 4, Disorders of Coagulation. The topics addressed here include the following:

- Inherited platelet disorders
- Idiopathic thrombocytopenic purpura (ITP)
- Thrombotic thrombocytopenic purpura (TTP)–hemolytic
- Uremic syndrome [TTP–hemolytic uremic syndrome (HUS)]
- Disseminated intravascular coagulation (DIC)
- Heparin-induced thrombocytopenia (HIT)
- Essential thrombocytosis

INHERITED ABNORMALITIES OF PLATELETS

Although inherited abnormalities of platelets are quite rare, they deserve brief mention because of their historical significance and importance in understanding platelet function. **Glanzmann's thrombasthenia** is an autosomal recessive disorder caused by a defect in GpIIb-IIIa—an important glycoprotein involved in binding fibrinogen—forming the primary hemostatic plug and activating platelets. A defect in GpIIb-IIIa due to any number of possible mutations leads to the typical mucosal bleeding pattern seen in acquired platelet disorders. Mild to severe bleeding may be seen. **Bernard-Soulier syndrome** is characterized by giant platelet forms (up to 20 μm) and thrombocytopenia. It is due to a defect in GpIb-IX, and this is significant because it is the receptor for von Willebrand factor (vWF). This autosomal recessive bleeding disorder is due to this improper platelet-vWF binding. **Pseudo-vWD,** or "platelet type vWD," is due to an abnormality in GpIb that has increased affinity for vWF. Abnormal platelet binding leads to increased clearance of vWF from the plasma. The **May-Hegglin** anomaly is an autosomal dominant disorder characterized by giant platelets and thrombocytopenia like Bernard-Soulier syndrome. There are a number of other inherited disorders associated with platelet defects, and these should be distinguished from acquired platelet abnormalities. A key distinguishing feature is giant platelets seen on peripheral blood smear. Also be aware that chronic ITP in children (the age when most of these inherited disorders are discovered) is rare. Many of these disorders are treated with platelet transfusions.

IDIOPATHIC THROMBOCYTOPENIC PURPURA

ITP is defined as thrombocytopenia in a patient with no clinically apparent associated conditions or factors that can cause thrombocytopenia. It is now thought that the etiology of thrombocytopenia is an antibody directed against platelets, which leads to platelet clearance and destruction by the reticuloendothelial system (most notably in the spleen). It tends to be classified into childhood and adult variants. In childhood, ITP usually is a self-limited disease, whereas in adults it tends to run a more chronic course. A rough estimate suggests an incidence of 100 cases/1 million person years, with approximately 50% found in children. Review of the literature documents significant deviation from this estimate, and, thus, the actual incidence is unknown. In adults, it is most common between ages 18 and 40. It tends to have a 2–3:1 female to male predominance.

Pathophysiology

Antibodies to platelet surface GpIIb/IIIa, -Ib/IX, -Ia/IIa and others have been identified as the likely causes of ITP. It is unclear why the immune system develops antibodies to these markers, but the process appears to be related to antigen-presenting cell-processing of the platelet glycoproteins and stimulation of T cells similar to foreign antigen processing. It also appears to be a polyclonal process, but the number of B-cell clones may be limited. These antibodies bind to intact platelet surface glycoproteins, which in turn bind to Fc-gamma receptors on macrophages, leading to clearance by the reticuloendothelial system, especially in the spleen. The body does try to compensate, and the platelets subsequently produced tend to be somewhat larger and more effective than typical platelets of the average population. The disease has been noted after viral infection, especially in children, which may initiate the malfunction in the immune system. There also appears to be a possible genetic predisposition, although more work is needed to assess the full role of genetics.

History and Physical

- Some cases of ITP are picked up as an incidental finding of a low platelet count on a screening CBC, but many will be discovered because of bleeding or purpura. Once thrombocytopenia has been identified, ITP is a diagnosis of exclusion of other causes. The history and physical must be directed at identifying other sources of thrombocytopenia. Key history questions are shown in Table 8-1. The workup of thrombocytopenia is addressed in Chap. 6, Evaluation of Complete Blood Count Abnormalities.
- Bleeding that is associated with ITP is usually cutaneous or mucosal. Petechiae and purpura with easy bruising are commonly seen. Epistaxis, mouth lesions, conjunctival hemorrhages, and menorrhagia are also frequently seen. Other types of bleeding are less common. Deep hematomas and hemarthrosis are more typical of clotting deficiencies. Intracranial hemorrhage is the most feared type of bleeding. Although rare, when it occurs, it has a high mortality and accounts for most of the fatal hemorrhages. Older reports note <5% mortality, but with treatment it is probably <1%. GI bleeding is uncommon, especially in younger patients, but can be a serious problem in older patients.
- Other findings such as splenic sequestration should always be assessed by looking for splenomegaly that is only noted in 3% of ITP patients. Alloimmune thrombocytopenia can be a real problem in patients that have received transfusions. Palpable lymph nodes suggest systemic disease and are not characteristic of ITP. Systemic infection can lead to DIC that usually has multiple signs inconsistent with ITP. Other history and physical findings, as noted, can elucidate other causes of thrombocytopenia.
- ITP can occur in pregnancy, but gestational thrombocytopenia and thrombocytopenia associated with preeclampsia and HELLP syndrome (*h*emolysis, *e*levated *l*iver enzymes, and *l*ow *p*latelets) should be ruled out.

Lab Evaluation

Once the history and physical are complete, thrombocytopenia is established, and there are no other obvious sources of this thrombocytopenia, ITP should be further assessed with only a few standard tests. Closely following the **CBC**—if the patient is actively bleeding or undergoing treatment for presumed acute ITP—is essential. A **peripheral**

TABLE 8-1. HISTORY AND PHYSICAL EXAM ELEMENTS IN THE EVALUATION OF IDIOPATHIC THROMBOCYTOPENIC PURPURA

History	Physical exam
Significant ethanol history	Petechiae (especially on the lower extremities)
Liver disease	Purpura
Drug history	Conjunctival bleeding
Bleeding and bruising	Retinal hemorrhages
Family history of bleeding disorders or thrombocytopenia	Lesions on mucosal membranes
	Enlarged liver or spleen
Risk factors for HIV or hepatitis C and/or B symptoms	Lymph nodes
	Signs of sepsis, DIC, or other severe systemic abnormalities
Symptoms of a myelodysplastic syndrome	
SLE or other autoimmune disorders	
Recent viral infection (especially in children)	
History of transfusions	
Lifestyle (vigorous vs sedentary)	

smear should be examined for schistocytes or signs of a marrow abnormality, which are not characteristic of ITP. The platelets may appear large but are not usually "giant" platelets described in other disorders. Pseudothrombocytopenia can be ruled out when platelet clumps are noted, and it occurs in 0.1% of the population. A **bone marrow biopsy** is not recommended except in patients >60 yrs. This is done to rule out myelodysplastic syndromes in atypical cases, in patients with disease that persist >6–12 mos, or in patients who will undergo a splenectomy. An HIV test should be done if the patient has risk factors. Thyroid function tests are indicated in patients that will get a splenectomy. In instances in which splenomegaly is suspected, a CT may be appropriate.

Management

- Practice guidelines have been established by the American Society of Hematology. The management of the disease depends on the patient's platelet count and whether the patient is bleeding. Childhood ITP has a somewhat different set of recommendations and is beyond the scope of this text. The ITP practice guidelines recommend the following (Table 8-2):
  - Patients with platelet counts >20,000/μL without bleeding should not be hospitalized.
  - Patients with platelet counts >50,000/μL without bleeding do not need to be treated.
  - Patients with platelet counts of <50,000/μL with mucosal bleeding or counts <30,000/μL should be treated.
  - Patients with platelet counts of <50,000/μL and risk factors for bleeding are also appropriate to treat.
  - Splenectomy should not be performed as initial therapy, but only after treatment failure.
  - In pregnant women, treatment is required with platelets <10,000/μL and for those in their second and third trimester with counts of 10,000–30,000/μL.
  - Treatment is indicated in any patient who has significant bleeding that is related to their diagnosis of ITP.
  - All patients who are to undergo splenectomy should have vaccinations for *Haemophilus influenzae*, *Staphylococcus pneumoniae*, and *Neisseria meningitidis* 2 wks before the operation. (For the complete guidelines, see reference 1.)

TABLE 8-2. TREATMENT REGIMENS FOR IDIOPATHIC THROMBOCYTOPENIC PURPURA

Initial treatment in noncritical cases with platelets <30,000/μL

1. Prednisone, 1–2 mg/kg/day (to be tapered slowly after count recovery)

2. IV Ig, 1 g/kg for 2–3 days is the initial treatment in pregnancy

Treatment in cases of significant/life-threatening bleeding and platelets <50,000/μL

1. High-dose steroids: methylprednisolone, 30 mg/kg/day or 1 g/day for 3 days

2. IV Ig, 1 g/kg for 2–3 days

3. Platelet transfusions

4. Other standard critical care treatments as needed

Treatment of refractory cases (treatment may take 4–6 wks)

1. IV Ig (should be considered before splenectomy if not previously tried)

2. Splenectomy

- **Serious spontaneous bleeding** is rare in patients with platelet counts >10,000/μL but is seen in up to 40% of patients with counts <10,000/μL. For this reason, patients with counts <10,000 should be treated more aggressively.
- **Other treatment modalities** include Anti-(Rh) D that is only effective in Rh-positive patients with spleens. It causes alloimmune hemolysis, which can cause a 2-g/dL drop in the Hgb concentration and is generally not recommended, although it may be appropriate at times. Azathioprine (Imuran), cyclophosphamide (Cytoxan, Neosar), danazol (Danocrine), and vinca alkaloids have been used in refractory cases.
- **Splenectomy** leads to platelet count recovery in two-thirds of patients, and count recovery is usually in the first week. It is now possible to do laparoscopic splenectomy that decreases the morbidity of the procedure in experienced hands. Accessory splenectomies, after identification by technetium scans, have been attempted after failed response to splenectomy.

THROMBOTIC THROMBOCYTOPENIC PURPURA AND HEMOLYTIC UREMIC SYNDROME

TTP and HUS are clinically similar disorders that are often grouped together and called *TTP-HUS*. They are classically defined by **thrombocytopenia** and **microangiopathic hemolytic anemia** (MAHA). Neurologic and renal impairment are also characteristic. Neurologic impairment is prominent in TTP, whereas HUS has many of the same clinical findings as TTP, but its major clinical feature involves acute renal failure. They both involve microvascular damage and platelet destruction. Recent work on the pathophysiology does distinguish the two, but they continue to be discussed together because of their clinical similarities. HUS has two forms—a sporadic form more typical of adults and a form associated with verotoxin and *Escherichia coli* O157:H7, which usually occurs in children. Both cause thrombocytopenia with MAHA but are distinct entities. TTP has an incidence of approximately 3.7 cases/100,000 persons. TTP-HUS once had a 90% mortality until the development of plasma exchange. Now its mortality is <30% with treatment. Therefore, treatment should be initiated in anyone with thrombocytopenia and MAHA without other cause.

Pathophysiology

Microvascular damage and platelet aggregation appears to be key in the development of these disorders. High shear stress and damage to endothelial cells are also noted as causative factors. Platelet thrombi subsequently form in the vasculature.

Thrombotic Thrombocytopenic Purpura

The importance of unusually large vWF molecules (ULvWF) has been clarified recently in TTP. A protease normally processes vWF, cleaving these ULvWF molecules that are normally produced by endothelial cells into their typical length multimers. In TTP, there is either a deficiency or inhibitor of this protease. There is evidence that a deficiency in this protease can be inherited through recessive inheritance, which is characteristic of enzymatic deficiencies. Antibodies (IgG) to this protease that act as inhibitors are also associated with TTP and may be induced by some drugs. When these ULvWF molecules persist, it is thought that they are associated with abnormal platelet aggregation in the microcirculation in which there is high shear stress. This leads to the platelet consumption and the fragmenting and destruction of RBCs. These ULvWF molecules also disappear in acute episodes of TTP, suggesting their consumption in an abnormal proteolytic process.

Hemolytic Uremic Syndrome

Although HUS has long been thought to be related to TTP, the protease involved in TTP does not appear to be the etiology of HUS. HUS appears to be related to selective endothelial damage in the organs most often affected, namely the kidneys and the brain. CD36 is thought to play a role. Heredity has been identified as the cause in <5% of the cases of HUS. Factor H is a complement regulatory protease that appears to be involved. Factor H mutations have been linked to familial forms of the disease, although it is not clear how these mutations predispose patients to HUS. As mentioned earlier, the childhood HUS variant is associated with Shiga verotoxin and is frequently seen after an episode of hemorrhagic diarrhea. Outbreaks have been documented in children secondary to *E. coli* O157:H7, but it is also seen in adults.

History and Physical Exam

- The **classic findings** of TTP-HUS include a pentad of physical exam and lab findings as shown in Table 8-3. The complete pentad does not have to be present for the diagnosis, and HUS often presents without fever or neurologic dysfunction. TTP may be preceded by a few weeks of malaise, but neurologic symptoms, including headache, confusion, vision changes, tinnitus, and seizures, are frequently the first characteristic symptoms with which patients present. Some patients may progress to coma. Although fever is part of the pentad, it should also prompt workup of sources of infection. Bleeding problems are commonly seen (90%). Abdominal pain, nausea/vomiting, and diarrhea are also frequently noted. Urine output can drop off dramatically, and weakness is a common complaint.
- **Various drugs** have been associated with thrombotic microangiopathy such as that of TTP-HUS. Most notable of these is quinine (Quinamm). Others include chemotherapeutic agents such as mitomycin C (Mutamycin), bleomycin (Blenoxane), and cisplatin (Platinol); immunosuppressive agents such as cyclosporine (Neoral, Sandimmune); or antiplatelet drugs such as ticlopidine (Ticlid) and clopidogrel (Plavix). A TTP-HUS–like picture may also be seen in patients with HIV infections, SLE, and adenocarcinoma. These should be considered when evaluating patients for

TABLE 8-3. THROMBOTIC THROMBOCYTOPENIC PURPURA–HEMOLYTIC UREMIC SYNDROME (HUS): THE CLASSIC PENTAD OF FINDINGS

1. Thrombocytopenia
2. Microangiopathic hemolytic anemia
3. Neurologic changes
4. Renal dysfunction (predominates in HUS)
5. Fever

TTP-HUS. DIC is another important disorder in the differential diagnosis, and lab evaluation is important to assess this.

Lab Evaluation

A **CBC** often shows anemia and thrombocytopenia (mean, <40,000/μL in TTP). The thrombocytopenia tends to be worse in TTP than HUS. A normal WBC is frequently seen, but severe neutrophilia may occur. An elevated **lactate dehydrogenase (LDH), indirect bilirubin,** and decreased **haptoglobin** will help identify hemolysis associated with the disorder, but a **peripheral blood** smear will help confirm the diagnosis by identifying schistocytes consistent with MAHA. A **direct Coombs** test is negative. The reticulocyte count should be elevated, but coagulation studies (PT/INR, PTT) are usually within normal limits. A DIC panel, including fibrinogen, fibrinogen degradation products (FDP), and D-dimer is useful to evaluate DIC as an alternate diagnosis. If the patient's **creatinine** is significantly elevated, HUS is suggested. Acute anuric renal failure is often present. The UA may be unimpressive with only mild findings, but proteinuria and red cells are typical when there are abnormalities. With fever, blood cultures should be drawn to evaluate for sepsis. Some, in cases that are unclear, have suggested a renal biopsy, but this is problematic in patients with thrombocytopenia.

Management

- The primary treatment for TTP-HUS is **plasma exchange** (plasmapheresis) with one estimated plasma volume being exchanged daily, although some patients require plasma exchange two times a day in severe cases or cases that progress despite daily treatments. Because of the high mortality of untreated TTP-HUS, thrombocytopenia and MAHA are all that is required to initiate plasma exchange if no other cause can be identified. Plasma exchange has also shown benefits in other thrombotic microangiopathies, so it should not be withheld in urgent cases. Plasma exchange carries a high complication rate, so a specialist in hematology should be involved in the decision to initiate it. The goal of daily plasma exchange should be to reverse the thrombocytopenia and hemolysis. This can be monitored with LDH and CBC measurements and typically takes 1–2 wks of plasma exchange but can take considerably longer. The frequency of plasma exchange is typically decreased to taper the treatment after the LDH and platelets are within normal limits. Some patients require dialysis if the renal failure is severe. Platelet transfusions are relatively contraindicated, except in cases of life-threatening bleeding. After remission, exacerbations due to discontinuing plasma exchange (<30 days) should lead to immediate retreatment with plasma exchange. With remission, neurologic symptoms often improve dramatically, but renal problems frequently persist. The childhood variant associated with verotoxin is not typically treated with plasmapheresis, and supportive treatment is often all that is necessary.
- In patients who appear **resistant to plasma exchange** at a frequency that has increased to twice a day, attempts with the cryosupernatant portion of plasma may be attempted. Solu-Medrol (methylprednisolone), 125 mg PO bid should also be added. Splenectomy is controversial. Drug-induced forms caused by agents like mitomycin C and cyclosporine often will not respond well and have a poor prognosis.
- After **remission,** approximately one-third of patients will relapse (having recurrent disease >30 days after completion of treatment) in 10 yrs, and routine follow-up is required. LDH levels should be monitored. Chronic renal insufficiency is a frequent problem, but if the disease is quickly identified, mortality and this long-term complication may be avoided.

DISSEMINATED INTRAVASCULAR COAGULATION

Although DIC is usually considered a malfunction in coagulation or secondary hemostasis, it is discussed here because it may have findings similar to disorders previously mentioned, especially the TTP-HUS spectrum. Rapid onset of thrombocytopenia or a significant drop in platelet count can be a clue that a patient with certain predisposing conditions is developing DIC (Table 8-4).

TABLE 8-4. CONDITIONS ASSOCIATED WITH DISSEMINATED INTRAVASCULAR COAGULATION

Systemic infection

Gram-negative sepsis related to endotoxin

Gram-positive organisms may also cause sepsis and DIC

Cancer

Solid tumors, including pancreatic, prostate, breast, and others that are usually malignant at the time

Hematologic malignancy, most notably acute promyelocytic leukemia (AML-M3)

Trauma

Head injury: usually life threatening

Serious burns involving large parts of the body

Serious crushing injuries with substantial tissue damage

Serious fractures, most notably a femur fracture with fat embolism

Obstetric complications

Amniotic fluid embolism related to giving birth

Placental abruption: often related to significant abruption

Vascular disorders

Aortic aneurysm

Hemangiomas: usually giant

Immune-mediated reactions

Anaphylaxis: mediated by cytokine release

Transfusion reactions

Transplant rejection

Toxins

Snake venom

IV drugs: possibly related to a drug affect, but IV drug abuse–associated systemic infections should be considered

Pathophysiology

DIC is an acquired disorder of hemostasis that involves **inappropriate thrombosis systemically** but is most notable in the small and mid-sized vessels. DIC evolves from a condition in which the patient is hypercoagulable, damaging organs by thrombosis and ischemia, to one in which the clotting factors are depleted, and the patient may develop bleeding problems and life-threatening hemorrhage. As noted earlier, there are many associated conditions, but the unifying cause appears to be *widespread endothelial damage and/or extensive release of inflammatory cytokines*, most notably interleukin-6, tumor necrosis factor-alpha, and interleukin-1. This exposes tissue factor, which interacts with factor VII, initiating the coagulation cascade. Subsequent to this is the generation of thrombin molecules and, therefore, the *consumption of the coagulation factors* involved in their production, specifically factors V and VIII and fibrinogen. The increased thrombin generation leads to release of tissue plasminogen activator from endothelial cells, as well as the generation of fibrin. This results in the proteolysis of plasminogen to plasmin, which ultimately leads to secondary fibrinolysis. The net result is systemic thrombosis and hemorrhage. Antithrombin III (ATIII), proteins C and S, and tissue factor pathway inhibitor are also affected by DIC. These factors become depleted or are inhibited in various ways. ATIII may be the most important of these, and low levels due to consumption and degradation by elastase from neutrophils are associated with increased mortality. The net result of all these processes is systemic thrombosis and hemorrhage.

History and Physical Exam

As noted previously, these patients are usually gravely ill, and the history should be focused on assessing the patient for a condition or disease that is associated with DIC.

Lab Evaluation

Although the lab evaluation should be customized to the patient, there are a number of useful lab tests in assisting in the diagnosis of DIC. A **CBC** to follow the platelet count and **PT/INR** and **PTT** are usually the first tests that indicate DIC is a potential problem. The platelets will usually show a substantial drop or a count of $<100,000/\mu L$. The coagulation studies are typically abnormal. The CBC may also be useful to identify a high WBC often seen in sepsis. So-called **DIC panels** often measure fibrinogen, FDP, and D-dimers. Fibrinogen may be low from its consumption. The FDP and D-dimers are markers of clot dissolution and are usually elevated at the time of diagnosis, but because fibrinogen is an acute phase reactant, the levels may remain normal. A **peripheral smear** may be useful in determining the diagnosis. Schistocytes are often seen owing to destruction of red cells.

Management

The overriding and most important treatment for DIC is **treatment of the initiating condition.** Antibiotics in sepsis, for example, are more important than any direct intervention related to coagulation. There has been considerable work on treating the coagulation or bleeding problems associated with DIC. Critical care support should be tailored to the patient. In patients with high bleeding risk or active bleeding, fresh frozen plasma and platelet **transfusions** are recommended. Platelet counts of $>50,000$ are preferable. In patients predominantly in the thrombotic phase of DIC, **heparin** has been suggested, but this is controversial. The dose is typically a 300–500 units/hr infusion. Low-molecular-weight heparin (LMWH) may have less risk for bleeding, and some consider it an alternative. In cases in which the patient has low ATIII levels and severe DIC, some consider ATIII replacement a reasonable option. The goal of this therapy should be to achieve normal or supranormal levels. A formula for achieving this has been given by de Jonge E et al. [2]:

$$\text{Dose (units)} = (100 - \text{measured ATIII activity}) \times \text{body weight (kg)}$$

HEPARIN-INDUCED THROMBOCYTOPENIA

HIT has been a well-known phenomenon seen with heparin therapy for many years, and its consequences can be devastating. It has been noted in up to 3% of people treated with typical IV doses. Thrombosis has been noted in 30% of those who develop HIT, with 25% of these thromboses being arterial. As a result, these patients are at increased risk for pulmonary embolus, stroke, and myocardial infarction, making it essential to consider HIT in any patient having even a moderate reduction in platelets (50,000–100,000) with a history of heparin treatment within the previous 5 days.

Pathophysiology

Some authors note that two forms of HIT exist (HIT I and HIT II). HIT I, or type I, is defined as nonimmune HIT, and it is a self-limited form that does not lead to significant thrombocytopenia. It is not a reason for discontinuing heparin therapy, and it is not usually associated with problems. Some note that this type of HIT should be called *nonimmune heparin–associated thrombocytopenia* and that the designation of HIT be limited to type II that is associated with an immune response to platelets and carries the risk of severe thrombotic complications. This is how it will be used here.

The designation HITTS—HIT and thrombosis syndrome—is used when thrombotic complications develop in HIT. HIT develops when **antibodies** are produced by the immune system **to platelet factor IV bound to heparin.** As with many primary specific immune responses, it has a delayed onset of at least 5 days after administration of heparin or LMWH. If the patient has been exposed previously, however, the thrombocytopenia can develop in hours. HIT is not usually seen after a patient has been on heparin for >2 wks. The HIT-IgG antibody (HIT-Ab) can activate platelets, generate platelet-derived micro-particles, as well as promote tissue factor expression, and this combination can lead to significant thrombosis that can threaten limb circulation and even lead to DIC. Although LMWH is associated with HIT, the incidence appears to be less than that of unfractionated heparin.

History and Physical Exam

Bleeding complications are not common with HIT, and these patients do not usually present with purpura or mucosal bleeding. They have a significantly elevated risk of thrombotic complications, and as many as 30% will develop thrombosis. Among these, deep vein thrombosis and pulmonary embolism are common, so questions about lower-extremity pain and swelling and shortness of breath are key. Thromboemboli are also complications of HIT, and 25% of thromboses are arterial. Thrombosis of limb arteries, myocardial infarctions, strokes, and bilateral adrenal gland involvement can all occur.

Lab Evaluation

When a patient is on heparin, he or she should have daily **platelet counts** (CBC). The platelet count will drop substantially if HIT develops, but a patient may not be thrombocytopenic with the initial drop. At least a 50% reduction in the platelet count or new absolute thrombocytopenia <100,000/μL in the 5- to 14-day treatment window should make one suspect HIT. Platelet counts of 20,000–150,000 are typical, and the median is approximately 50,000/μL. In general, the suspicion of the diagnosis should lead to the discontinuation of heparin, as specific tests for HIT typically take several days for their results. **Functional assays** have been designed to diagnose HIT. The ^{14}C-serotonin release assay uses donor platelets with ^{14}C-serotonin and heparin in combination with the patient's plasma. Platelet release of the radioactive marker is sensitive and specific for HIT. An assay for HIT-Ig (Ab) has been developed using an ELISA and is the more common test. This test has become favored, but the specificity is not as good as the functional assays.

Management

The first step in treating HIT is the **discontinuation of heparin.** Because of 90% cross-reactivity to the HIT-Ab, LMWH should not be substituted. Patients with persistent thrombocytopenia after the discontinuation of heparin, patients with thrombosis, and patients who were receiving heparin for significant anticoagulation needs should be treated with an alternative anticoagulant agent. **Lepirudin (Refludan)** is a recombinant form of hirudin and is a good treatment option but should be avoided in patients with renal disease. Dosing is complex, and detailed information may be found at http://www.refludan.com. **Argatroban** is an effective thrombin inhibitor but should be used cautiously in patients with liver problems. Monitoring levels is possible by monitoring the aPTT, with 1.5–2.5 times normal as the goal. Danaparoid (Organan) is another treatment option, but it has 15% cross-reactivity with HIT-Ig.

ESSENTIAL THROMBOCYTOSIS

Essential thrombocytosis is a chronic myeloproliferative disorder characterized by platelet counts >600,000/μL, but counts can be well >1,000,000/μL. Patients may develop thromboses with some of the associated symptoms, including painful ischemic changes in the limbs. Because the platelets in this disorder are abnormal and do not function well, patients may also have bleeding complications. See Chap. 10, Myeloproliferative Disorders, for a complete discussion.

KEY POINTS TO REMEMBER

- ITP is a diagnosis of exclusion.
- ITP is generally treated with steroids, and IV Ig is added in serious cases.
- TTP-HUS is a disease that can be identified by MAHA and thrombocytopenia without other cause.
- TTP-HUS should be treated with plasma exchange.
- DIC is a condition of abnormal coagulation due to another underlying condition.
- The primary treatment for DIC is treating the underlying condition.
- HIT typically occurs 5–14 days after starting heparin initially and has only been seen in <5 days in cases in which heparin had been used before.
- LMWHs [e.g., enoxaparin (Lovenox)] and warfarin should not be used in patients with HIT.
- HIT is seen ≥ 5 days after exposure unless there has been prior exposure.
- Lepirudin and argatroban are effective treatment options for HIT.

SUGGESTED READING

The American Society of Hematology ITP Practice Guideline Panel. Diagnosis and treatment of idiopathic thrombocytopenic purpura: recommendations of the American Society of Hematology. *Ann Intern Med* 1997;126:319–326.

Cines DB, Blanchette VS. Immune thrombocytopenic purpura. *N Engl J Med* 2002;346:995–1008.

Favaloro EJ. Laboratory assessment as a critical component of the appropriate diagnosis and sub-classification of von Willebrand's disease. *Blood Rev* 1999;13:185–201.

George JN. (Multiple titles): 1. Clinical manifestations and the diagnosis of idiopathic thrombocytopenic purpura; 2. Treatment and prognosis of idiopathic thrombocytopenic purpura; 3. Drug-induced thrombocytopenia. In: Rose BD, ed. *UpToDate*. Wellesley, MA: UpToDate, August 2002.

George JN. How I treat patients with thrombotic thrombocytopenic purpura-hemolytic uremic syndrome. *Blood* 2000;96:1223–1229.

George JN. Platelets. *Lancet* 2000;355:1531–1539.

George JN, Raskob GE, Shah SR, et al. Drug induced thrombocytopenia: a systematic review of the published case reports. *Ann Intern Med* 1998;129:886–890.

George JN, Shattil S. The clinical importance of acquired abnormalities of platelet function. *N Engl J Med* 1991;32:27–39.

Greinacher A, Volpel H, Janssens U, et al. Recombinant hirudin (lepirudin) provides safe and effective anticoagulation in patients with heparin-induced thrombocytopenia. *Circulation* 1999;99:73–80.

Harrington WJ, et al. Demonstration of a thrombocytopenic factor in the blood of patients with thrombocytopenic purpura. *J Lab Clin Med* 1951;38:1–10.

Hatem CJ, Kettyle WM (Co-editors in Chief) with contributions by: Williams ME, Epstein PE, Kickler TS, et al. (Multiple Titles) MKSAP 12, (American College of Physicians–American Society of Internal Medicine). *Hematology* 2001;32–82.

Lämmle B, Furlan M. New insights into the pathogenesis of thrombocytopenic purpura. *Hematology* 1999;243–248.

Levi M, Ten Cate H. Disseminated intravascular coagulation. *N Engl J Med* 1999;341:586–592.

Lewis BE, Walenga JM, Wallis DE. Anticoagulation with Novastan (argatroban) in patients with heparin-induced thrombocytopenia and heparin-induced thrombocytopenia and thrombosis syndrome. *Semin Thromb Hemost* 1997;23:197–202.

Mannucci PM. How I treat patients with von Willebrand disease. *Blood* 2001;97:1915–1919.

Nurden AT. Inherited abnormalities of platelets. *Thromb Haemost* 1999;82:468–480.

Rock GA, Shumak KH, Buskard NA, et al. Comparison of plasma exchange with plasma infusion in the treatment of thrombotic thrombocytopenic purpura. *N Engl J Med* 1991;325:393–397.

Rose BD, George JN, Kaplan AA. on #3. (Multiple Titles): 1. Causes of thrombotic thrombocytopenic purpura-hemolytic uremic syndrome; 2. Diagnosis of thrombotic thrombocytopenic purpura-hemolytic uremic syndrome; 3. Treatment of thrombotic thrombocytopenic purpura-hemolytic uremic syndrome. In: Rose BD, ed. *UpToDate*. Wellesley, MA: UpToDate, August 2002.

Sadler JE, et al. Hemostasis/platelets. Hematology (Education Program of the American Society of Hematology) 1996;79–87.

Warkentin TE. Heparin-induced thrombocytopenia: a ten-year retrospective. *Annu Rev Med* 1999;50:129–147.

Warkentin TE, Chong BH, Greinacher A. Heparin-induced thrombocytopenia: towards consensus. *Thromb Haemost* 1998;79:1–7.

REFERENCES

1. George JN, Woolf SH, Raskob GE, et al. Idiopathic thrombocytopenic purpura: a practice guideline developed by explicit methods for the American Society of Hematology. *Blood* 1996;88:3–40.
2. de Jonge E, Levi M, Stoutenbeek CP, et al. Current drug treatment strategies for disseminated intravascular coagulation. *Drugs* 1998;55:767–777.

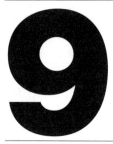

Myelodysplasia

Sarah Waheed

INTRODUCTION

Myelodysplastic syndromes (MDS) are heterogeneous clonal hematopoietic stem cell disorders grouped together because of the presence of the dysplastic changes in one or more of the cell lineages. They are associated with inappropriate apoptosis and excessive marrow proliferation, resulting in peripheral cytopenias in combination with a hypercellular bone marrow exhibiting dysplastic changes, which are the hallmarks of the disease.

Epidemiology and Risk Factors

There are approximately 7000–20,000 new cases in the United States annually, with a prevalence of 10,000–25,000 cases total. The mean age of diagnosis is 68 yrs, although they can be seen in children and young adults. There is a slight male preponderance. Environmental links include smoking, benzene, organic chemicals, heavy metals, herbicides, pesticides, fertilizers, and petroleum and diesel derivatives. Other predisposing factors include prior therapy with chloramphenicol, radiation, and chemotherapeutic agents such as melphalan, chlorambucil, cyclophosphamide, or procarbazine. The effects of these exposures are synergistic.

Classification

MDS falls into one of several different categories based on features of peripheral blood and bone marrow biopsy, by the WHO classification (Table 9-1). These categories have prognostic significance. The WHO classification has replaced the FAB (French-American-British) classification scheme.

CAUSES

Pathophysiology

The underlying mechanism of MDS is not entirely clear. One mechanism postulated is abnormal control of apoptosis, leading to ineffective RBC and WBC synthesis. Genes responsible for this may include protooncogenes bcl-2, c-myc, and p53. Also noted is that the intracellular ratio of c-myc:bcl-2 oncoproteins is increased in MDS.

PRESENTATION

Clinical Manifestations and Syndromes

MDS generally presents as refractory cytopenias. Anemia and fatigue are present in nearly all of the patients; however, patients can also be asymptomatic at diagnosis. Patients can also present with pallor, infections, and bleeding. However, lymphadenopathy and hepatosplenomegaly are uncommon, and CNS involvement is rare. Infection is the principal cause of death, of which bacterial is the most common. Although very rare, **Sweet syndrome** is a cutaneous form of MDS and heralds acute leukemia transformation.

TABLE 9-1. WHO CLASSIFICATION OF MYELODYSPLASTIC SYNDROMES

Category	Peripheral blood	Bone marrow
Refractory anemia (RA)[a]	Anemia No blasts	<5% blasts <15% ringed sideroblasts
RA with ringed sidero-blasts (RARS)[a]	Anemia No blasts	<5% blasts ≥ 15% erythroid ringed sidero-blasts
RA with excess blasts-1 (RAEB-1)	Cytopenias <5% blasts Absence of Auer rods	5–9% blasts Absence of Auer rods
RA with excess blasts-2 (RAEB-2)	Cytopenias <5% blasts Auer rods may be present <1000/μL monocytes	10–19% blasts Auer rods may be present
MDS, unclassified (MDS-U)	Cytopenias No blasts Absence of Auer rods	Dysplasia in granulocytes or megakaryocytes <5% blasts Absence of Auer rods
MDS with isolated del(5q)	Anemia <5% blasts Absence of Auer rods	Normal or increased megakaryo-cyte number Absence of Auer rods del(5q) as the only cytogenetic abnormality

[a]This is the classification of RA and RARS *only* if there are anemia and erythroid dysplasia on bone marrow exam (i.e., *only* the RBC line is affected). If RA and RARS are associated with more than one cell line affected (i.e., a bicytopenia or pancytopenia in peripheral blood is present and has dysplasia on bone marrow in >10% of cells in two or more cell lines), the phrase "with multilineage dysplasia" is added to the classification.
Adapted from Vardiman J, Harris N, Brunning R. The World Health Organization classification of the myeloid neoplasms. *Blood* 2002;100:2292–2302.

5q- Syndrome
5q- syndrome is characterized by progression to overt leukemia in only 25% of the patients. There is a marked predominance of cases in women (up to 70%). Red cell transfusion is the principal treatment of these patients.

Hypoplastic Myelodysplasia
Only a minority of MDS patients have hypoplastic syndrome. The natural history of the hypocellular or hypoplastic myelodysplasia seems to be similar to that of normo-cellular and hypercellular myelodysplasia, described previously.

Childhood Myelodysplasia
MDS is uncommon in children, but when it occurs, its clinical manifestations are similar to that of the adults. Median age of onset is age 6 yrs. Down's syndrome is present in one-third of the pediatric patients.

Myelodysplasia with Bone Marrow Fibrosis
Patients with myelodysplasia with bone marrow fibrosis are found to have a substantial amount of reticulin fibers in the marrow but can be differentiated from the myelofibrosis by the presence of trilineage dysplasia and absence of hepatosplenomegaly.

Myelomonocytic Leukemia

Absolute monocytic count is $>1 \times 10^9/L$. There is prominent splenomegaly (38%), hepatomegaly, and skin or visceral infiltration at diagnosis or that develops during the course of the disease.

Therapy-Related Myelodysplasia

Exposure to ionizing radiation or certain myelotoxic drugs is associated with substantially increased risk of acute myeloid leukemia or myelodysplasia. Risk is greatest in patients who have received alkylating agents or ionizing radiation to the pelvis. Procarbazine (Matulane, Natulan) and nitrosoureas are strongly mutagenic. Patients with therapy-related myelodysplasia are more likely to have a karyotypic abnormality that is associated with poor prognosis. Cases develop 4–7 yrs after treatment of primary cancer. Risk is 1–1.5% per year, with no increased risk after 11 yrs. Prior splenectomy also increases the risk for developing MDS.

MANAGEMENT

Diagnosis

The diagnosis of myelodysplasia rests largely on morphologic findings in a patient with clinical evidence of impaired hematopoiesis as manifested by anemia, neutropenia, thrombocytopenia, or a combination of cytopenias. The CBC often reveals macrocytic anemia and low reticulocyte count. On peripheral smear, there may be oval macrocytic red cells, hypogranular granulocytes with pseudo–Pelger-Huët anomaly (neutrophils with only two nuclear lobes), and giant platelets.

Bone marrow biopsy is needed for diagnosis and has normal or increased cellularity. Morphologic abnormalities include megaloblastic red cell precursors with multiple nuclei or asynchronous maturation of the nucleus and the cytoplasm. Ringed sideroblasts—erythroid precursors with iron-laden mitochondria—are occasionally identified. There is often a predominance of immature myeloid cells, and granulocytic precursors may show asynchronous maturation of the nucleus and the cytoplasm. Mature granulocytes are often hypogranular and hypolobulated. Megakaryocytes may have few nuclear lobes and are often small (micromegakaryocytes).

Treatment

Standard of care is generally accepted to be supportive (see Supportive Therapy). Patients with an indolent course make up the majority of cases and may have long asymptomatic survival. Rarely, some patients with a poor prognosis may have a survival of <1 yr, similar to patients with AML.

Supportive Therapy

Blood transfusions should be given when symptoms develop, and if the frequency of transfusions increases to 1–2 every mo, a trial of vitamins, androgens, or erythropoietin alone or in combination with immunomodulatory therapy may be indicated. Transfuse platelets if platelets are <10,000 or if the patient experiences bleeding. Therapy using vitamins, such as B_6 and retinoids, has a low response rate. Hematopoietic growth factors are often used to stimulate blood cell production. Erythropoietin has improved anemia and decreased the need for transfusion in 16–25% of selected patients, and granulocyte colony-stimulating factor (G-CSF) and granulocyte-macrophage colony-stimulating factor (GM-CSF) has improved neutropenia in 70–80% patients in some series, but there has been no significant impact on survival found with its use.

Chemotherapy

Low-dose cytarabine (Cytosar-U) has been used and has a response rate of 10–15%, although survival is not improved. AML-like regimens typically have a remission rate of 40–60%, with mortality of 20–40%. Complete responses are noted in 70–80% in favorable karyotype and 40–50% in unfavorable karyotypes. Patients most likely to benefit from AML-like regimens are younger than 50 yrs, have normal karyotype, and

TABLE 9-2. *INTERNATIONAL PROGNOSTIC SCORING SYSTEM FOR MDS*
RISK FACTOR CATEGORIES[a]

Points	Bone marrow blasts (%)	Karyotype	Cytopenias
0	<5	Good	0 or 1
0.5	5–10	Intermediate	2 or 3
1.0		Poor	
1.5	11–20		
2.0	21–30		

[a]%Marrow blasts, karyotype, and cytopenias are each assigned point values. These are then added together to come up with a patient's risk score.
Note: Good prognosis—normal, –Y only, del (5q) only, del (20q) only; intermediate—trisomy 8; poor—complex defects, monosomy 7.
Hemoglobin <10 g/dL; absolute neutrophil count, $<1.5 \times 10^9$; platelet count, $<100 \times 10^9$/L.
Modified from Greenberg P, Cox C, LeBeau MM, et al. International Scoring System for evaluating prognosis in myelodysplastic syndromes. *Blood* 1997;89:2079–2088.

refractory anemia with excess blast (RAEB) transformation. Ara-C plus doxorubicin are most commonly used. Novel agents such as topotecan (Hycamtin) can be used and have a role in poor prognosis patients (older patients with poor cytogenetics).

Bone Marrow Transplantation

Allogeneic stem cell transplantation is the only hope for cure in MDS in a small subset of patients. Use is restricted only to patients <50 yrs with HLA-matched donors. Greatest application is in patients with secondary MDS. However, most patients do not qualify because of age or comorbidities. It should be noted that the mortality rate is 40%. The disease-free period is estimated at 45% at 3 yrs.

Immunotherapy, such as antithymocyte globulin and cyclosporin (Neoral, Sandimmune), may be used for hypoplastic MDS, and monoclonal antibodies directed against surface antigens in MDS (CD33 and CD45) may be beneficial.

Prognosis

Evolution to AML occurs in 10–50% of all cases of MDS. In RAEB, the rate is approximately 20–55%, whereas with refractory anemia and refractory anemia with ringed sideroblasts, it occurs in 0–29%. RAEB typically has a median survival of 5–12 mos, whereas refractory anemia (RA) or refractory anemia with ringed sideroblasts (RARS) has a median survival of 3–6 yrs. Prognosis can also be roughly gauged by the *International Prognostic Scoring System for MDS* (Tables 9-2 and 9-3). This system assigns

TABLE 9-3. *INTERNATIONAL PROGNOSTIC SCORING SYSTEM BY MDS*
RISK LEVEL

Risk level (total points)	Median survival (yrs)
Low (0)	5.7
Intermediate-1 (0.5–1.0)	3.5
Intermediate-2 (1.5–2.0)	1.2
High (≥2.5)	0.4

Adapted from Greenberg P, Cox C, LeBeau MM, et al. International Scoring System for evaluating prognosis in myelodysplastic syndromes. *Blood* 1997;89:2079–2088.

points to certain lab features. The patient's total point score can then be used as a rough gauge of risk level.

KEY POINTS TO REMEMBER

- MDS are one of the most common causes of peripheral cytopenias among the elderly and patients with preexisting bone marrow injury.
- Among age-comparable groups, 3-yr complete response and survival rates were similar with intensive chemotherapy vs allogeneic stem cell transplant.
- Treatment is largely supportive.

REFERENCES AND SUGGESTED READINGS

Besa EC. Myelodysplastic syndromes(refractory anemia). A perspective of the biologic, clinical, and therapeutic issues. *Med Clin North Am* 1992;76(3):599–617.

DeVita VT, Rosenberg SA, Hellman S. *Principles and practice of oncology*, 6th ed. Philadelphia: Lippincott Williams & Wilkins, 2000.

Greenberg P, Cox C, LeBeau MM, et al. International Scoring System for evaluating prognosis in myelodysplastic syndromes. *Blood* 1997;89:2079–2088

Heaney ML, Golde DW. Myelodysplasia. *N Engl J Med* 1999;340(21):1649–1660.

Hofmann WK, Ottmann OG, Ganser A, et al. Myelodysplastic syndromes: clinical features. *Semin Hematol* 1996;33(3):177–185.

Koeffler HP. Introduction: myelodysplastic syndromes. *Semin Hematol* 1996;33(2):87–94.

Mijovic A, Mufti GJ. The myelodysplastic syndromes: towards afunctional classification. Haematological oncology. *Blood Rev* 1998;12:73–83.

Vallespi T, Imbert M, Mecucci C, et al. Diagnosis, classification, and cytogenetics of myelodysplastic syndromes. *Haematologica* 1998:83:258–275.

Vardiman J, Harris N, Brunning R. The World Health Organization classification of myeloid neoplasms. *Blood* 2002;100:2292–2302.

Myeloproliferative Disorders

Holly M. Magiera

INTRODUCTION

Myeloproliferative disorders are characterized by increased cellularity of the bone marrow with the result of increased peripheral blood cell counts. Polycythemia vera (PV), essential thrombocythemia (ET), chronic myelogenous leukemia (CML), and idiopathic myelofibrosis (IMF) are the disorders that are recognized as myeloproliferative. It may be difficult to differentiate the disorders because they have similar features and can lack distinguishing morphologic or lab characteristics. Some patients may have clinical findings that overlap among the myeloproliferative disoders. CML is also a myeloproliferative disorder, but because of its unique chromosomal abnormality, clinical course, and treatment, it is reviewed in Chap. 30, The Leukemias.

PATHOPHYSIOLOGY

Myeloproliferative disorders arise from abnormal stem cell proliferation. The stem cell abnormality is recognized as clonal, and autonomous growth appears to be a general feature. Clonally derived cells include erythrocytes, granulocytes, and platelets. Lymphocytes have been seen to be clonal occasionally but are more typically polyclonal. Fibroblasts may also be increased and are polyclonal (i.e., they are not the neoplastic cells). The neoplastic clone appears to have a survival advantage relative to normal cells, as it proliferates independently of growth factors and leads to increased cell counts. Additionally, cytokines may be elaborated by the neoplastic cells that may alter the microenvironment in the bone marrow, resulting in fibroblast proliferation and myelofibrosis. However, the exact role of growth factors in these disorders is not completely understood.

POLYCYTHEMIA VERA

PV is a clonal stem cell disease characterized by proliferation of a multipotent stem cell with expansion of the erythron. Erythropoietin (EPO) levels are generally low or low-normal, in contrast to the elevated EPO levels frequently seen in secondary polycythemia. Initially, the erythrocyte precursors in the marrow are both of neoplastic and normal origin, but ultimately the neoplastic clone dominates.

Epidemiology

PV is the most common of the myeloproliferative disorders, with an incidence of approximately 2/100,000 people. The average age of PV patients is 60 yrs, but it occurs across all age groups, with a slight male predominance. There are a number of reports of PV clustering in families, giving rise to a possible genetic basis for the disease; however, most cases are not familial.

Clinical Manifestations

Patients are commonly asymptomatic at presentation; however, they may present with symptoms related to increased RBC mass and hyperviscosity. These may include headache, weakness, peptic ulcer disease, hyperhydrosis, vision changes, tinnitus, and vertigo. In addition, many patients experience pruritus, especially with exposure to hot water. Erythromelalgia, due to microarteriolar occlusion, is characterized by a burning sensation in the digits and may be severe. Patients are also predisposed to thrombosis and, less often, hemorrhage and may present with these complications. Physical exam findings include splenomegaly, hepatomegaly, hypertension, and plethora.

Diagnosis

- The diagnosis is suspected when a blood count reveals an **elevated Hct.** These patients also have an elevated RBC mass as demonstrated by ^{51}Cr labeling of RBCs and isotope dilution. In addition, approximately 60% of patients have elevated granulocyte counts, and 50% have thrombocytosis. The EPO level is low (<20 mU/mL) and often undetectable. Leukocyte alkaline phosphatase scores, vitamin B_{12}, and uric acid levels may be elevated but are nonspecific findings.
- The **peripheral smear** may show microcytic, hypochromic RBCs with anisocytosis and poikilocytosis, reflecting exhaustion of iron stores due to increased Hgb synthesis. The WBCs generally have normal morphology, but there are often increased basophils, eosinophils, and immature forms. Platelets occasionally have abnormal morphology with megathrombocytes seen on the smear.
- On **bone marrow biopsy,** the findings are not diagnostic of PV but include hypercellular marrow with trilineage hyperplasia and clustered megakaryocytes with hypolobulated nuclei. Iron stores are decreased or absent in most patients, and they often have iron-limited hematopoiesis. Fibrosis is often noted in the bone marrow of some patients. Approximately 10–20% of PV patients will have an abnormal karyotype.

Diagnostic Criteria

- The PV Study Group established criteria >30 yrs ago for the diagnosis of PV, and these are generally reliable today. However, no set of criteria is foolproof. Major (or category A) criteria variables include increased red cell mass, normal O_2 saturation, and splenomegaly. If splenomegaly is absent, two minor (or category B) variables must be present. Minor criteria variables include thrombocytosis, leukocytosis, elevated leukocyte alkaline phosphatase score, and elevated vitamin B_{12}.
- **Secondary erythrocytosis must be excluded.** It is associated with increased RBC mass and increased EPO levels. Causes include chronic hypoxemia, heavy smoking, renal disease, and malignancies such as renal cell cancer, hepatocellular cancer, and hemangioblastoma. Relative polycythemia, or pseudopolycythemia, is associated with normal red cell mass and decreased plasma volume secondary to causes such as dehydration, diuretics, and burns.
- Alternate diagnostic schemes include the one proposed by Pearson [1]. According to this criteria, PV is diagnosed in the presence of elevated red cell mass or very elevated Hgb, absence of secondary causes, and either splenomegaly or a clonality marker. In the absence of splenomegaly or clonality, two of the following criteria must be met: elevated platelets, elevated neutrophil count, splenomegaly by U/S, low EPO levels, or endogenous erythroid colonies grown from the blood.
- CML must be ruled out, as it may present with many of the same features.

Clinical Course

PV is a chronic disorder and may be characterized as having phases during its course. The preerythrocytic phase is generally asymptomatic and is characterized by isolated increase in platelets or in RBCs. Patients may experience trivial pruritus and may have mild splenomegaly. This progresses to an erythrocytic phase, characterized by erythrocytosis requiring regular phlebotomy as well as increased granulocytes and platelet counts. Splenomegaly, pruritus, thrombosis, and hemorrhage may be present. This may last for a number of years. A "spent phase" is characterized by a reduced need for phlebotomy. Thrombocytosis and leukocytosis persist, and splenomegaly is progressive.

Up to 50% of patients may progress to a clinical picture difficult to differentiate from idiopathic myelofibrosis. Anemia develops, and the peripheral smear shows a leukoerythroblastic picture with teardrop poikilocytes, nucleated red cells, and anisocytosis. Immature granulocytes are seen with a slight increase in basophils. and platelets are often abnormal in morphology. Splenomegaly worsens, and there are increased systemic symptoms. Acute myeloid leukemia may occur in up to 20% of patients, and the risk is increased in patients treated with alkylating agents. Progression to acute myeloid leukemia is higher in patients with myelofibrosis.

Management

The goals of treatment are to reduce blood volume to normal and to prevent complications such as thrombosis and hemorrhage. Agents such as radioactive phosphorus and alkylating agents are associated with increased transformation to acute myeloid leukemia and are rarely used today. **Reduction to a Hct of <45% by phlebotomy** is the principal treatment for PV. After an initial reduction of HCT has been achieved, maintenance phlebotomy is then performed as needed. Iron deficiency is a goal of treatment. This may be adequate in patients without risk factors for thromboembolism for many years. However, thrombotic episodes may still occur secondary to elevated platelet counts, and platelet-lowering agents may be needed. Low-dose ASA (325 mg PO qd) is considered a helpful adjunct in patients with recurrent thromboses.

Pharmacologic Agents

Hydroxyurea, interferon-alpha, and anagrelide have efficacy in lowering counts and are commonly used. These agents have distinctive mechanisms of action and side effect profiles, and these determine which agent is chosen. Hydroxyurea may have benefit over phlebotomy, particulary in patients with extensive pruritis. **Symptomatic treatment** can be helpful. Hyperuricemia may be associated with symptoms, which can be managed with allopurinol. Erythromelalgia may be treated with ASA or other NSAIDs. Hemorrhage should be managed with platelet transfusion, since platelets have abnormal function in PV. Pruritus is often poorly responsive to antihistamines but may respond to cimetidine or cyproheptadine. If these agents fail, interferon-alpha or other myelosuppressive agents may be needed.

Surgery

Elective surgery should be avoided in patients with poorly controlled polycythemia, as 75% will have hemorrhagic or thrombotic complications, and mortality is high. Platelet counts and Hct should be controlled for at least 2 mos before surgery, if possible. Thromboembolic prophylaxis should be used as well. Splenectomy is rarely recommended in PV patients because of the high risk of surgical complications.

Polycythemia Vera and Pregnancy

There is an increased incidence of premature births, preeclampsia, and hemorrhage in PV patients. Management should include phlebotomy and low-dose ASA. If cytotoxic treatment is needed, interferon-alpha is the agent of choice, as it has not been shown to be teratogenic or leukemogenic.

Prognosis

Treated patients with PV have a mortality rate similar to age-matched controls. Death is secondary to thrombosis in 30–40% of patients. Myelofibrosis is the cause of death in approximately 15% of patients, and hemorrhage is the cause in 2–10% of patients.

ESSENTIAL THROMBOCYTHEMIA (OR ESSENTIAL THROMBOCYTOSIS)

ET is a clonal stem cell disorder whose distinguishing characteristic is markedly elevated platelet count caused by excessive megakaryocyte proliferation. As with all myeloproliferative diseases, the erythrocyte and granulocyte lineages are also derived from the neoplastic clone. The neoplastic stem cells are increased in number and grow autonomously without growth factors, similar to what is seen in PV.

Epidemiology

ET occurs with an incidence between 1.5 and 2.5/100,000. This myeloproliferative disorder has generally been described in a older population, with most patients >50 yrs and with an equal male:female distribution. However, there is a bimodal distribution with a second population of patients who are affected being younger and predominantly female. No external agent has been identified to be a causative factor for ET. There have been few case reports of familial occurrence.

Clinical Manifestations

Most patients are asymptomatic when their disease is diagnosed. A small percentage of patients may experience pruritus. Symptoms that may be experienced are related to the hemorrhagic manifestations and vasoocclusive manifestations. Bleeding is generally experienced from the mucous membranes, skin, and GI tract and is rarely life-threatening. Vasoocclusive symptoms include erythromelalgia (burning pain, increased skin warmth, and erythema of the feet and hands), transient ischemic attacks, visual disturbances, headache, seizures, and dizziness. Large vessel involvement has also been reported with MI and cerebrovascular accidents. Signs are generally limited to splenomegaly and signs of easy bruising.

Diagnosis

Patients have an elevated platelet count with large platelets visible on peripheral smear. Many patients have a microcytic, hypochromic anemia, and iron deficiency is common. Granulocytes may be increased with mild basophilia and rare early forms. Serum B_{12} and leukocyte alkaline phosphatase scores are generally normal. Bone marrow findings are commonly nondiagnostic and include hypercellularity with granulocyte hyperplasia and increased megakaryocytes. The megakaryocytes are large, often clustered, and may exhibit mild atypia.

Diagnostic Criteria

- The PV Study Group established criteria including a platelet count >600,000 with no history of splenectomy and no secondary cause. In addition, bone marrow exam shows no tumor infiltration, and iron stores are present. If iron stores are absent, iron replacement is initiated, which may uncover PV in some patients. Additional criteria that are often used but that are not part of the original criteria include normal red cell mass, absence of the Philadelphia chromosome, absent to minimal fibrosis, and no cytogenetic or morphologic evidence of a myelodysplastic disorder.
- *Reactive (secondary) thrombocytosis must be ruled out*. Its causes include splenectomy, trauma, cancer, acute and chronic inflammation, infection, and iron deficiency. The other myeloproliferative disorders, myelodysplastic disorders, and CML are also on the differential.

Clinical Course

The natural history of untreated patients with ET is frequently benign but may include recurrent thrombotic and hemorrhagic events for some high-risk patients. However, many patients will remain asymptomatic for many years and may have a relatively benign course with few events.

Management

The goals of treatment in ET include control of the platelet count to minimize thrombotic and hemorrhagic events, supportive care, and avoidance of agents that may increase the risk of leukemia.

Treatment to decrease platelet count most often involves use of cytotoxic agents such as hydroxyurea. Alternative agents include interferon-alpha and anagrelide (Agrylin), which appear to lower platelet counts without increasing leukemia rates. These treatments are generally used only in patients at higher risk of events. Rapid reduction of platelet counts to normal values can be achieved with plateletpheresis in the event of life-threatening complications. This effect is transient, however, and, therefore, is used only in emergency situations.

Patients may be treated with allopurinol (Zyloprim) if they develop symptoms of gout. Vasoocclusive symptoms may respond to ASA alone. Pruritus can be managed with cimetidine (Tagamet) or cyproheptadine (Periactin).

Surgery

Splenectomy poses high risk for increases in platelet counts for ET patients and is contraindicated.

Essential Thrombocythemia and Pregnancy

Pregnant patients are at higher risk of early miscarriage complications and are often treated with ASA. As the pregnancy progresses, the platelet count usually decreases toward the normal range but may rebound quickly after delivery.

Prognosis

Patients generally have an excellent prognosis and appear to have median survivals similar to age-matched controls. Morbidity and mortality are related to thrombotic and hemorrhagic events. Patients with higher risk include those with prior thrombotic events, those >60 yrs, and those with cardiovascular risk factors. Platelet counts >1,000,000/μL and with long-term thrombocytosis may also have greater risk of developing complications. Transformation to acute myeloid leukemia is relatively rare, but risk is increased in patients treated with multiple cytotoxic drugs.

IDIOPATHIC MYELOFIBROSIS (ANOGENIC MYELOID METAPLASIA)

IMF is a stem cell disorder characterized by clonal expansion of hematopoietic stem cells with hypercellularity of the marrow, abnormal megalokaryocytes, and variable degrees of marrow fibrosis and extramedullary hematopoiesis. The fibroblasts are increased in this disorder and have been shown to be polyclonal. Increased cytokine expression, angiogenesis, and matrix proteins have also been observed, and it is believed that the environment created by the clonal hematopoietic cells favors fibroblast proliferation and fibrosis.

Epidemiology

IMF is the least common of the myeloproliferative disorders, with an incidence of 0.5–1.5/100,000 people. The median age of diagnosis is 60 yrs, although there are a substantial number of younger patients. Radiation exposure has been associated with IMF.

Clinical Manifestations

Many patients initially have "B" symptoms, including weight loss, night sweats, and fever, as well as symptoms related to the severity of the anemia and splenomegaly, such as fatigue and abdominal fullness. Bone pain may also be a prominent feature.

Physical exam findings include hepatosplenomegaly. Patients may also have pete-chiae, lymphadenopathy, and peripheral edema, but these are more common later in the course of the disease.

Diagnosis

At presentation, patients have a macrocytic anemia of variable severity, granulocy-tosis or granulocytopenia, and variable platelet counts. The peripheral smear shows a leukoerythroblastic picture with teardrop poikilocytes, nucleated red cells, and aniso-cytosis. Immature granulocytes are seen with modest basophilia. Large platelets are often abnormal in morphology. Abnormalities in immunologic studies are found in 50% of patients and include autoantibodies, polyclonal hyperglobulinemia, a positive Coombs test, and monoclonal antibodies. During bone marrow biopsy, marrow may not be attainable by aspiration secondary to fibrosis, resulting in a "dry tap." Findings on marrow exam include increased cellularity, granulocyte hyperplasia, and mega-karyocyte dysplasia. Reticulin staining is increased, and variable degrees of fibrosis are present.

Diagnostic Criteria

- Diagnostic criteria consist of splenomegaly, a leukoerythroblastic smear, normal red cell mass, bone marrow with fibrosis that is not secondary to an identifiable cause, and absence of the Philadelphia chromosome.
- Other causes of bone marrow fibrosis, including cancers metastatic to the marrow, CML, myelodysplasia with fibrosis, other myeloproliferative disorders, infection, and lymphoma, must be ruled out. In addition, the marrow may not be fibrotic early in the course of the disease, further complicating the diagnosis. Careful mor-phologic exam of the bone marrow, as well as cytogenetic studies, may help to dif-ferentiate among these disorders.
- The diagnosis of *osteosclerosis* is made when sclerotic lesions by x-ray are present along with the criteria for IMF. These lesions occur in up to 50% of patients and may cause severe pain.

Clinical Course

The course of IMF is highly variable but is generally characterized by progressive marrow failure with transfusion-dependent anemia and worsening organomegaly. Approximately 7% of patients will develop portal hypertension related to increased portal flow from massive splenomegaly as well as intrahepatic obstruction related to thrombosis in small portal veins. Associated ascites and variceal bleeding may occur. Progressive splenomegaly may lead to infarction, which presents acutely with fever, nausea, and left upper quadrant pain. Patients may develop neutrophilic dermatoses, which appear as tender plaques. Extramedullary hematopoiesis may develop in many sites, including the spleen, liver, lymph nodes, serosal surfaces, paraspinal or epidural spaces, or the urogenital system.

Management

- Conventional therapy for IMF, including **supportive care,** does not prolong sur-vival. Patients are managed with blood and platelet transfusions and folic acid for anemia and antibiotics for infections. Androgens, erythropoietin, or corticosteroids may improve anemia, potentially decrease the need for transfusion, as well as improve systemic symptoms in some patients. Hydroxyurea has generally been used for the control of leukocytosis, thrombocytosis, and organomegaly. Interferon-alpha may also be used instead of hydroxyurea, although it is not as well tolerated.
- Traditionally, **stem cell transplantation** has not been part of the treatment for IMF, given concerns that stem cells would be unable to engraft in the fibrotic marrow, as well as concern with the advanced age of most patients. However, recent studies

have suggested that selected patients may benefit from transplantation and that fibrosis is reversible with successful transplant. It should be considered in young patients with a poor prognosis and a histocompatible donor.

- **Splenectomy** has often been undertaken in patients with mass-related symptoms, portal HTN, refractory anemia, and thrombocytopenia. Prolonged benefit has been seen; however, serious periop complications, including bleeding, thrombosis, and infection, may occur. Therefore, it should be reserved for patients who have not responded to more conservative management for these symptoms. The median survival for patients undergoing splenectomy is 2 yrs.
- Splenic irradiation is an option for controlling pain and other symptoms related to splenomegaly. Severe cytopenias may develop in up to 25% of patients and are not related to radiation dose, so blood counts must be monitored closely with treatment. In addition, radiation therapy does not improve the anemia and, therefore, is generally used for patients who are not surgical candidates.
- Control of blood counts is not as successful in this disease compared to PV and ET, so additional approaches have been considered, including stem cell transplant, thalidomide to control angiogenesis, and experimental agents to control fibroblast proliferation.

Prognosis

IMF carries the worst prognosis of the myeloproliferative disorders, with a median survival of approximately 3 yrs. However, the prognosis is quite variable and ranges from <3 yrs to >10 yrs. Poor prognostic features include advanced age and level of anemia. Additional findings that indicate a poor prognosis include thrombocytopenia, leukocytosis, systemic symptoms, immature granulocytes, and immature blasts, as well as karyotype abnormalities. The degree of fibrosis does not appear to be related to prognosis. Patients with IMF die of infection, hemorrhage, heart failure, and leukemic transformation. The transition rate to acute leukemia is approximately 20% over 10 yrs.

KEY POINTS TO REMEMBER

- The myeloproliferative syndromes are a heterogeneous group of clonal stem cell disorders that can have significant clinical overlap.
- The diagnosis of PV and ET requires the exclusion of secondary causes.
- Phlebotomy is the primary treatment for PV. Hydroxyurea, interferon, and anagrelide for cytoreduction are reserved for patients with persistent thrombocytosis or at increased risk for thromboembolic events.
- ET patients require cytoreductive treatment to prevent the complications of thrombocytosis.
- Myelofibrosis carries the poorest overall prognosis of the myeloproliferative syndromes.
- The diagnostic criteria for the myeloproliferative syndromes are not absolute rules, and the patient's entire clinical picture should be taken into consideration.

SUGGESTED READING

Bench AJ, Cross NC, Huntly BJ, et al. Myeloproliferative disorders. *Best Pract Res Clin Haematol* 2001;14(3):531–551.

Briere J, Guilmin F. Management of patients with essential thrombocythemia. *Pathol Biol (Paris)* 2001;49:178–183.

Gilbert H. Current management in polycythemia vera. *Semin Hematol* 2001;38(1):25–28.

Guardiola P, et al. Allogeneic stem cell transplantation for agnogenic myeloid metaplasia. *Blood* 1996;88:1013–1018.

Hoffman R. Agnogenic myeloid metaplasia. In: Hoffman R, Benz EJ Jr, Shattil SJ, et al., eds. *Hematology: basic principles and practice*, 3rd ed. Philadelphia: Churchill Livingstone, 2000:1172–1188.

Hoffman R. Polycythemia vera. In: Hoffman R, Benz EJ Jr, Shattil SJ, et al., eds. *Hematology: basic principles and practice*, 3rd ed. Philadelphia: Churchill Livingstone, 2000:1130–1155.

Hoffman R. Primary thrombocythemia. In: Hoffman R, Benz EJ Jr, Shattil SJ, et al., eds. *Hematology: basic principles and practice*, 3rd ed. Philadelphia: Churchill Livingstone, 2000:188–204.

Murphy S, Peterson P, Iland H, et al. Experience of the polycythemia study group with essential thrombocythemia. *Semin Hematol* 1997;34(1):29–39.

Smith BD, Moliterno AR. Biology and management of idiopathic myelofibrosis. *Curr Opin Oncol* 2001;13:91–94.

Tefferi A. Myelofibrosis with myeloid metaplasia. *N Engl J Med* 2000;341:1255–1265.

REFERENCE

1. Pearson TC. Evaluation of diagnostic criteria in polycythemia vera. *Semin Hematol* 2001;38:21–24.

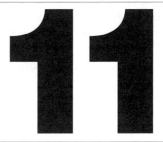

Transfusion Medicine

Geoffrey L. Uy

INTRODUCTION

Blood product transfusion can be lifesaving in the appropriate situation. However, these products are a limited resource that should be given only in specific indicated situations. The physician ordering a blood product should have a thorough understanding of what is being transfused to ensure the appropriate use of resources.

PRETRANSFUSION TESTING

All donors and recipients of blood products are required to undergo testing to help protect against adverse transfusion reactions. **Donors** must meet minimum requirements for weight, BP, and Hct. Before donation, individuals are screened for high-risk behavior that may put them at risk for transfusion-associated diseases such as Creutzfeldt-Jakob disease, HIV, and hepatitis. Donor units are screened for hepatitis B surface antigen, hepatitis B core antibody, hepatitis C virus antibody, HIV-1 and HIV-2 antibody (anti–HIV-1 and anti–HIV-2), HIV p24 antigen, human T-cell leukemia virus (HTLV)-I and HTLV-II antibody (anti–HTLV-I and anti–HTLV-II), and syphilis. Table 11-1 lists the approximate risks of infection from blood transfusion. **Compatibility testing** of blood products is comprised of blood typing, an antibody screen, and crossmatch. Donor and recipient blood are classified by ABO group and Rh blood types. Naturally occurring IgM antibodies against red cell antigens of the ABO system are capable of fixing complement and lead to immediate hemolytic reactions when ABO-incompatible blood is transfused. Before red cell transfusions, an *antibody screen* is performed in which the patient's serum is screened against a panel of red cells containing antigens responsible for most hemolytic reactions via an indirect antiglobulin test. Most alloantibodies are IgG antibodies and result from previous exposure via transfusion or pregnancy and include antibodies to Duffy, Kell, Kidd, and Rh red cell antigens. A *major crossmatch* is an indirect antiglobulin test in which the patient's serum is incubated with donor blood cell to establish compatibility. Historically, a major crossmatch was performed on all donors but now is reserved only for individuals with an alloantibody detected on the antibody screen or a history of transfusion reaction suggestive of RBC incompatibility. For individuals without clinically significant alloantibodies, an *immediate spin crossmatch* is performed instead, in which the patient's serum is mixed with donor red cells. The tube is spun and read immediately. The lack of agglutination demonstrates ABO compatibility. As an alternative to the immediate spin crossmatch, a computer crossmatch may be used if the recipient's ABO blood type has been determined on two separate occasions.

RED CELL TRANSFUSIONS

Indications

The indication for RBC transfusion is the augmentation of O_2 delivery to tissues when O_2 delivery is impaired by anemia. Guidelines for blood transfusion have been issued by several organizations. These guidelines recommend that, among patients without known cardiac risk factors, the threshold for transfusion should be a Hgb level of 6–8 g/dL. They also indicate that patients with Hgb levels >10 g/dL are unlikely to benefit from blood transfu-

TABLE 11-1. APPROXIMATE RISKS OF INFECTION FROM BLOOD TRANSFUSION

	Risk factor (per million)	Estimated frequency (per unit)	No. of deaths/ million units
Hepatitis A	1	1/1,000,000	0
Hepatitis B	7–32	1/30,000–1/250,000	0–0.14
Hepatitis C	4–36	1/30,000–1/150,000	0.5–17.0
HIV	0.4–5.0	1/200,000–1/2,000,000	0.5–5.0
HTLV-I and -II	0.5–4.0	1/250,000–1/2,000,000	0
Parvovirus B19	100	1/10,000	0

HTLV, human T-cell leukemia virus.
Adapted from Goodnough LT, Brecher ME, Kanter MH, et al. Transfusion medicine. First of two parts—blood transfusion. *N Engl J Med* 1999;340:438–447.

sion. Guidelines advocating a uniform "transfusion trigger" are unrealistic, as the measurement of the Hgb and Hct are imprecise measures of the O_2-carrying capacity of blood, and the decision for transfusion is dependent on variables such as the patient's cardiopulmonary reserve and O_2 consumption in addition to the rate and magnitude of blood loss.

Red Cell Products

- **Whole blood** contains physiologic amounts of RBCs, platelets, and plasma proteins. Whole blood is rarely used, because whole blood units are usually divided into their individual components to maximize the use of available blood resources.
- **Packed RBCs** are composed of approximately 200 mL of red cells suspended in plasma and additives to a final volume of 225–350 mL. Each unit is predicted to raise the Hgb of a 70-kg adult by approximately 1 g/dL.
- **Gamma-irradiated products** are used to prevent graft vs host disease and are used for immunocompromised patients receiving blood transfusions from family members.
- **CMV-negative** products are indicated in individuals who are CMV negative and in whom infection with CMV may produce adverse consequences (e.g., transplant recipients, pregnant women, and other immunocompromised individuals). As an alternative, because CMV is highly associated with white cells, leukoreduction (i.e., leukocyte-depletion or leukopoor) is also considered effective at reduction of transmission of CMV. Leukocyte depletion may prevent alloimmunization to platelets and should be used in patients who are expected to need platelet transfusions during multiple courses of chemotherapy and do not have preexisting HLA antibodies.
- **Washed RBCs** that are processed with normal saline have reduced content of plasma proteins. Washed blood is indicated (a) if the plasma contains antibodies known to be harmful for the intended recipient or (b) to remove constituents to which the intended recipient is known to have severe side effects. These components are indicated when the removal of antibodies such as anti-IgA or anti-HPA-1 is needed. *The most common indication for washed RBCs is IgA deficiency in the recipient.* Washed blood is also indicated in rare recipients experiencing anaphylactic reactions to plasma components.

Dosing and Administration

Packed RBCs are stored at 1–6°C for up to 42 days. Red cell transfusions are given over a maximum of 4 hrs through a standard 170- to 260-μm filter. Premedication with acetaminophen, 650 mg PO or PR, and diphenhydramine, 25–50 mg PO or IV, is used for many patients to reduce the frequency and severity of urticaria and febrile nonhemolytic reactions. Hydrocortisone, 50–100 mg IV, may benefit patients with recurrent febrile nonhemolytic reactions. Each unit of blood will typically **raise Hgb by 1 g/dL** or **Hct by 3%**. Whenever possible, transfusion should be withheld until blood typing and antibody screens are performed. In **emergency situations,** type O, Rh-negative red cells may be used when a type and screen are not available.

Complications

- **Viral infection** via blood transfusion has been a great concern even before the identification of HIV in 1982. The development of highly sensitive screening assays has greatly reduced the frequency of viral transmission via transfusion over the past 20 yrs. All blood products are now screened for the *hepatitis B virus, hepatitis C virus, HIV-1, HIV-2, HTLV-I and HTLV-II*, and *syphilis*. Current rates of transmission for viral infections are too low to be measured directly and are estimated using mathematic models based on the window period in which the donor is infectious, but screening tests are negative (Table 11-1). A number of other agents, which are not routinely screened for, may be transmitted via blood transfusion, including CMV, parvovirus B19, and Creutzfeldt-Jacob Disease.
- **Bacterial contamination** can result in fever, chills, and hypotension during or immediately after transfusion. The most commonly implicated organism is *Yersinia enterocolitica*, but other gram-negative organisms have been reported. The risk of infection is related directly to the length of storage.
- **Simple allergic reactions** occur from transfused allergens in the plasma, leading to local or generalized urticaria. These reactions are common and usually respond to treatment with diphenhydramine (20–50 mg IV q4–6hrs).
- **Acute hemolytic reactions** occur as a result of IgM antibodies against ABO-incompatible donor red cells. Approximately one-half of acute transfusion reactions are due to clerical error and occur with frequencies estimated at 1 in 250,000–1,000,000. Patients complain of chills, dyspnea, back pain, and chest pain, which may begin immediately after starting transfusion. Initial signs include fever and tachycardia with severe reactions resulting in hypotension, disseminated intravascular coagulation (DIC), and renal failure from acute tubular necrosis. Nonimmunologic hemolysis can rarely occur from hypotonic fluids, coadministered drugs, bacterial toxins, or thermal injury. When an acute hemolytic transfusion is suspected, the **transfusion must be stopped immediately.** The blood product and patient ID should be rechecked and the blood bank notified. Blood should be sent for direct antibody testing and urine sent for free Hgb. Lab tests for DIC and hemolysis should be ordered including PT, PTT, fibrinogen, and fibrinogen degradation products, as well as bilirubin, lactate dehydrogenase, and haptoglobin. Therapy consists of aggressive hydration to maintain a urine flow >1 mL/kg/hr and may require the use of loop diuretics and/or mannitol.
- **Delayed hemolytic reactions** result from reactions to minor red cell antigens in alloimmunized individuals when circulating antibodies from an amnestic response react with circulating donor red cells. Hemolysis occurs at a much slower rate than in acute reactions with a delay of 2–14 days posttransfusion. Signs include an unexpected decrease in the Hgb concentration with evidence of hemolysis and development of a positive direct antibody test. Treatment is supportive, with minimal adverse effects in most patients.
- **Febrile nonhemolytic reaction** manifests as a temperature elevation occurring during or shortly after a transfusion and in the absence of any other pyrexic stimulus. It may reflect the action of antibodies against WBCs or the action of cytokines either present in the transfused component or generated by the recipient in response to transfused elements. Febrile reactions may accompany approximately 1% of transfusions; they occur more frequently in patients previously alloimmunized by transfusion or pregnancy. No routinely available pre- or posttransfusion tests are helpful in predicting or preventing these reactions. Antipyretics usually provide effective symptomatic relief. Patients who experience repeated, severe, febrile reactions benefit from receiving leukocyte-reduced components.
- **Transfusion-related acute lung injury** is a poorly understood and infrequently recognized form of acute respiratory distress syndrome. Donor anti-HLA, antineutrophil antibodies, or lipid products from donor red cell membranes have been postulated to react with recipient neutrophils to damage pulmonary epithelium. Transfusion-related acute lung injury is characterized by dyspnea, hypotension, and fever with bilateral

pulmonary infiltrates within 1–8 hrs of transfusion without evidence of cardiac compromise or fluid overload. Therapy is supportive, but be aware that the patient may require intensive monitoring and support that necessitates transfer to the ICU.

- **Iron overload:** One unit of packed RBCs contains 200–250 mg of elemental iron. In patients with thalassemia or bone marrow suppression, chronic transfusion saturates macrophages from the reticuloendothelial system, resulting in iron deposition in the liver, myocardium, and endocrine tissues, leading to organ dysfunction. Concern is typically after approximately 100 units.
- **Transfusion-associated graft vs host disease** results when donor lymphocytes remain viable in an immunocompetent host and react with host tissue. The reaction occurs in HLA homozygous haplotype–identical donors or in immunocompromised recipients. Rash, fever, cytopenias, and GI symptoms appear 4–10 days after transfusion. This condition is almost universally fatal. Gamma irradiation of blood products effectively inactivates immunocompetent lymphocytes in the blood products in at-risk patients.
- **Other adverse effects** associated with red cell transfusions include volume overload, especially in patients with congestive heart failure or renal failure. In these patients, frequent respiratory exams and inquiries to breathing status should be assessed. The clinician should have low threshold for furosemide administration in these patients with any suspicion of fluid overload. Hypothermia may occur, particularly in the elderly in the setting of massive transfusion. Hyperkalemia is a consideration as RBCs leak potassium during storage.

PLATELET TRANSFUSIONS

Indications

Platelet transfusions reduce the risk of spontaneous hemorrhage in individuals with thrombocytopenia secondary to impaired bone marrow function or in those with dilutional thrombocytopenia secondary to the massive transfusion of red cells. In general, transfusions are *not indicated* in conditions in which there is increased platelet destruction, such as ITP, TTP, and DIC, except in the presence of bleeding. In stable patients with acute leukemia or stem cell transplant, applying a transfusion threshold of <10,000 cells/μL is similar in outcome to <20,000 cells/μL with respect to bleeding complications. In contrast, patients with myelodysplasia or aplastic anemia can often be observed without transfusion. Therapeutic transfusions are *indicated* in individuals with bleeding secondary to thrombocytopenia. In surgical patients, transfusion triggers at 50,000 cells/μL are adequate for most surgical and invasive procedures, and a trigger at 100,000 cells/μL for neurosurgical procedures is generally accepted. The trigger for platelet transfusion must be considered within the clinical context of each individual patient and factors such as fever, infection, qualitative platelet defects [e.g., von Willebrand disease (vWD), uremia, cirrhosis], a precipitous drop in platelet count, or planned procedures, all can contribute to the decision for transfusion.

Platelet Products

- **Pooled platelets** or **random donor platelets** are concentrates of platelets separated from single units of whole blood and suspended in 40–70 mL of the original plasma. Random donor units are required to contain >5.5 × 10^{10} platelets in 75% of tested units. Usually, six donor platelet units (often called a six-pack) are used at a time.
- **Single donor platelets** or **apheresis platelets** are produced by cell separator systems that remove platelets and cellular components while returning blood and plasma to the donor. One single donor unit replaces 4–8 units of random donor platelets and is suspended between 100 and 500 mL of plasma. Units are required to contain >3 × 10^{11} platelets in 75% of tested units and have been shown to be equivalent to pooled platelets. The use of apheresis platelets may reduce disease transmission by reducing the number of donor exposures but costs 50–100% more than pooled platelets.
- **Leukocyte-reduced platelets** are derived from either a single or random donor source and contain <5 × 10^6 leukocytes. As with red cell transfusions, leukocyte-reduced platelets are indicated for the prevention of recurrent febrile, nonhemolytic transfusion reaction, HLA alloimmunization, and transfusion-transmitted CMV infection.

Dosing and Administration

Platelets are stored at room temperature for a maximum of 5 days. Crossmatching is generally not required. Premedication is not necessary, and each unit must be transfused over a maximum of 4 hrs. The usual dose in an adult patient is 4–8 units of pooled platelets or 1 apheresis platelet unit. In general, 1 unit of random donor platelets is expected to increase the platelet count of a 70-kg adult by 5000–10,000 cells/μL for a period of 2–3 days. Dosing of platelets is often imprecise, because the number of platelets contained within each unit is not standardized.

Complications

- **Platelet-related sepsis** results from bacterial contamination of platelet products. As a consequence of storage at room temperature, the incidence is much higher than in red cell transfusion and is estimated to be 1 in 12,000 with a mortality rate of 26%. Implicated organisms include *Staphylococcus aureus*, *Klebsiella pneumoniae*, *Serratia marcescens*, and *Staphylococcus epidermidis*. No accepted method exists for identifying contaminated products, but it should be considered in individuals who develop fever within 6 hrs of transfusion.
- **Platelet refractoriness** results in a platelet response less than predicted and is thought to be the result of HLA alloantibodies in transfusion recipients. Platelet response is assessed by measuring the platelet count before and 10–60 mins after transfusion. A corrected count increment (CCI) of <5000 is indicative of platelet refractoriness.

$$CCI = (posttransfusion\ platelet\ count - pretransfusion\ platelet\ count)/number\ of$$
$$platelets\ transfused \times body\ surface\ area$$

Platelet transfusions from HLA-matched donors or platelet crossmatching techniques may reduce refractoriness in selected patients.

PLASMA PRODUCTS

Indications

Plasma products contain various amounts of the coagulation factors necessary for hemostasis. Plasma products are available for use in replacement of some or all plasma proteins. In addition, a number produced by recombinant DNA technologies are available for the replacement of factors VIII and IX in patients with hemophilia.

Whole Plasma Products

- **Fresh frozen plasma** (FFP) consists of the fluid portion of blood that is separated and placed at –18°C or below for ≤ 1 yr and is available in units of approximately 200 mL. By definition, each milliliter of undiluted plasma contains 1 IU of each coagulation factor.
- **Donor-retested FFP** is produced from single units of plasma, and the donor must come back and test negative on a second donation 112 days later before the first donation is released. The practice reduces the risk of viral transmission, because testing spans the window period in which an individual may be infected but possess negative serologies.
- **Solvent/detergent-treated plasma** is produced from single units of FFP that are pooled in lots of 2500 units and treated with the solvent tri-*N*-butyl phosphate and the detergent Triton X-100 to destroy any lipid-bound viruses, including HIV, hepatitis B virus, hepatitis C virus, and HTLV-I and -II. The process does not destroy nonenveloped viruses such as parvovirus and hepatitis A.
- **Transfusion of FFP** is indicated in patients for the management of preop or bleeding patients who have clinically significant coagulation abnormalities requiring replacement of multiple plasma coagulation factors, patients on warfarin (Coumadin) who

require immediate reversal, patients with thrombotic thrombocytopenic purpura, and patients with factor deficiencies for which no concentrates are available. The initial transfusion is 2 U followed by lab measurement of the patient's PT/PTT.

Fractionated Products

- **Cryoprecipitate** is prepared by thawing FFP at 1–6°C and recovering the cold-insoluble precipitate. Each unit of cryoprecipitate should contain 80 IU factor VIII:C units and 150 mg of fibrinogen in approximately 15 mL of plasma and is a source of factor VIII, fibrinogen, von Willebrand factor, and factor XIII. Cryoprecipitate is indicated in bleeding associated with fibrinogen deficiency and factor XIII deficiency. After administration of cryoprecipitate, periodic measurement of the fibrinogen level should be performed. Prophylactic fibrinogen administration is typically not performed until the fibrinogen level is <100. The component may be used as second-line therapy for vWD and hemophilia A if virally inactivated factor concentrates are unavailable.
- **Factor VIII** and **factor IX concentrates** are available from a number of different manufacturers and differ in the method of preparation and activity. Plasma-purified products are virally inactivated in some manner (pasteurization, solvent-detergent treatment, immunoaffinity purification) to reduce the risk of transmission of HIV and hepatitis B and C. Factor concentrate products produced by recombinant technology are also available and, therefore, seem to pose no risk for viral transmission.
- **von Willebrand factor–containing factor VIII concentrates** are indicated in type 2B, 2N, and type 3 vWD. In addition, these products may be used in type 1 or 2A vWD, unresponsive to desmopressin (DDAVP). Only humate-P has been licensed by the FDA for use in vWD. Alphanate or Koate DVI are factor VIII concentrates that are not specifically licensed for vWD but also contain von Willebrand factor.
- **Prothrombin complex concentrates** can be used to treat patients with deficiencies of factors II, VII, and X. These products vary considerably in the amounts of these factors that they contain—between the different preparations and even between individual lots.

GRANULOCYTE TRANSFUSIONS

Granulocytes collected by pheresis are rarely indicated or used because of the availability of granulocyte colony-stimulating factor and granulocyte-macrophage colony-stimulating factor. Because these products contain lymphocytes that can cause graft vs host disease, they are typically gamma irradiated. Granulocytes must be transfused as soon as possible after collection, as their function deteriorates rapidly with storage. Indications for granulocyte transfusions include patients with severe neutropenia and infection who do not respond to antibiotic treatment.

BLOOD CONSERVATION

Autologous Blood Donations

Autologous blood donation may be used in patients having elective surgical procedures for which blood is usually crossmatched. Patients donate a unit of blood 1–2 times/wk before surgery. Advantages of autologous donation include the prevention of transfusion-transmitted disease and red cell alloimmunization. Disadvantages include substantially higher costs over allogeneic donations and the discarding of blood that is not transfused. In addition, many transfusion-associated risks, such as clerical error, bacterial contamination, and volume overload, are still present with autologous transfusions.

Acute Normovolemic Hemodilution

Acute normovolemic hemodilution is the removal of blood with the simultaneous infusion of acellular solutions to maintain intravascular volume before surgical blood loss. Hemodilution reduces RBC loss because of the blood lost during surgery as the result of preop lowering of the Hct. The removed blood is held in the OR and is reinfused during or after surgery to maintain the desired Hgb concentration.

Intraop Blood Recovery

Intraop recovery of blood involves the collection and reinfusion of red cells lost during surgery using cell-washing devices. Contraindications for the use of devices include bacteria or other contaminants in the operative field, as they are not completely removed by the washing devices. Cancer is a relative contraindication because of the potential for aspiration and dissemination of malignant cells. Although recovery of blood has not been shown to reduce transfusion requirements in several controlled trials, blood salvaged during surgery is readily available and less costly than donor units.

KEY POINTS TO REMEMBER

- Blood products are a limited resource and should be infused only when clinically indicated.
- The most common indication for washed RBCs is IgA deficiency in the recipient.
- Although there are some guidelines regarding red cell transfusions, they are imprecise and consideration must be given to the clinical situation of each individual patient.
- Infectious complications from blood products are exceedingly rare today, but these risks must still be weighed when deciding to transfuse the patient.
- When an acute hemolytic transfusion is suspected, the transfusion must be stopped immediately.
- When a plasma product is indicated, the product most directly targeted to the hematologic defect should be used.

REFERENCES AND SUGGESTED READINGS

American College of Physicians. Practice strategies for elective red blood cell transfusion. *Ann Intern Med* 1992;116:403–406.

Circular of information for the use of human blood and blood components. American Association of Blood Banks. Available at: http://www.aabb.org. Last accessed: March 25, 2003.

College of American Pathologists. Practice parameter for the use of red blood cell transfusions. *Arch Pathol Lab Med* 1998;122(2):130–138.

Consensus Conference. Perioperative red blood cell transfusion. *JAMA* 1988;260:2700–2703.

Expert Working Group. Guidelines for red blood cell and plasma transfusions for adults and children. *CMAJ* 1997;156(Suppl 11):S1–S25.

Goodnough LT, Brecher ME, Kanter MH, et al. Transfusion medicine—blood transfusion—first of two parts. *N Engl J Med* 1999;340:438–447.

Goodnough LT, Brecher ME, Kanter MH, et al. Transfusion medicine—blood conservation—second of two parts. *N Engl J Med* 1999;340:525–533

Hébert PC, Wells G, Blajchman MA, et al. A multicenter, randomized, controlled clinical trial of transfusion requirements in critical care. *N Engl J Med* 1999;340:409–417.

Practice guidelines for blood component therapy. A report by the American Society of Anesthesiologists Task Force on Blood Component Therapy. *Anesthesiology* 1996;84:732–747.

Rebulla P, Finazzi G, Marangoni F, et al. The threshold for prophylactic platelet transfusions in adults with acute myeloid leukemia. *N Engl J Med* 1997;337:1870–1875.

Sazaama, K, DeChristopher PJ, Dodd R, et al. Practice parameter for the recognition, management, and prevention of adverse consequences of blood transfusion. *Arch Pathol Lab Med* 2000;124:61–70.

Schiffer CA, Anderson KC, Bennett CL, et al. Platelet transfusion for patients with cancer: clinical practice guidelines of the American Society of Clinical Oncology. *J Clin Oncol* 2001;19:1519–1538.

Silliman C. Transfusion-related acute lung injury. *Transfusion* 1999;13:177–186.

Wu W-C, Rathore SS, Wang Y, et al. Blood transfusion in elderly patients with acute myocardial infarction. *N Engl J Med* 2001;345:1230–1236.

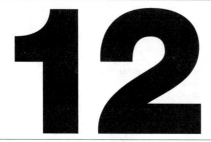

Sickle Cell Disease

Marcia L. Chantler

INTRODUCTION

Sickle cell disease is a term for a group of genetic disorders characterized by the predominance of Hgb S. In the United States, these disorders are most commonly observed in African Americans and Hispanics from the Caribbean, Central America, and parts of South America and less commonly in Mediterranean, Indian, and Middle Eastern populations. The two hallmark pathophysiologic features of sickle cell disorders are chronic hemolytic anemia and vaso-occlusion, resulting in ischemic tissue injury. Examples of sickle cell disorders include sickle cell anemia (Hgb SS), sickle beta-thalassemia syndromes (Hgb S-beta$^+$ or S-beta^0), and Hgb SC disease. There is tremendous variability among disease groups and among individual patients with the same Hgb abnormalities regarding clinical severity.

CAUSES

Pathophysiology

Hemoglobin S

Normal Hgb is a tetramer consisting of two alpha and two beta chains. Hgb S is a result of a single adenosine to guanine nucleotide substitution in the sixth codon of the beta-globin gene, resulting in the substitution of valine for glutamic acid on the outer surface of the Hgb molecule. The change in the molecular structure of Hgb S results in the polymerization of the Hgb tetramers when deoxygenated, which leads to the sickled shape of the RBC. The poor deformability of the RBC containing Hgb S causes occlusion of the microvasculature and ischemic tissue injury.

Sickle Cell Trait

Sickle cell trait (Hgb AS) has a prevalence of approximately 8–10% in African Americans. Sickle cell trait is a **benign carrier condition** with no hematologic manifestations. Red cell morphology, red cell indices, and the reticulocyte count are normal. Clinical complications of sickle cell trait have been reported, most typically splenic infarction occurring at high altitudes, hematuria, and a mild defect in ability to concentrate urine. Sickle cell trait is also associated with a 30-fold increased incidence of sudden death during basic training of African American military recruits. This unexplained death is apparently related to exercise-induced vaso-occlusion and rhabdomyolysis. In individuals who appear to have sickle cell trait but are symptomatic, the lab diagnosis must be verified. Hgbs other than S that polymerize may account for reports of "sickle cell trait" associated with clinical problems.

Hemoglobin SC disease

Hgb SC is approximately one-fourth as frequent among African Americans as Hgb SS. Although oxygenated Hgb C forms crystals, Hgb C does not participate in polymerization with deoxy–Hgb S. This results in a disease that is less severe than homozygous Hgb SS disease. Splenomegaly may be the only physical finding, and clinical complication may be less frequent than in sickle cell anemia. Hgb SC red cells have a longer circulatory survival of 27 days vs 17 days in Hgb SS red blood cells. The degree of anemia and leukocytosis is frequently mild. The predominant red cell abnormality on the peripheral smear is an abundance of target cells and crystal-containing cells. The frequency of acute painful episodes is approximately one-half that of sickle cell anemia, and the life expectancy is two decades longer. However, there is a higher incidence of peripheral retinopathy in Hgb SC disease than Hgb SS disease.

PRESENTATION

Clinical Manifestations

The clinical manifestations of sickle cell disease **vary tremendously** both within and among the major genotypes. Even within genotypes regarded as being the most severe for patients with sickle cell anemia, some patients are entirely asymptomatic, whereas others are disabled by recurrent pain and chronic complications. Sickle cell disease is associated with a **shortened life expectancy** due to the multisystem failure from acute and chronic vaso-occlusion associated with the disease. In 1973, the mean survival was only 14.3 yrs. Currently, it is reported that the life expectancy is 42 yrs for men and 48 yrs for women with sickle cell anemia. The remarkably prolonged survival over the past 20 yrs is more the result of improved general medical care, rather than antisickling therapy.

Diagnosis

All newborn infants born in the United States are **screened** for sickle cell disease. When a newborn's screening test indicates sickle cell disease, a definitive diagnosis is established through further blood testing. Sickle cell disease is identified through lab testing alone. There are no findings on physical exam that suggest the presence or absence of Hgb S. In adults, there may be findings that correlate with the long-term complications of the disease. The **diagnosis** of sickle cell syndromes involves examination of the peripheral smear and Hgb electrophoresis. The peripheral smear is normal in sickle cell trait (Hgb S), but sickle cells are seen in each of the major sickle cell disease syndromes. Solubility testing is abnormal in all syndromes having at least one sickle cell gene and thus detects all carriers of the Hgb S gene, as well as those with the SS phenotype. *Hgb electrophoresis* is able to provide the clinician with the exact phenotype of sickle cell disease. Typical electrophoretic profiles are listed in Table 12-1.

ACUTE MANAGEMENT

Hematologic Complications

Acute exacerbations of anemia in the patient with sickle cell disease are a significant cause of morbidity and mortality. The most common causes of these exacerbations are splenic sequestrations and aplastic crises.

- **Acute splenic sequestration** of blood is characterized by acute exacerbation of anemia; persistent reticulocytosis; a tender, enlarging spleen; and sometimes hypovolemia. It is associated with a *15% mortality rate*. Patients susceptible to splenic sequestration are those whose spleens have not undergone fibrosis (i.e., young patients with sickle cell anemia and adults with Hgb SC disease or S-beta⁺ thalassemia). The basis of therapy is to **restore blood volume** and **red cell mass.** Because splenic sequestration recurs in 50% of cases, splenectomy is recommended after the event has abated. Other common sites of acute sequestration include the liver and possibly the lung.

- **Aplastic crises** are transient arrests of erythropoiesis characterized by abrupt falls in Hgb levels and reticulocytosis. *Parvovirus B19* accounts for the majority of aplastic crises in children with sickle cell disease, but the high incidence of protective antibodies in adults makes parvovirus a less frequent cause of aplasia in this age group. Other reported causes of transient aplasia are infections caused by *Staphylococcus pneumoniae,* salmonella, streptococci, and Epstein-Barr virus. Aplastic crisis can also be the result of bone marrow necrosis, which is characterized by fever, bone pain, reticulocytopenia, and a leukoerythroblastic response. The mainstay of treating aplastic crises is **red cell transfusion.** Often, transfusion is necessitated by the degree

TABLE 12-1. CLINICAL AND HEMATOLOGIC FINDINGS IN THE COMMON VARIANTS OF SICKLE CELL DISEASE[a]

Morphology	Clinical severity	Hemoglobin electrophoresis					Hematologic values		
		S (%)	F (%)	A$_2$ (%)	A (%)	Hgb (g/dL)	MCV (fL)	RBC	
SS	Usually marked	>90	<10	<3.5	0	6–11	>80	Sickle cells Nrbc Normochromia Target cells Howell-Jolly bodies	
SC	Mild to moderate	50	<5	[b]	0	10–15	75–95	Sickle cells Target cells	
AS	None	40–50	<5	<3.5	50–60	12–15	>80	Normal	
S-beta[0]	Marked to moderate	>80	<20	>3.5	0	6–10	<80	Sickle cells Nrbc Microcytosis Target cells	
S-beta[+]	Mild to moderate	>60	<20	>3.5	10–30	9–12	<80	No sickle cells Microcytosis Target cells	

MCV, mean corpuscular volume; Nrbc, nucleated RBC.
[a]Hematologic values are approximate.
[b]50% Hgb C.
Adapted from NIH Guidelines. National Institutes of Health, National Heart, Lung, and Blood Institute. Revised December 1995. NIH Publication No. 95-2117.

of anemia or cardiorespiratory symptoms. A single transfusion will usually suffice, because reticulocytosis resumes spontaneously within 2–3 days. A useful guideline for transfusion is the reticulocyte count. A patient having an exacerbation of a chronic anemia with an elevated absolute reticulocyte count is less likely to require urgent transfusion than one with a normal or low absolute reticulocyte count.

- **Hyperhemolytic crisis** is the sudden exacerbation of anemia with increased reticulocytosis and elevated bilirubin level. The onset of chronically more severe anemia may be due to developing renal insufficiency or the deficiency of folic acid or iron. Chronic hemolysis results in increased use of folic acid stores and can lead to megaloblastic crises if nutritional supplementation is not undertaken. The usual therapy for a hyperhemolytic crisis is transfusion of packed RBCs. Most of these patients usually recover within 14 days. Despite increased intestinal iron absorption in sickle cell disease, the combination of nutritional deficiency and increased urinary iron losses results in iron deficiency in 20% of patients with sickle cell disease. The diagnosis of a delayed hemolytic transfusion reaction should be considered in any patient receiving a recent blood transfusion.

Acute Painful Crisis

Acute pain is the first symptom of disease in >25% of patients. There is *tremendous variability of painful episodes* within genotypes and within the same patient over time. In one large study of patients with sickle cell anemia, one-third rarely had pain, one-third were hospitalized for pain approximately 2–6 times/yr, and one-third had >6 hospitalizations/year. More frequent pain crises are associated with higher mortality rates. Pain episodes may be *precipitated* by events such as heat or cold, dehydration, infection, hypoxia, acidosis, stress, menses, and alcohol consumption. In addition, patients may cite that anxiety, depression, or physical exhaustion may be precipitants. In many instances, no precipitating factors can be identified. The painful episodes can occur in any area of the body, most commonly the back, chest, extremities, and abdomen. Severity can be described from trivial to excruciating. In approximately 50% of painful episodes, patients will present with objective clinical signs such as fever, joint swelling, tenderness, tachypnea, hypertension, nausea, and vomiting.

Management of the Acute Painful Episode

- The acute painful episode is the most frequent reason for which patients with sickle cell disease seek medical attention. In general, the management of acute painful crises includes the identification and treatment of possible precipitating factors, IV fluid hydration, and analgesics. When a patient presents complaining of pain, the physician is charged with **ruling out etiologies other than vaso-occlusion.** There is no clinical or lab finding that is pathognomonic for painful crises. The diagnosis of a painful crisis is based on the medical history and physical exam. Hospitalization and IV administration of fluid and narcotics are quite often needed for the treatment of these patients' severe pain. Acute painful episodes generally last 4–6 days but may vary in intensity and duration. Sometimes the episode may last for weeks.
- The possibility that the pain is **precipitated by a concurrent medical condition,** such as an infection, should be considered, and the physician should search for a precipitating illness in every instance. When abdominal or visceral pain is present, care should be taken to exclude sequestration syndromes or other acute conditions, such as appendicitis, pancreatitis, etc. *Pneumonia develops during the course of 20% of painful events* and can present as abdominal pain.
- If a **fever** is present, an aggressive evaluation should be done to look for the appropriate source. If pulmonary symptoms are present, a chest x-ray should be obtained, and the measurement of an ABG should be considered. If osteomyelitis or a septic arthritis is suspected, an aspiration of the suspected joint should be performed. X-rays, bone scans, and MRI scans may help separate infarction from infection, but these exams are not always reliable. Serum electrolytes and pH levels should be obtained in those patients who are severely ill, as there is a relatively high incidence of electrolyte disorders in patients with sickle cell disease.

- Providing aggressive relief of pain often requires the use of **parenteral narcotics,** adjuvant analgesics, or occasionally other modalities. Patient regimens are very individualized. They will often be aware of the dosages, and medications that have provided adequate relief in the past. **Patients are often undertreated for pain,** because many physicians and other health care providers are unfamiliar with the pharmacology of analgesia and are overly concerned with the potential for addiction. Patients with sickle cell disease do not respond to conventional doses of analgesia, as these patients more rapidly metabolize narcotics than other individuals. They typically are on chronic PO narcotics at home and may have developed a tolerance to conventional doses of narcotics that most physicians feel comfortable prescribing. Those on chronic PO narcotics may need medications such as methadone, MS Contin, or duragesic patches during an acute pain crisis. Additional medications such as percocet, MSIR, and OxyIR may provide immediate relief. Appropriate conversion between chronic PO medications and IV doses of narcotics must be used to ensure adequate and prompt pain relief. In cases in which there is no nausea or vomiting, patients are continued on the regimen prescribed for continuous relief at home and patient-controlled anesthesia (PCA)-demand only doses will be added. **PCA pumps** are effective in the treatment of an acute painful crisis. Appropriate continuous narcotic infusions, as well as effective bolus dosing, are typically required for more effective and immediate analgesia. Morphine and Dilaudid can be used. Doses vary widely from a 1 mg/hr basal rate + 1-mg demand rate up to several mg/hr for both. Demerol may be used occasionally but should be avoided if possible. When used with IV diphenhydramine (Benadryl), it can produce a better "high" for some patients. Taken PO, Benadryl, 25–50 mg PO q6hrs, has sometime provided relief for pruritus. Patients should be monitored frequently and objective pain scores followed closely for titration of effective analgesia.
- Painful events are not commonly associated with changes in the patient's Hgb levels. Low reticulocyte counts are occasionally seen. The WBC count may be recorded as high. The Coulter counter often counts nucleated RBCs as monocytes, based on the similar size and nuclear characteristics. It is important to look at the WBC differential and look for nucleated RBCs on the peripheral smear. An elevated WBC count with a left shift may be an indication of an underlying infection as the etiology of the acute painful crisis.

Neurologic Complications

Neurologic complications occur in 25% of patients with sickle cell disease, including TIAs, cerebral infarction, cerebral hemorrhage, seizures, spinal cord infarction or compression, CNS infections, vestibular dysfunction, and sensory hearing loss. Ischemic strokes are common in children and those >30 yrs, whereas hemorrhagic stroke is more common between ages 20 and 30. *Risk factors* for strokes include severe anemia, low reticulocyte counts, low Hgb F levels, higher WBC counts, the Hgb SS genotype, and systolic HTN. Strokes are fatal in approximately 20% of initial cases, and 70% of patients will have a recurrence within 3 yrs. Patients with symptoms and signs of an *acute stroke* should be *evaluated immediately* using CT scanning or MRI to distinguish TIA, cerebral thrombosis, and hemorrhage. In those with hemorrhage, angiography is indicated—after partial exchange transfusion is performed to avoid complications associated with the injected contrast material. In those with thrombosis, *prompt partial exchange transfusion* is performed, and chronic transfusion therapy to maintain Hgb S levels below 30% is shown to prevent recurrent thrombosis.

Pulmonary Complications

- Tachypneic patients should be evaluated with an ABG to differentiate between metabolic acidosis, hypoxemia, and anxiety. If a PaO_2 of 70 mm Hg cannot be maintained by O_2 inhalation, the patient should be transferred to the ICU, where an emergency partial exchange transfusion can be performed. Improvement in oxygenation may precede any changes in radiographic abnormalities. Severe episodes may not respond to transfusion therapy and require support with mechanical ventilation. Acute chest syndrome occurs less commonly during chronic transfusion programs and is often preceded by a vaso-occlusive pain crisis in adults.

- **Acute chest syndrome** consists of dyspnea, chest pain, fever, tachypnea, pulmonary infiltrates on radiography, and leukocytosis. It affects approximately 10% of patients with sickle cell disease and may be life-threatening. The usual etiology is believed to be vaso-occlusion or infection, or both simultaneously. Therefore, antibiotics are often indicated as initial therapy. Acute chest syndrome, in which common pathogens are not cultured, may be due to "atypical" agents such as *Mycoplasma*, *Legionella*, and *Chlamydia*. Antibiotic therapy should include antibiotics directed at atypical infectious agents, in addition to the major infectious etiologic organisms. Empiric therapy consisting of the combination of ceftriaxone and a macrolide such as azithromycin is appropriate in these patients. Acute chest syndrome has a *mortality rate of approximately 10%*. The major danger of the acute chest syndrome is **hypoxemia** and its resultant widespread sickling and vaso-occlusion, creating the risk of multiorgan system failure.
- **Chronic pulmonary status** in patients with sickle cell disease reveals restrictive and obstructive lung disease patterns, hypoxemia, and pulmonary HTN. Pulmonary disease is more common in those with a history of acute chest syndrome. High-resolution CT scanning of the lungs may reveal chronic interstitial fibrosis. Pulmonary HTN usually occurs in adults and carries a poor prognosis. The condition can be diagnosed with cardiac catheterization or echocardiogram-Doppler study. There is no efficacious treatment, and these patients may be considered for hydroxyurea, vasodilators, anticoagulation, and home O_2 therapy.

Hepatobiliary Complications

- The prevalence of **pigmented gallstones** in sickle cell disease is directly related to the rate of hemolysis. In sickle cell anemia, gallstones occur in children as young as 3–4 yrs and are eventually found in approximately 70% of patients. It is currently recommended to undergo the surgical removal of asymptomatic gallstones with the availability of laparoscopic cholecystectomy.
- **Hepatomegaly and liver dysfunction** in sickle cell disease can be caused by multiple etiologies, including intrahepatic sequestration, transfusion-acquired hepatitis, transfusion-related hemosiderosis, and autoimmune liver disease. There are other acute hepatic syndromes that are unique to sickle cell disease. In all of these, the combination of hemolysis, hepatic dysfunction, and renal tubular defects results in strikingly high serum bilirubin levels, sometimes >100 mg/dL.
- **Benign cholestasis of sickle cell disease** results in severe, asymptomatic hyperbilirubinemia without fever, pain, leukocytosis, or hepatic failure. A far more serious event is the **hepatic crisis** associated with sickle cell disease, in which hepatic ischemia results in fever, right upper quadrant pain, leukocytosis, severe hyperbilirubinemia, and abnormal liver function tests. It may progress to fulminant liver failure, which is associated with a dismal prognosis. Because of the nearly uniform mortality of this type of hepatic crisis, exchange transfusion, plasmapheresis, and liver transplantation have been used as therapy, but no controlled data are available to support this approach.

Obstetric and Gynecologic Complications

Delayed menarche, dysmenorrhea, ovarian cysts, pelvic infection, and fibrocystic disease of the breast are more common in women with sickle cell disease. However, the major reproductive concern in these patients is *pregnancy*. The fetal complications of pregnancy, most of which are related to compromised placental blood flow, are increased. The incidence of spontaneous abortion, intrauterine growth retardation, preeclampsia, low birth weight, and intrauterine fetal death are higher in women with sickle cell disease. Maternal complications during pregnancy include increased rates of acute painful episodes, severe anemia, infections, and even death. The course of pregnancy is more benign in Hgb SC disease. The improvement in fetal and maternal outcomes in recent years is largely due to improved prenatal and obstetric care. The role of transfusions in pregnancy remains largely controversial. There is a very high incidence of acute painful episodes associated with *therapeutic abortions*. Inpatient IV hydration immediately before the procedure and for the 24 hrs after the procedure is recommended. PO contraceptives containing low-dose estrogen are a safe, recommended method of birth control in women with sickle cell disease.

Renal Complications

- The kidney is particularly vulnerable to complications of sickle cell disease with manifestations that result from medullary, distal and proximal tubular, and glomerular abnormalities leading to the *inability to concentrate the urine*. Papillary infarction with hematuria, renal tubular acidosis, and abnormal potassium metabolism occur more commonly in patients with sickle cell disease or sickle cell trait. Patients with **hematuria** should be evaluated with U/S.
- Patients with sickle cell disease cannot excrete acid and potassium normally but usually do not develop systemic acidosis or hyperkalemia without an additional acid load such as in the setting of renal insufficiency. **Chronic renal insufficiency** may be predicted by albuminuria and should be suspected in the setting of HTN and a worsening anemia. Risk factors for the development of chronic renal failure include essential HTN or the use of antiinflammatory drugs. The average age of onset of chronic renal failure is 23 yrs in sickle cell anemia and 50 yrs in Hgb SC disease. The use of ACE inhibitors were found to diminish proteinuria but did not improve glomerular filtration rate. Renal transplantation is recommended for patients with end-stage renal failure.

Priapism

Priapism affects nearly two-thirds of males with sickle cell disease. It peaks in frequency between the ages of 1 and 5 yrs and 13 and 21 yrs. Priapism is most likely to develop in patients with lower Hgb F levels and reticulocyte counts, increased platelet counts, and the Hgb SS genotype. First-line therapy is conservative, increasing PO intake of fluid and analgesia. If the episode persists 3 hrs, the patient should seek medical care. IV fluids, parenteral narcotics, and a Foley catheter to promote bladder emptying are the initial treatments for acute priapism. If the event lasts >12 hrs, *partial exchange transfusion* is performed to reduce the Hgb S level to <30%. If no resolution ensues within 12–24 hrs of transfusion, the use of *alpha-adrenergic agents* is recommended. If there is still no response after conservative measures or alpha-adrenergic medications, *surgery* may be recommended. In this case, a penile aspiration should be attempted first. If this is not successful, a spongiosum-cavernosum shunt is recommended. Despite interventions, impotence remains a frequent complication of priapism. For incapacitating recurrent priapism, chronic transfusion therapy may be beneficial.

Ocular Complications

Anterior chamber ischemia, retinal artery occlusion, proliferative retinopathy, and retinal detachment and hemorrhages are common in sickle cell disease. Routine retinal exam is a part of routine health care maintenance in these patients. Patients should undergo a *yearly retinal exam* performed by an ophthalmologist. Sickle cell retinopathy may require vision-improving therapy with laser photocoagulation.

Bone Complications

- Bone disease is the result of an extended hematopoietic marrow causing widening of the medullary space, thinning of trabeculae, and cortices. **Osteonecrosis** occurs in all sickle cell disease phenotypes but most frequently in sickle cell anemia with coexistent thalassemias. Osteonecrosis occurs with equal frequency in the femoral and humeral heads. The femoral heads more commonly undergo progressive destruction as a result of chronic weightbearing. Decompression surgery to relieve increased intraosseous pressure can be used in early-stage osteonecrosis to prevent further disease progression. A patient with more advanced disease is a candidate for major reconstructive therapy. This decision must take into account the likelihood that a second hip revision will be required within 4–5 yrs of prosthetic hip placement in patients with sickle cell disease.

- **Osteomyelitis** must be differentiated from the more common bone infarction, because the two syndromes present with similar clinical and imaging findings but are treated very differently. *Staphylococcus* and salmonella are common pathogens for osteomyelitis in sickle cell patients. Increasing antibiotic resistance to salmonella is a major problem in sickle cell disease. Surgical débridement in osteomyelitis is not commonly performed and should be based on individual clinical judgment. Septic arthritis must also be distinguished from the more common joint effusion associated with acute painful episodes. It is essential to establish a bacterial diagnosis before starting long-term antibiotics.

Dermatologic Complications

Skin ulcers are major causes of morbidity in sickle cell disease. Ulcers occur commonly near the medial or lateral malleolus and are frequently bilateral. Ulcers may begin spontaneously or as a result of trauma. They are commonly infected by *Staphylococcus aureus*, *Pseudomonas*, streptococci, or *Bacterioides* species. Males have a threefold greater risk of developing leg ulcers. Treatment of leg ulcers requires persistence and patience, as the resolution usually requires weeks. Therapy with gentle débridement, wet-to-dry dressings, and DuoDERM hydrocolloid pads is typically effective. Topical antibiotics may be beneficial in some cases but are not routinely recommended.

Cardiac Complications

An important cardiac consideration in the management of patients with sickle cell disease is *high cardiac output* related to chronic anemia. The chronic high cardiac output can result in four-chamber enlargement and cardiomegaly. Age-dependent loss of cardiac reserve can lead to a greater risk of heart failure in adult patients during fluid overload, transfusion, or other reduced O_2-carrying capacity states. Acute myocardial infarction in the absence of coronary disease has been reported but is rare.

CHRONIC MANAGEMENT

Many patients can live for long periods without experiencing acute or severe exacerbations of the disease. Increased awareness of the disease and its long-term complications, along with the availability of health care, are contributing to the prolonged survival seen in sickle cell patients today.

Routine Patient Visits

- All patients with sickle cell disease should have **routine office appointments** to establish baseline physical findings, lab data, and a healthy relationship between the patient and treating physician. Patients with Hgb SS should have regular medical evaluations every 3–6 mos or sooner, depending on symptoms or manifestations of the disease.
- On an **initial visit,** a complete medical history, with particular attention to the complications of sickle cell disease, number of hospital admissions, number of blood transfusions, and other important health history, should be obtained. A patient should have a CBC, reticulocyte count, and Hgb electrophoresis if this information is not readily available. Other lab tests to obtain include urinalysis, liver function tests, creatinine, serum electrolytes, and a chest x-ray. These should be followed on a routine basis to monitor for long-term complications of the disease.
- **Preventive care should be initiated and maintained.** A vaccination history should also be maintained. Adults should have seasonal influenza vaccines. If the patient

TABLE 12-2. RED FLAGS FOR PATIENTS WITH SICKLE CELL DISEASE THAT REQUIRE MEDICAL ATTENTION

Fever >101°F

Lethargy

Dehydration

Worsening pallor

Severe abdominal pain

Acute pulmonary symptoms

Neurologic symptoms

Pain associated with extremity weakness or loss of function

Acute joint swelling

Recurrent vomiting

Pain not relieved by conservative measures or home medications

Priapism lasting >3 hrs

has never received the pneumococcal vaccination, it should be offered and given at further intervals based on the recommendations of the American Association of Family Physicians. Daily folic acid (1 mg PO qd) is given for the prevention of folate deficiency in the chronic hemolytic state. Retinal evaluation is begun at school age and should be continued routinely to monitor for evidence retinopathy by an ophthalmologist.

- Patients should be counseled during routine clinic visits as to **red flags** for which they should seek further medical attention (Table 12-2).

Surgery and Anesthesia

- Surgery and anesthesia are stress states that can provoke a painful sickle crisis. Currently, it is recommended for all patients with sickle cell disease to be **conservatively transfused** to a Hgb of 10 mg/dL before elective surgery. Studies comparing aggressive transfusion (Hgb S levels <30%) vs conservative transfusion (Hgb S <60%; Hgb = 10 mg/dL) showed no benefit to the more aggressive regimen. In healthy patients with stable Hgb SC disease, current data do not support preoperative transfusion. There are no definitive data available to recommend no preoperative transfusion, even in healthy Hgb SS patients.
- Intraoperative overexpansion of blood volume should be avoided, particularly in patients with decreased cardiac function. Hypothermia must also be avoided in the OR to prevent sickling. After surgery, IV fluid management must ensure adequate hydration with the avoidance of volume overload and pulmonary complications. Minor hyponatremia (sodium, 130–140 mEq/L) is common and can be tolerated, but hypernatremia should be avoided. Incentive spirometry is effective in ensuring deep breathing and avoiding atelectasis.
- **Dental procedures** requiring local anesthesia can be performed in the dentist's office. However, any dental procedure requiring general anesthesia warrants hospital admission. The use of nitrous oxide in patients with sickle cell disease remains controversial. It is customary to administer concentrations of 50% oxygen with nitrous oxide to alleviate the risk of sickling. Prophylactic antibiotics should be given with tooth extractions or root canals in patients with orthopedic prostheses.

Transfusion Therapy

- **Transfusion of RBCs** has been used for almost every implication of sickle cell disease, but its value has been demonstrated for few. Indications for transfusion include the need to improve O_2-carrying capacity (as in aplastic crisis or acute chest syndrome), increase blood volume (as in splenic sequestration), or improve blood rheology (to prevent stroke recurrence, leg ulcers, priapism). Simple transfusion can be sufficient to improve O_2-carrying capacity and blood volume. Partial exchange transfusion is recommended for acute indications and for chronic programs, in which avoiding hyperviscosity and iron overload are important. The goal of transfusion is to raise the Hgb to a level of approximately 10 g/dL. Levels >10 g/dL can lead to hyperviscosity and increased vaso-occlusion.
- **Transfusion complications** in sickle cell patients are common and include alloimmunization, iron overload, and transmission of viral illness. 30% of alloimmunization in transfused sickle cell patients is due in part to minor blood group incompatibilities due to racially mismatched blood. Antibodies against the Rh, Kell, Duffy, and Kidd antigens present the greatest problem in transfusing these adults.
- **Iron overload** and its complications of end-organ damage become a problem in those patients who are chronically transfused. Chelation with desferrioxamine is recommended when the total body iron level is elevated, and serum ferritin levels should not be allotted to exceed 1000 g/dL. Chelation therapy is extremely time consuming and inconvenient therapy for the patient in addition to being very expensive. This is one of the motivating factors for trying to reduce the amount of transfusions in patients with sickle cell disease. However, attempts to reduce the number of yearly transfusions are not always successful, and serum ferritin levels should be monitored on a regular basis.

Hydroxyurea

Hydroxyurea is a drug that has been used with some success in the treatment of patients with sickle cell disease. Hydroxyurea causes a significant increase in Hgb F synthesis. Higher levels of Hgb F have been found to have significant clinical advantages with decreased rates of acute painful episodes, longer intervals between acute painful episodes, fewer episodes of acute chest syndrome, and a diminished number of transfusions. The mechanism by which hydroxyurea influences sickle cells and vaso-occlusion remains unknown. Some hypotheses include changes in sickle erythrocytes such as increased water content, improved deformability, and decreased adherence to the endothelium.

KEY POINTS TO REMEMBER

- Sickle cell disease is a group of genetic disorders characterized by the presence of Hgb S.
- Hgb S is the result of a single nucleotide substitution (adenosine to guanine) on the beta-globin gene that results in the polymerization of Hgb tetramers when deoxygenated, leading to the sickled RBC.
- Sickle cell trait has a prevalence of 8–10% in the African-American population and is a benign carrier condition with no associated hematologic abnormalities.
- The two hallmark features of sickle cell disease are a chronic hemolytic anemia and vaso-occlusion resulting in ischemic tissue injury.
- There is a tremendous variability of acute painful crises, even within the same patient over time. There is no pathognomonic clinical or lab finding for acute painful crisis, and the diagnosis is based on history and physical exam.
- The acute management of painful crises is IV fluid hydration, analgesia, and treatment of identifiable precipitating factors such as infection.
- Aplastic crisis is the transient arrest of erythropoiesis characterized by abrupt falls in Hgb and reticulocytosis. The most common causes are infections (e.g., parvovirus B19) and bone marrow necrosis.

- Acute chest syndrome is characterized by dyspnea, chest pain, fever, tachypnea, pulmonary infiltrates, and leukocytosis and may be indistinguishable from acute painful crisis. However, acute chest syndrome must be considered in sickle cell patients with the clinical features listed, as it is associated with a 10% mortality rate due to multisystem organ failure.
- The management of acute chest syndrome is O_2, antibiotics, and partial-exchange transfusion to decrease the amount of Hgb S in the patient.
- All patients with sickle cell disease should be transfused to a Hgb of 10 mg/dL before all elective surgery to decrease the risk of perioperative complications from sickling.

REFERENCES AND SUGGESTED READINGS

Bunn HF. Pathogenesis and treatment of sickle cell disease. *N Engl J Med* 1997;337:762–769.

Embury SH, Vichinsky EP. Sickle cell disease. In: Hoffman R, Silberstein LE, Banz EJ, et al., eds. *Hematology: basic principles and practice*, 3rd ed. New York: Churchill Livingstone, 2000:510–554.

Reid CD, Charache S, Lubin B, eds. Management and therapy of sickle cell disease. *NIH publication 96-2117*. 1995:1–114.

Serjeant GR, Ceulaer CD, Lethbridge R, et al. The painful crisis of homozygous sickle cell disease: clinical features. *Br J Haematol* 1994;87:586–591.

Vichinsky EP, Haberkern CM, Neumayr L, et al. A comparison of conservative and aggressive transfusion regimens in the perioperative management of sickle cell disease. *N Engl J Med* 1995;333:206–213.

Wayne AS, Kevy SV, Nathan DG. Transfusion management of sickle cell disease. *Blood* 1993;81:1109–1123.

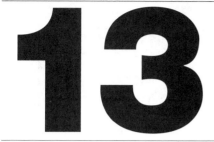

Hematologic Drugs

Shachar Peles and
Giancarlo Pillot

INTRODUCTION

Anticoagulant drugs are widely used to treat or prevent thromboembolic diseases. There are also additional choices for active clot lysis. Each of these medications has serious potential for harm and should be used only after the risks and benefits have been thoroughly pondered. However, there are fewer drugs available for a procoagulant effect. These medications and their mechanism of action are also briefly reviewed in this chapter. Specific indications are not discussed here, and the reader is referred to other chapters in the series regarding treatment of conditions such as deep vein thrombosis, pulmonary embolism (PE), myocardial infarction, acute arterial thrombosis, atrial fibrillation.

COAGULATION CASCADE

The coagulation cascade is separated into intrinsic and extrinsic pathways, as seen in Fig. 13-1. The end result of activation of coagulation by either pathway is the activation of factor X to factor Xa, which, in turn, converts prothrombin to thrombin. Thrombin is the enzyme that converts fibrinogen to fibrin, thus forming a clot. Any process that interferes with the intrinsic pathway interferes with aPTT; the extrinsic pathway; PT; and the common pathway, both aPTT and PT. This model of the coagulation cascade, although incomplete, aids in the understanding of bleeding disorders and explains the lab tests affected by the anticoagulant drugs.

ANTICOAGULANTS

- **Heparins** are a group of molecules comprised of long, negatively charged chains of polysaccharide. These negatively charged moieties bind to antithrombin III, activating it. This complex then inactivates factor Xa, thrombin, and other proteins in the clotting cascade. Heparins are a naturally occurring biologic product prepared from porcine intestine or bovine lung. Treatment with unfractionated heparin involves an initial bolus followed by a continuous infusion. This infusion needs to be continually adjusted according to the aPTT, as heparin has a narrow therapeutic range and large variability with regard to patient response. The target aPTT should be 1.5–2.5 times the control value. Use of heparin nomograms may assist in maintaining therapeutic heparin levels.
- **Low-molecular-weight heparins** (LMWHs) are a group of medications derived from heparin. They are typically produced by degradation of standard heparin and fractionation into a product having a mean polysaccharide chain size of approximately one-third that of standard heparin. The resulting mix of molecules has greater anti-Xa compared to factor IIa activity. They have several advantages over standard unfractionated heparin in that they have longer half-lives and a more predictable dose response. Lab monitoring is therefore not necessary. It is also possible that they are associated with fewer bleeding complications, while having equivalent anticoagulant effect. However, the LMWHs have not been tested in every indication for which standard heparin is indicated. They also are not appropriate for patients with impaired renal function. Another drawback to this class of heparins is that they are difficult to reverse and typically long acting, which can be troublesome when bleeding does occur.

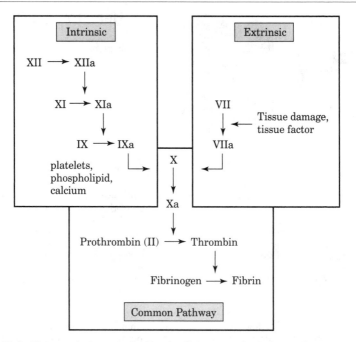

FIG. 13-1. The coagulation cascade. For simplicity, several cofactors and some potential steps in the cascade have been left out of this diagram. (Modified from Cotran RS, Kumar V, Robbins SL. *Robbins pathologic basis of disease*, 5th ed. Philadelphia: WB Saunders, 1994:103.)

Coumadin

Long-term anticoagulation is achieved with **oral coumarins.** These are vitamin K antagonists, warfarin being the most widely used. They act by interfering with gamma carboxylation of factors II, VII, IX, and X and proteins C and S. Warfarin results in a rapid decrease in factor VII and protein C levels, as these have the shortest half-lives of all the clotting factors. Thus, it induces a transient hypercoagulable state due to the low protein C levels. Therefore, anticoagulation with heparin should be continued for at least 4 days and until the patient has been therapeutically anticoagulated for at least 2 days. Monitoring is via the **international normalized ratio,** which is a method of standardizing between different PT assays. Regular monitoring of the INR and dose adjustment are required because of variations in patient response over time and interpatient variation in requirements. The target level of anticoagulation and duration of therapy is dependent on the indication for initiating therapy.

One must be cautious when initiating new medications to patients already on warfarin therapy. Many drugs, including some antifungals (miconazole, fluconazole), antibiotics (metronidazole, quinolones, sulfonamides), antiarrhythmics (amiodarone, quinidine), acute alcohol ingestion, aspirin, and acetaminophen, have been shown to increase warfarin levels and subsequently the INR (Table 13-1).

Direct Thrombin Inhibitors

The direct thrombin inhibitors are a relatively new class of drugs, actively being developed. An example of this drug is **hirudin,** which has its origins in leech saliva (although manufactured from recombinant DNA technology). As a direct thrombin inhibitor, it causes inhibition of factor II and elevated PT, PTT, and thrombin time in the lab. Its

TABLE 13-1. DISEASE-SPECIFIC ANTITHROMBOTIC THERAPY

Indication	First-line Rx	Alternate Rx	Comment and duration
AF			
Low risk (i.e., no risk factors[b]) Typical patient	ASA INR 2.5	INR 2.5 ASA	Duration: lifelong[a]
DVT/PE	INR 2.5[c] and UFH or LMWH	INR 2–5[c] and pentasaccharide	LMWH options: dalteparin, 100 units/kg SC q12h; dalteparin, 200 units/kg SC qd; enoxaparin, 1.0 mg/kg SC q12h; enoxaparin, 1.5 mg/kg SC qd; nadroparin, 90 units/kg q12h; tinzaparin, 175 units/kg SC qd
			Duration for warfarin: 6 mos typically, but shorter for postoperative DVT and longer for multiple events or ongoing risk factors
Ischemic stroke (secondary prophylaxis)			
Noncardioembolic stroke	ASA 81–325 mg	Ticlopidine, 250 mg bid; clopidogrel, 75 mg qd; or ASA, 25 mg, + dipyridamole, 200 mg bid	In patients taking ticlopidine, check CBC q2wk for 3 mos
Cardioembolic stroke, MS, or history of AF	INR 2.5	—	Use warfarin in patients with AF, MS, or acute cardioembolic stroke (rule out hemorrhage with CT first)
			Duration: lifelong
Post-MI			
Typical patient	ASA 81–325 mg	INR 2.5	Duration for ASA: lifelong
High risk for embolism (e.g., anterior MI, severe LV dysfunction, AF, mural thrombosis, or history of embolism)	INR 2.5 or 3.0	ASA ± warfarin	Except for chronic embolic risk factors (e.g., AF), warfarin duration: 3 mos; then substitute ASA

continued

TABLE 13-1. CONTINUED

Indication	First-line Rx	Alternate Rx	Comment and duration
Heart valve replacement			
Tissue	INR 2.5	ASA 325 mg	Duration, tissue: 3 mos for warfarin; subsequently, ASA can be used lifelong
Mechanical			Duration, mechanical: lifelong warfarin
Low risk (i.e., aortic St. Jude valve)	INR 2.5	INR 3.0	Can add ASA or use INR >3 for patients with CAD, caged-ball, or caged-disk valves (e.g., Bjork-Shiley), or prior embolism
Typical patient	INR 3.0	INR 3.0 + ASA 81 mg	—

AF, atrial fibrillation; CAD, coronary artery disease; DVT, deep venous thrombosis; LMWH, low-molecular-weight heparin; LV, left ventricular; MS, mitral stenosis; PE, pulmonary embolus; UFH, unfractionated heparin.

[a]Warfarin for cardioversion should begin 3 wks before cardioversion and can be stopped once sinus rhythm has been maintained for >4 wks.

[b]Risk factors for stroke: history of stroke, transient ischemic attack, hypertension, diabetes mellitus, CHF, MS, or age >75 yrs.

[c]Higher INR may be needed for patients who had a DVT or PE with an INR of 2–3 or who have the antiphospholipid antibody syndrome.

Adapted from J Hirsh, J Dalen, DR Anderson, et al. Oral anticoagulants: mechanism of action, clinical effectiveness, and optimal therapeutic range. *Chest* 2001;119:8S–21S.

major use is for anticoagulation in the setting of heparin-induced thrombocytopenia when further use of heparin is contraindicated but anticoagulation is desired. Other agents that have been used include agratroban and danaparoid sodium.

Complications of Treatment

- **Bleeding complications** are present in 5% of patients treated with unfractionated heparin. Predictors for this complication include recent surgery, liver disease, thrombocytopenia, and antiplatelet medications. Bleeding risk is lower with LMWH. Risk factors for bleeding associated with warfarin include a history of GI bleeding, atrial fibrillation, renal disease, liver disease, and concurrent antiplatelet therapy. Every patient beginning warfarin therapy needs to be warned about the complications of concurrent aspirin therapy.
- **Management of bleeding** associated with anticoagulant therapy should be individualized, with treatment depending on severity of hemorrhage, lab test results, and risk of recurrence of thromboembolism. Anticoagulant therapy should be discontinued, and local measures to stop bleeding should be instituted as a first step. Protamine should be administered to heparin-treated (unfractionated and LMWH) patients who have a prolonged aPTT with a serious bleed. In the case of warfarin-related bleeding, Table 13-2 describes an algorithm to aid in management. It should be noted that although warfarin therapy prolongs the PT/INR primarily, the PTT can also become elevated at very high levels of warfarin anticoagulation.

TABLE 13-2. TREATMENT GUIDELINES FOR PATIENTS ON WARFARIN THERAPY

High INR—no bleeding

INR >5

    Hold warfarin

    Search for occult bleed

    Evaluate for food or drug interactions

    Follow INR

5<INR<10

    Vitamin K, 1.0–2.5 mg PO

    Document fall in INR within 48 hrs

    Redose vitamin K if INR remains high

INR ≥ 10

    Vitamin K, 3 mg SC

    Follow INR q8h, repeat vitamin K if needed

Minor bleeding

    Hold warfarin

    Vitamin K, 1–5 mg SC

    Follow q8–24h, repeat vitamin K as needed

    If bleeding not readily controlled, treat as for major bleeding

Major bleeding—admit to hospital if not already there

    Hold warfarin

    Vitamin K,[a] 10 mg SC or 10 mg IVPB over 20 mins and fresh frozen plasma

    Follow INR q6–24h and repeat vitamin K until INR normal and bleeding has stopped

    Control bleed—surgical consultation, transfusion

[a]Vitamin K administration via the IV route does carry a risk of anaphylaxis, which does not occur when given by PO or SC routes. There is some evidence that the PO route results in faster reversal of warfarin-induced hypercoagulability than the SC route.

- **Heparin-induced thrombocytopenia** occurs in approximately 3% of heparin-treated patients and is an immune IgG-mediated decrease in platelets. It may be complicated by extension of venous thrombus or development of new arterial thrombus. It should be suspected if the platelet count drops to <100,000/μL or to <50% of the baseline platelet count. This drop typically occurs 5–15 days after heparin is begun or sooner if there is a history of recent exposure to heparin. It should be differentiated from the early, benign, transient thrombocytopenia that can occur with heparin therapy as a nonspecific reaction. LMWH may cross-react immunologically with unfractionated heparin, and treatment of this complication therefore involves using hirudin. See Chap. 8, Disorders of Platelets and Primary Hemostasis, for a complete discussion.
- **Warfarin-induced skin necrosis** is seen in patients with protein C or protein S deficiency. It is caused by thrombotic occlusion of small vessels occurring between 3 and 8 days after warfarin therapy is initiated and results from a decrease in protein C that precedes reduction in factors IX and X. This skin necrosis occurs most often in the patient's extremities, trunk (the breast in particular), and penis (in males) and marginates very quickly from the initial lesion site. Biopsies from these lesions show fibrin thrombi within local vessels with interstitial hemorrhage often occurring. This complication is avoided by starting warfarin therapy after a therapeutic aPTT is achieved with heparin.

HEMOSTATIC DRUGS

Aminocaproic Acid

Aminocaproic acid is a derivative of lysine. Its major effect is in inhibiting the transformation of plasminogen to plasmin by blocking its binding to fibrin. It can be used in the setting of **mucosal bleeding** (upper GI tract or oral cavity). It can be useful in dental procedures in those with coagulation disorders (congenital or acquired) or with low platelet counts. Aminocaproic acid is also used for menorrhagia when other measures are ineffective or contraindicated. Other indications, such as use in the setting of bleeding complications from thrombolytics, cardiac surgery, joint replacement, and liver transplant have not been accepted. Most side effects are GI—nausea, vomiting, and diarrhea. No major thrombotic complications have been noted during trials. Typical dosing for chronic bleeding is 5–30 g IV or PO in divided doses at 3- to 6-hr intervals. For acute bleeding in the setting of elevated fibrinolytic activity, dosing is 5 g during the first hr, followed by 1–1.25 g for approximately 8 hrs or until bleeding stops, either PO or IV.

Desmopressin

Arginine vasopressin (desmopressin or DDAVP) increases tissue release of von Willebrand factor and factor VIII. It is a transient **increase in the clotting factors** and occurs in any patient **capable** of synthesizing them. (Note that those with hemophilia A often synthesize **some** factor VIII and may have some benefit.) It is given SC or IV as a 0.3-μg/kg dose or 300 μg nasally (in adults). The dose can be repeated in 24 hrs, but exhaustion of stored pools causes this treatment to lose its efficacy after a few doses. Desmopressin is also used in the setting of bleeding in uremic patients to counteract platelet dysfunction by increasing available von Willebrand factor. Side effects are related to the physiologic action of desmopressin, namely, water retention and hyponatremia. There are reports of arterial thromboses that have occurred with its use.

THROMBOLYTICS

Compared to the anticoagulant drugs, which express most of their activity by interfering with clot formation, thrombolytics play an active role in **clot dissolution**. However, they have a high incidence of bleeding side effects, the most serious being intracranial hemorrhage—thus, their indications are typically for serious indications such as hemodynamically significant PE or acute myocardial infarction or for localized use. Major formulations include streptokinase (derived from bacterial cell products), urokinase (from renal tubular epithelial cells), and recombinant tissue plasminogen activator. All have the same mechanism of action in that they cleave plasminogen to form plasmin, which actively lyses clot and other procoagulant proteins. Recombinant tissue plasminogen activator has more clot specificity *in vitro*, but this does not appear to translate into major differences in bleeding complications *in vivo*. Furthermore, as streptokinase is a bacterial product, it is antigenic, and, therefore, antibodies may form after its administration, limiting repeat future use in a patient. The use of thrombolytics should only be undertaken by those experienced in their use.

KEY POINTS TO REMEMBER

- The first step in treating anticoagulant-related bleeding is stopping the anticoagulant and performing local measures if possible.
- Most stable, nonbleeding patients with an elevated INR may be treated by simply withholding their warfarin dose.
- HIT should be suspected in any patient whose platelet count has dropped to <100,000 cells/μL or >50% after being initiated on heparin.
- Low-molecular-weight heparins may be used in certain instances when heparin is indicated, but each product should only be used for its approved uses.

REFERENCES AND SUGGESTED READINGS

Cotran RS, Kumar V, Robbins SL. *Robbins pathologic basis of disease*, 5th ed. Philadelphia: WB Saunders, 1994:100–104.

Fauci, et al. *Harrison's principles of internal medicine*, 14th ed. New York: McGraw-Hill, 1998:744–747.

Mannucci PM. Hemostatic drugs. *N Engl J Med* 1998;339:245–253.

USP DI, 1997 publication, The United States Pharmacopeial Convention.

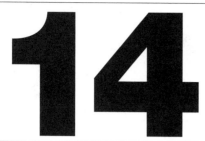

Plasma Cell Disorders

Judah D. Friedman

INTRODUCTION

Gammopathy refers to the production of a monoclonal protein (called **M-protein** or **paraprotein**) by a clone of malignant lymphoid or plasma cells. These M-proteins are detectable as a peak or "spike" on serum or urine protein electrophoresis (SPEP or UPEP) in the gamma or beta region, and are Igs or components of Igs. The detection of M-protein may be due to a spectrum of diseases from a stable production of low levels of monoclonal protein (called a **monoclonal gammopathy of undetermined significance,** or **MGUS**) to multiple myeloma. IgM production is usually produced in Waldenström's macroglobulinemia. IgG and IgA are usually seen in multiple myeloma. Rarely, IgD and IgE can be seen as well. Some gammopathies result from either heavy chain or light chain (lambda or kappa) Ig production. Monoclonal light chains found in the urine are referred to as **Bence-Jones proteins.**

MONOCLONAL GAMMOPATHY OF UNDETERMINED SIGNIFICANCE

MGUS is defined by the presence of a serum monoclonal protein at a concentration of <3 g/dL and the absence of light chains in the urine (usually <1 g/24-hr collection). *Patients with MGUS also lack findings of multiple myeloma*, including hypercalcemia, lytic bone lesions, anemia, and renal insufficiency due to gammopathy. In addition, the proportion of plasma cells in the bone marrow should be <10%. MGUS occurs in 2% of those older than 50 yrs and 3% of those older than 70 yrs.

Evaluation

Clinical Manifestations
Patients are typically asymptomatic and are often diagnosed by SPEP and UPEP in the evaluation of other organ dysfunction.

Diagnosis
If suspected (during the workup of renal insufficiency, proteinuria, or elevated total protein on chemistry profile, for example), obtain a SPEP and UPEP along with immunofixation to identify the monoclonal protein type. UPEP can detect light chains or monoclonal proteins concentrated in urine that could be missed on SPEP. However, the UPEP would miss larger proteins that may not be excreted (whole Ig and especially IgM), and very often it just detects overall presence. The SPEP on the other hand, gives you a sense of the total amount of monoclonal fraction, which can be used to follow response to therapy. Light chains are usually not detected in the serum, as they are rapidly excreted by the kidney. Because some patients may produce only light chains, it is essential to obtain both an SPEP and UPEP in the workup of a gammopathy. The main diagnostic objective in MGUS is to ascertain whether multiple myeloma or another serious lymphoproliferative disorder is present. When a monoclonal protein is identified, it is generally recommended to obtain a CBC, peripheral smear, and basic metabolic panel. It is usually not necessary to obtain a bone marrow biopsy unless the monoclonal protein is >2 g/dL, the patient has unexplained anemia, renal insufficiency, hypercalcemia, or bone pain (see Multiple Myeloma). In most cases, one should obtain a skeletal survey to rule out lytic bone lesions.

Management

No treatment is usually necessary, and patients usually remain asymptomatic. The risk of progression of MGUS to a plasma cell disorder or related lymphoid malignancy is approximately 1%/yr. A large long-term study of the prognosis in MGUS found the cumulative probability of progression was 12% at 10 yrs, 25% at 20 yrs, and 30% at 25 yrs. An increased risk of progression was seen in those patients with IgM and IgA (as compared with those with IgG) and in those with a higher initial monoclonal protein level. Although monitoring may not increase survival, it is recommended that patients with MGUS are usually monitored yearly (with CBC, BMP, SPEP, and UPEP) to detect evolution to multiple myeloma to prevent complications. Rapid increases in the M-component may warrant therapy (see Multiple Myeloma).

MULTIPLE MYELOMA

Introduction

Multiple myeloma results from a clonal proliferation of plasma cells that produce a monoclonal protein that is detectable by protein electrophoresis. This monoclonal protein on electrophoresis is referred to as the **M-protein.** Multiple myeloma accounts for 1% of all cancer-related deaths, and is two times more likely in African Americans. In addition, exposure to radiation, benzene, herbicides, and insecticides may play a role, but at present the data is sparse, and the case numbers are few. The average age of diagnosis is 60 yrs, and incidence increases with age. Myeloma is a monoclonal disease, and cells can secrete IgG (50%), IgA (20%), light chain only (20%), or IgD (2%) but only one type in any given individual patient (all the myeloma cells secrete an identical product in a given patient, as the cells are monoclonal). Approximately 5% of patients have no detectable monoclonal antibody but usually have a hypogammaglobulinemia. IgM secretion is usually associated with Waldenström's macroglobulinemia.

Evaluation

Clinical Manifestations

Patients with overt multiple myeloma may present with **bone pain** (most commonly involving the spine and ribs), **weakness, anemia, abnormal bleeding** (secondary to platelet dysfunction), or **infection.** Bone marrow infiltration results in a normocytic, normochromic anemia; thrombocytopenia; and leukopenia. In one-half of multiple myeloma patients, rouleaux formation is found on the peripheral smear. Bone resorption causes osteopenia and hypercalcemia. There are osteolytic lesions on x-rays. Sufficient monoclonal protein may accumulate to result in proteinuria renal failure. The disease may also be associated with plasmacytomas—collections of malignant plasma cells—which may result in conditions such as vertebral collapse or spinal cord compression. Chronic infections and autoimmune diseases, as well as chronic lymphocytic leukemia, lymphoma, and cirrhosis may also be associated with an M-protein spike.

Diagnosis

- **Initial testing** should include both a SPEP and UPEP, as 20% of patients secrete only light chains. Light chains are rapidly cleared from the serum. Immunoelectrophoresis determines the identity and quantity of the monoclonal protein.
- A **bone marrow biopsy** should be obtained to quantitate the degree of plasmacytosis.
- Obtain a **CBC, ESR, peripheral smear, UA** (proteinuria but negative dipstick because not usually spilling albumin) and **blood chemistries** to assess extent of tumor burden (anemia, renal failure, hypercalcemia).
- A **skeletal survey** identifies lytic bone lesions. A radionucleotide bone scan is typically not helpful, as the lesions of myeloma are purely lytic, which are not detected on this study.
- A **beta$_2$-microglobulin** level (the light chain of the HLA antigen) is a useful marker and provides prognostic information (see Prognosis).

- The diagnosis of multiple myeloma is usually made in the presence of one major and one minor criterion or three minor criteria.
  The **major criteria** for diagnosis of multiple myeloma include the following:
  - Plasmacytoma
  - Bone marrow plasmacytosis with >30% plasma cells
  - High levels of monoclonal protein (>3 g/dL for IgG, >2 g/dL for IgA, and >1 g/dL for kappa or light chains in the urine)
  The **minor criteria** for diagnosis of multiple myeloma include the following:
  - Bone marrow plasmacytosis of 10–30%
  - Monoclonal protein levels of less than above
  - Lytic bone lesion
  - Hypogammaglobulinemia or suppression of antibody production

Staging

The stage of multiple myeloma correlates with tumor burden and median survival (Table 14-1).

Patients are also subclassified based on renal function:

- a: creatinine <2 g/dL
- b: creatinine >2 g/dL

For example, a patient with stage III disease is designated IIIb if the serum creatinine is >2 g/dL.

Management

- Patients with **MGUS, indolent** or **smoldering myeloma,** or **stage I multiple myeloma** require close monitoring with a paraprotein measurement q6–12mos. Treatment is largely palliative. Therapy is indicated if there is doubling of the M-protein in <1 yr or progressing bone lesions. Immediate treatment is necessary with bone pain, elevated serum calcium, or progressive renal failure. Cord compression requires radiation, and pathologic fractures of long bones require orthopedic intervention with internal fixation. Pain resulting from compression fractures of the vertebral bodies may be relieved by vertebroplasty.
- Two common **chemotherapy** regimens are as follows:
  - M&P: melphalan (Alkeran) and prednisone (Deltasone, Sterapred) q4–6wks
  - VAD: vincristine (Oncovin, Vincasar), doxorubicin (Adriamycin), and dexamethasone (Decadron)

TABLE 14-1. DURIE-SALMON STAGING SYSTEM

Stage	Criteria	Median survival (mos)
I	Hemoglobin >10 g/dL	60
	Calcium <12 mg/dL	
	0–1 lytic lesions	
	IgG <5 g/dL, IgA <3 g/dL, or ULC <4 g/24 h	
II	Between stages I and III criteria	55
III	Hemoglobin <8.5 g/dL	15
	Calcium >12 mg/dL	
	>5 lytic bone lesions	
	IgG >7 g/dL, IgA >5 g/dL, or ULC >12 g/24 h	

ULC, urine light chain.
Adapted from NCI Web site. Multiple myeloma. Available at: http://www.cancer.gov/cancerinfo/pdq/treatment/myeloma/healthprofessional#Section_18. Accessed August 8, 2003.

- A response rate of 40–50% can be achieved with these regimens. Treatment should be discontinued once the paraprotein level reaches a plateau phase for several mos. The addition of a maintenance dose of **daily prednisone** has been shown to improve survival and progression-free survival.
- Patients who do not respond to M&P may show a response to VAD or another course of M&P. Originally, VAD was used for those who failed M&P. However, VAD often is used as initial therapy for those who will be treated with high-dose therapy followed by autologous bone marrow transplantation.
- As another option, some patients may respond to **thalidomide** (Thalomid), an anti-angiogenesis agent.
- **Supportive measures,** including aggressive hydration to delay renal insufficiency, are essential to improving quality of life. Bisphosphonates, such as pamidronate (Aredia) or zoledronic acid (Zometa), have been shown to delay skeletal disease in multiple myeloma patients, decrease bone pain, and improve quality of life and are generally recommended.
- In suitable candidates, **high-dose chemotherapy followed by autologous stem cell transplant** has resulted in a higher rate of complete response and overall survival compared to standard dose chemotherapy. Interferon-alpha is used posttransplant to help maintain remission. Allogeneic bone marrow transplant has the potential for curative therapy but is associated with significant treatment-related mortality.

Prognosis

The median survival for patients with multiple myeloma is approximately 3 yrs. Without treatment, the median survival for patients is 6 mos. As shown earlier, patients with advanced stage have a shorter survival. In addition, a higher beta$_2$-microglobulin level has been shown to correlate with shorter survival times.

Stage I: 5-yr survival rate is approximately 50%. Median survival time is >60 mos (or 5 yrs).
Stage II: 5-yr survival rate is approximately 40%. Median survival time is approximately 41 mos (or nearly 3.5 yrs)
Stage III: 5-yr survival rate is 10–25%. Median survival time is approximately 23 mos (or nearly 2 yrs).

Although chemotherapy and supportive measures improve overall quality of life, the effects on improving survival are limited.

WALDENSTRÖM'S MACROGLOBULINEMIA

Macroglobulinemia occurs in disorders in which there is proliferation of B-lymphocytes and plasma cells that produce an IgM monoclonal protein. Physical findings include excessive weakness, fatigue, weight loss, and chronic oozing of blood from the nose and gums. Lab findings are commonly anemia and rouleaux formation on the blood smear. The complications of the disease are usually hyperviscosity syndrome related to the overproduction of IgM proteins by the malignant plasma cells, in addition to the lymphoproliferative process itself.

KEY POINTS TO REMEMBER

- The diagnosis of MGUS requires the exclusion of features of multiple myeloma.
- The risk of progression of MGUS to a plasma cell disorder or related lymphoid malignancy is approximately 1%/yr.
- Multiple myeloma should be considered in any case of anemia, recurrent infections, hypercalcemia, or bone pain.
- Multiple myeloma is two times more common in African Americans, and additionally may be associated with environmental exposure to radiation, benzene, herbicides, or insecticides.

- Multiple myeloma requires a SPEP, UPEP, and immunoelectrophoresis. A 24-hr protein is also needed to quantitate the presence of light chains in the urine.
- Patients with multiple myeloma may be eligible for autologous transplantation and improved survival.

REFERENCES AND SUGGESTED READINGS

American Cancer Society Web site. Detailed guide: multiple myeloma. How is multiple myeloma staged? Available at: http://www.cancer.org/docroot/CRI/content/CRI_2_4_3X_How_is_multiple_myeloma_staged_30.asp?sitearea. Accessed August 7, 2003.

Attal M, Harousseau JL, Stoppa AM, et al. A prospective, randomized trial of autologous bone marrow transplant and chemotherapy in multiple myeloma. *N Engl J Med* 1996;335:91.

Bataille R, Harousseau JL. Medical progress: multiple myeloma. *N Engl J Med* 1997;336:1657.

Casciato DA, Lowitz BB. *Manual of clinical oncology*, 4th ed. Philadelphia: Lippincott Williams & Wilkins, 2001.

De Vita VT, Hellman S, Rosenberg S. *Cancer: principles and practice of oncology*, 5th ed. Philadelphia: Lippincott Williams & Wilkins, 1996.

Durie BG, Stock-Novack D, Salmon SE, et al. Prognostic value of pretreatment serum beta 2 microglobulin in myeloma: a Southwest Oncology Group Study. *Blood* 1990;75(4):823–830.

Kyle RA, Therneau TM, Rajkumar SV, et al. A long-term study of prognosis in monoclonal gammopathy of undetermined significance. *N Engl J Med* 2002;346:564–569.

Murphy G, Lawrence W, Lenhard R. *American Cancer Society textbook of clinical oncology*, 2nd ed. Atlanta: The Society, 1995.

Saint S, Frances C. *Saint Frances guide to inpatient medicine*, 1st ed. Baltimore: Lippincott Williams & Wilkins, 1997.

Oncology

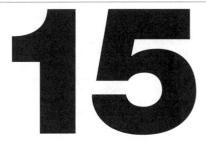

Introduction and Approach to Oncology

Marcia L. Chantler

INTRODUCTION

In the second half of the nineteenth century, cancer had been thought of primarily as a surgical disease. Cancer was believed to be a local process in the body and, therefore, amenable to surgical removal. Since the 1970s, cancer has been reconceptualized as a systemic disease amenable to medical treatments, as opposed to a solely surgical approach. This belief has led to the modern multidisciplinary approach to the diagnosis and treatment of the most common adult malignancies with medical, surgical, and radiation oncology. This manual focuses on the main elements related to medical oncology, including the diagnosis and treatment of adult malignancy.

APPROACH TO THE CANCER PATIENT

- All patients facing a cancer diagnosis have four basic questions. Answering these questions forms the basis of cancer management.
  - How much cancer is there?
  - What can be done about it?
  - Can it be cured?
  - How much time do I have?
- The treatment of a malignancy requires a *diagnosis based on tissue pathology*. In only the very rare case would treatment be started without a diagnosis. Consultation from the surgical, medical, and radiologic oncology team members is essential when an initial search for an area to biopsy to confirm the diagnosis of cancer is performed. These oncology professionals are crucial to include in cases in which prompt therapy should be delivered to the patient to reduce the risk of morbidity or mortality in certain oncologic emergencies.
- The coordination of the oncologist with the referring physician needs to be individualized in the best interest of the patient. A trusting relationship with both the patient and the referring physician is important in implementing future recommendations for the oncologist. Listening and taking the time to explain terminology, prognosis, and treatment options are key components to the relationship between an oncologist and the patient. Given that most advanced cancers cannot be cured, the oncologist's knowledge of and experience with the behavior of advanced malignancies combined with the use of complex medical regimens often lead to the role of the oncologist as the primary care physician during active treatment. Oncologists also are useful in providing optimal palliative care for symptom relief as well as assisting in the role of end-of-life discussions and care.

APPROACH TO DIAGNOSING A MALIGNANCY

Tumor Stage and Grade

- **Staging** describes the extent of the disease in an individual patient. Staging is essential to the treatment of cancer in that it enables the oncologist to provide optimal treatment strategies and discussion of outcomes or prognosis. In research studies, staging is used for comparison between cancer trials. Many tumors are associated with several staging systems. The most common staging system uses the **TNM classification system** developed by the American Joint Committee on Cancer. "T" represents the primary tumor characteristics. "N" represents the presence of nodal sites of disease. "M" represents metastatic or distant organ sites of spread. It is recommended that the reader consult an up-to-date staging manual when evaluating a patient because of frequent revisions for each individual malignancy. Clinical staging uses radiologic data to describe the extent of gross disease. Pathologic staging can identify microscopic foci of distant disease that may not be described on clinical staging exams.

- The **grade** of a tumor is a pathologic description of the cellular characteristics of any given malignancy. A *low-grade malignancy* retains many of the characteristics of the originating cell type. Low-grade malignancies tend to be associated with a less aggressive cell type and more favorable prognosis. A *high-grade malignancy* is characterized by the loss of the characteristics of the originating cell type and evidence of higher mitotic activity. High-grade malignancies are often associated with a poorer prognosis, given the more aggressive behavior of the cells.

Performance Status

Performance status describes the functional abilities of the oncology patient. It is frequently used to provide a standardized assessment of patients considered for inclusion in protocols or to characterize patients at diagnosis or during treatment or follow-up. The initial performance status score can hold prognostic implications for some malignancies such as brain and lung cancers. There are several different scales used by physicians, including the Karnofsky Performance Status and the Eastern Cooperative Oncology Group (ECOG) performance status scale (Table 15-1). Both are frequently used, but the ECOG performance status scale is easier to remember.

TABLE 15-1. KARNOFSKY AND EASTERN COOPERATIVE ONCOLOGY GROUP (ECOG) PERFORMANCE STATUS SCALES

- The *Karnofsky* scale runs in increments of 10 from 0 (death) to 100 (no impairment) and can be divided into three broad ranges:

  100–80: normal activity without the need of special assistance and no or minimal symptoms of disease.

  50–70: unable to work but able to live at home and capable of self-care, although varying levels of assistance may be required.

  10–40: incapable of self-care, requiring acute or chronic care in a hospital or institutional setting, with rapidly progressive disease process.

  0: death.

- The *ECOG* scale runs in increments of 1 from 0 (no impairment) to 5 (death):

  0: full activity, without symptoms.

  1: ambulatory, able to carry out light activity, minimal symptoms.

  2: unable to work, ambulatory >50% of daytime activity.

  3: in bed or chair >50% of daytime activity, limited self-care.

  4: completely disabled, confined to bed or chair, inability to do any self-care.

  5: death.

APPROACH TO ONCOLOGY TREATMENTS

The majority of adult solid malignancies are best managed through a multidisciplinary approach involving surgeons, radiation oncologists, and medical oncologists. There are often multiple different treatment options, and patients should be an active part of the decision-making process. An important element in the treatment of cancer patients is to *define the goals of treatment*, including cure, prolongation of survival, or improvement in quality of life. Treatment recommendations should be carefully tailored to the individual patient, taking into account comorbid conditions, performance status, and other psychosocial issues.

Surgical Approach to Cancer

Surgery still remains the most effective modality for curing cancer confined to a local site. In many instances, the surgical removal of the primary cancer also involves the removal of a regional node-bearing area. Appropriate patients can be identified for definitive or curative surgery. The goal is for the surgeon to remove all neoplastic cells and avoid implantation and dissemination of "loose" tumor cells. This involves the resection of a complete margin of normal tissue around the primary tumor. Depending on the tumor, patients with a solitary or limited number of metastases to sites, such as the brain, liver, or lung, can be cured by the surgical resection of the metastatic disease. Cytoreductive surgery or tumor debulking can facilitate subsequent radiation and/or chemotherapy in some malignancies such as ovarian cancer. Surgery may also be necessary in the palliative setting to relieve symptoms from the cancer in the absence of a cure. One such example is the relief of an intestinal obstruction from colon cancer.

Radiation Therapy Approach to Cancer

Radiation therapy is the treatment of choice for some cancers. The use of this treatment modality is based on the responsiveness of a cancer to ionizing radiation. Some cancers are extremely sensitive, including lymphomas and seminomas, whereas others are relatively resistant (Table 15-2). Radiation therapy can be the sole curative local modality in such malignancies as Hodgkin's disease, cervical cancer, or prostate cancer. It is also useful in the adjuvant setting to increase the likelihood of local or regional control after surgery. Radiation therapy also plays a key role in the palliation of symptoms from primary or metastatic tumor masses such as spinal cord compression or bone metastases. For more information regarding radiation therapy, see Chap. 17, Introduction to Radiation Oncology.

Systemic Therapy Approach to Cancer

- In contrast to surgery or radiation therapy, which has only local effects on the tumor, the role of systemic therapy is geared at treating both the local tumor and

TABLE 15-2. SENSITIVITY OF MALIGNANT TUMORS TO RADIATION

Very responsive	Moderately responsive	Poorly responsive
• Hodgkin's disease	• Head and neck cancer	• Melanoma
• Non-Hodgkin's lymphoma	• Breast cancer	• Glioblastoma
• Seminoma, dysgerminoma	• Prostate cancer	• Renal cancer
• Neuroblastoma	• Cervical cancer	• Pancreatic cancer
• Small-cell cancers	• Esophageal cancer	• Sarcoma
• Retinoblastoma	• Rectal cancer	
	• Lung cancer	

potential or actual areas of metastatic disease throughout the body. Before the initiation of chemotherapy, the **goal of treatment** must be clearly defined and discussed with the patient. Not all patients are candidates for chemotherapy. Potential risks as well as benefits must be considered when deciding to treat a patient with cytotoxic agents. The performance status and overall nutritional state of the cancer patient is extremely important when making the decision to use chemotherapy. Performance status scores of 3–4 on the ECOG scale are usually not candidates for systemic therapy unless they have previously untreated tumors known to be especially responsive to chemotherapy.

- **Adjuvant therapy** refers to the use of systemic therapy in conjunction with surgical curative therapy to improve both disease-free and overall survival. The goal is to eliminate undetected local and micrometastatic foci of tumor. There is no way to measure or follow response to therapy, and thus duration of treatment is determined empirically by clinical trials. Cancers for which adjuvant chemotherapy has proved to benefit survival include colorectal, breast, and ovarian cancers and osteosarcoma. Similarly, adjuvant hormonal therapy is effective in improving survival in breast cancer patients who are estrogen-receptor positive.

- **Neoadjuvant therapy** refers to systemic therapy that is administered before surgery. The goal of neoadjuvant therapy is to decrease the tumor burden for the definitive surgical procedure, thus minimizing complications and making organ preservation more feasible. In addition, the clinician can monitor the tumor response to a systemic agent for effectiveness. Neoadjuvant chemotherapy is used in breast, esophageal, rectal, lung, and bladder cancers, as well as osteosarcomas.

- **Combined modality therapy** refers to the combination of chemotherapy and radiotherapy used to treat bulky disease. The goal of combined modality therapy may be to decrease the size of the tumor for either a curative or salvage surgical procedure. Combined modality therapy improves survival for some patients with locally advanced lung, esophageal, head and neck, pancreatic, and cervical cancers. The combination can also be curative and organ-preserving in certain tumors such as laryngeal and anal cancers.

- **Induction chemotherapy** is used as the initial treatment of a malignancy to achieve complete remission or significant cytoreduction of disease. It is commonly used in the treatment of acute leukemias and lymphomas. **Consolidation chemotherapy** is given after a patient is in remission to prolong the duration of remission and overall survival in patients with acute leukemias. Consolidation chemotherapy is often the same drug or drugs that are not cross-resistant to the induction chemotherapy agents. **Maintenance chemotherapy** is the use of prolonged, low-dose chemotherapy to prolong the duration of remission and achieve a cure in those patients. **Salvage chemotherapy** is given with the intent to control disease or palliate symptoms after the failure of other known effective treatments.

- **High-dose chemotherapy** is typically used in the treatment of hematologic malignancies. The high doses of chemotherapy are used to ablate the bone marrow requiring rescue with **allogeneic** or **autologous** bone marrow or stem cell replacement to repopulate the marrow. Allogeneic transplants have been curative in selected patients with chronic myelogenous leukemia and acute myelogenous or lymphoid leukemias. Autologous stem cell transplants have been most successful for aggressive lymphomas. The use of bone marrow transplant in solid organ malignancies remains investigational.

- **Immunotherapy** refers to the use of pharmacologic agents that are intrinsic to the immune system. High concentrations of these biologic response modifiers stimulate the immune system to kill cancer cells. Examples include interferon-alpha, interleukin-2, or monoclonal antibodies. Toxicities can range from fevers and flulike symptoms to anaphylaxis and adult respiratory distress syndrome–like manifestations. Tumor vaccines and gene therapies remain experimental.

- Once a decision is made to administer chemotherapy, **response criteria** are used to measure the outcome of therapy. In general, responses to therapy are measured by objective changes in tumor size and increases in disease-free and overall survival. The single most important indicator of the effectiveness of chemotherapy is the complete response rate. No patient with advanced cancer can be cured without attaining a complete remission.

- A **complete response** is defined as the disappearance of disease on imaging studies for at least 1 mo duration.
- A **partial response** is the decrease of 50% or more in the sum of the products of the biperpendicular diameters of the measurable disease (as measured by radiology or physical exam), with no new sites of disease for at least 1 mo's duration. For example, if the oncologist is following a lung lesion measuring 3 cm × 2 cm and a liver lesion measuring 4 cm × 5 cm, then the sum of the products of the biperpendicular diameters in this example is $(3 \times 2) + (4 \times 5)$, which is 26. To document a partial response in this example, on follow-up measurements, the sum should be ≤ 13.
- **Progression** of a tumor is defined if the product of the biperpendicular diameters increases by >25% in one or more sites, new lesions appear, or the patient dies as a result of the tumor. Chemotherapy is discontinued in the setting of progression, and the patient is reevaluated. The term **stable disease** is used when the measurable disease does not meet the criteria for complete response, partial response, or progression. Stable disease represents a difficult challenge to oncologists. If therapy is tolerated with no significant side effects, it is often continued, provided it is recognized that progressive disease will eventually occur.
- An individual's **prognosis** is based on staging, comorbidities, performance status, and response to treatment. Although it is possible to predict curability or median survival, long-term follow-up is essential to get a more accurate sense of prognosis for any given patient. Even when the overall prognosis is poor, an honest and compassionate discussion with the patient and family members is essential. This is a key role of the medical oncologist. Up-front and honest answers to even the most difficult questions allow the patient and family to make realistic goals that will help guide future health care decisions. See Table 15-3 for a list of potentially curable malignancies.
- **Clinical trials** are available for many disease sites and stages. Because cancer treatment is far from ideal, clinical research is vital to test new strategies for improving survival and quality of life. Patients who participate in clinical trials receive treatments that are theorized to be at least as good as, if not better than, the current standard of care. Informed consent must always be obtained, and patients have the right to withdraw at any time. In general principle, patients should be offered enrollment in clinical trials whenever possible.
- **Palliative care** of cancer patients entails the management of all of the symptoms related to the cancer itself and the toxicities of treatment. It also includes the multidisciplinary care of psychosocial issues, with the primary goal of optimizing the quality of life and minimizing the morbidity and symptoms related to cancer and its

TABLE 15-3. CANCERS CURABLE OR OCCASIONALLY CURABLE WITH CHEMOTHERAPY ALONE

Curable with chemotherapy alone
- Gestational choriocarcinoma
- Hodgkin's disease
- Germ cell cancer of the testis
- Acute lymphoid leukemia
- Non-Hodgkin's lymphoma (some subtypes)
- Hairy cell leukemia

Occasionally curable with chemotherapy alone
- Acute myeloid leukemia
- Ovarian cancer
- Small-cell lung cancer

treatments. Prolongation of survival is a secondary goal, which may or may not be achieved, but cure is not the primary intent in palliative care. Chemotherapy, hormonal therapy, radiation, and surgery are still useful in palliation. Patient selection for interventions is crucial. For patients with advanced cancer and poor performance status, aggressive treatment may be detrimental rather than beneficial.

- **Hospice** is a philosophy of care based on a coordinated program of support services for terminally ill patients and their families. Palliative care is provided with the aim to improve quality of life and a comfortable death. Any patient with a limited life expectancy ($\leq$ 6 mos) may be eligible for hospice care. Although the majority of hospice patients have cancer, patients with other advanced diseases, such as Alzheimer's dementia or chronic obstructive pulmonary disease, may benefit from this health care approach. The interdisciplinary hospice team consists of nurses trained in pain and symptom management, home health aides, social workers, chaplains, and volunteers. The referring physician may remain involved in medical decisions unless transfer to the hospice medical director is desired. Care is generally given in the home but may be imparted in nursing homes or hospitals if necessary. Medicare hospice benefits also include complete coverage for all medications pertaining to the hospice diagnosis, durable medical equipment, and oxygen. Most hospice agencies will provide 24-hr on-call service, brief respite care, and bereavement counseling for up to 1 yr after the patient dies.

KEY POINTS TO REMEMBER

- A tissue diagnosis of a cancer is usually required before an oncology consult is appropriate.
- The oncologist often becomes a primary care giver to the patient during active treatment.
- Mutual goal setting between the patient and physician is an important part of the care of the oncology patient and should be reassessed frequently.
- Patients should be offered enrollment in clinical trials whenever possible, but respecting the patient's wishes regarding this is the first principle.
- The philosophy behind hospice is to provide patients who have limited life expectancy the care and support needed to improve their quality of life and ensure a comfortable death.

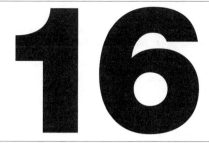

Cancer Biology

Holly M. Magiera

INTRODUCTION

The development of cancer is a multistep process in which a cell and its progeny gradually attain genetic changes leading to a survival advantage and the ability to invade and spread distantly. In general, cancer is a disease that increases in incidence with age, supporting the idea that multiple genetic "hits" must be accumulated over time for its development. The most common cancers occur in tissues that turn over rapidly and are exposed to environmental agents favoring genetic damage. This chapter briefly reviews the process of carcinogenesis and gives a brief overview of the inherited cancer syndromes.

CARCINOGENESIS

- Normal human cells behave in an orderly fashion. They populate specific areas of the body appropriate to their function, and they grow and divide in response to appropriate signals (i.e., growth factors) from the body. When their function is exhausted, they are shed or die in an orderly fashion. During their lifetime, they are subject to a wide variety of insults causing cellular and genetic damage. However, they also have repair mechanisms that detect when the signals within the cell have become deranged and attempt repair. There are also checkpoints in the cell growth cycle, leading to cell death in the event of severe damage that cannot be repaired.
- **Malignancy** occurs when cells develop genetic defects that make the normal cellular growth process described earlier impossible. Nonlethal alterations in DNA change the usual control mechanisms that tell a cell when to grow, divide, and die. The tumor cells lose their usual orderly growth pattern. They begin to divide in a less controlled fashion, either by no longer requiring exogenous growth factors or producing their own. They become resistant to cellular mechanisms that normally prevent uncontrolled cell growth and gain the ability to avoid programmed cell death. They may gain the ability to leave their usual site in the body, travel throughout the bloodstream or lymphatic system, grow in a new location, and stimulate normal tissues to grow blood vessels to support the new growth. As the tumor cells become more deranged, they may lose the ability to fix acquired DNA damage, causing further genetic defects to accumulate.
- The **principal genes** affected include oncogenes, tumor suppressor genes, and genes involved in apoptosis (programmed cell death). Mechanisms of damage to these genes include environmental insults from agents, such as radiation or chemicals, as well as intrinsic damage from faulty replication. There are many types of mutations, including point mutations and chromosomal aberrations. Chromosomal aberrations may consist of deletions, gene amplification, or translocation. Multiple mutations are typically required in a cell to transform it from a normally behaving cell into a cancer cell.

Oncogenes and Proliferation

- **Oncogenes** (i.e., cancer genes) are genes whose normal function involves promoting the growth and reproduction of cells in a regulated fashion. When these genes are activated in an uncontrolled manner, they lead to malignant transformation of cells. They were initially identified in retroviruses that were capable of inducing tumors in host species, but, subsequently, similar genes were identified in normal animal cells. They are initially present as proto-oncogenes (i.e., precancer genes) until a mutation renders them into active oncogenes. The products of oncogenes are involved in regulation of cell proliferation, and mutations make them independent of regulatory mechanisms. Oncoproteins (the products of oncogenes) may have a role in various parts of the cell cycle and proliferation. Growth factors and their receptors, signal-transducing proteins, nuclear transcription factors, and cyclins may all be affected by mutations.

- **Growth factors** are chemicals that normally act as signals to cells to divide, grow, or interact with nearby cells. These factors may become produced in an uncontrolled fashion, or genes controlling them may develop mutations that make them lose their ability to be regulated. Oncogenes involving growth factors such as c-sis (platelet-derived growth factor) and hst-1 (fibroblast growth factor) have been described in several GI and other tumor lines. It is also common for other oncoproteins to increase growth factor transcription and translation.
- Alternatively, oncogenes may code for **growth factor receptors.** Changes in receptors are common in cancers. This may entail overexpression of receptors or mutations, leading to continuous activation of the receptors independent of exogenous signals. For example, **C-erb B1,** the epidermal growth factor receptor, has been overexpressed in up to 80% of squamous cell cancers of the lung. **C-erb B2** or **c-neu** is amplified in breast cancers and other tumors and has provided a molecular target in treatment.
- Proteins involved in **signal transduction** from the receptors to the nucleus are also commonly mutated in malignancy. These proteins normally carry the signal to reproduce from the growth factor receptor on the cell to the nucleus. **Ras** is one such protein, and it is mutated in approximately 30% of human malignancies. Activated **ras** acts downstream to stimulate DNA that causes increased cell proliferation, and normally it can be inactivated by GTP hydrolysis. Mutant **ras** proteins cannot hydrolyze GTP and thus are always activated, leading to uncontrolled proliferation. The c-abl oncogene also encodes a signal-transducing tyrosine kinase that is important in chronic myelogenous leukemia in which a chromosome translocation causes its overactivity and the malignant phenotype.
- The final step in signal transduction is alterations in **nuclear transcription factors** that orchestrate the cell's progress through the cell cycle. These are the proteins that bind to the DNA and cause replication or protein synthesis to occur. Many mutations have been described in cancer affecting these genes. For example, c-myc is an oncogene whose presence is needed for cell division. In normal cells, the level of myc rapidly tapers off once the cell cycle is initiated. Amplification or dysregulation of myc is common in human cancer, including Burkitt's lymphoma, small-cell lung cancer, and neuroblastomas.
- **Cyclins** are important regulatory elements that control progress through the cell cycle. Different types of cyclin proteins are expressed during the various phases of cell cycle, and mutations involving cyclins are common in malignancy. For example, D cyclins are involved in the transition from growth to synthesis phases in the cell, and these genes are frequently dysregulated and overexpressed in esophageal, breast, and squamous carcinomas.

Tumor Suppressor Genes

- The products of tumor suppressor genes normally tend to stop cell proliferation. Loss of function of these genes may lead to unchecked cell growth. Multiple examples of tumor suppressor genes have been described, and the protein products may act at various points in growth regulation. The **Rb** gene was the first tumor suppressor gene to be discovered—in the setting of hereditary retinoblastoma. Loss of both normal Rb genes was found to be necessary to form tumors, leading to the "two-hit" hypothesis— that is, for tumor suppressor genes to be carcinogenic, both copies of the gene must be altered. This is unlike the situation with oncogenes, in which a single gene will have a defect that promotes carcinogenesis. Some hereditary cancer syndromes are associated with germline mutations of one copy of a tumor suppressor gene. This predisposes patients to malignancy if the second copy is altered through a somatic mutation. *Rb* has been well studied, and its gene product is known to be a cell cycle regulator. The *Rb* protein (pRb) exists in both active and inactive phases. In quiescent cells, *pRb* is unphosphorylated and active and sequesters transcription factors important for proliferation. Phosphorylation of *pRb* occurs when cells are stimulated by growth factors and results in release of transcription factors favoring replication. If *pRb* is inactive or mutated, it cannot provide a check against cell growth, and cancerous growth may result.

- Another well-studied tumor suppressor gene is **p53**. Loss of *p53* is found in almost every type of cancer. *P53* is also involved in cell cycle regulation. Normal *p53* protein accumulates when DNA is damaged and causes an arrest in the cell cycle. This allows for time to repair DNA damage. If the damage is too severe for repair, *p53* protein signals the cell to undergo apoptosis. If *p53* protein is lost, DNA damage is not repaired, and the cell continues through cell cycle. Mutations can become fixed in the DNA, and this can lead to malignant transformation.

Apoptosis

Mutations affecting apoptosis—programmed cell death—are common in malignancy. These genes normally function to cause cell death when cellular or DNA damage has occurred or when the cell's useful life has expired. Families of genes involved in this process have been identified. The *bcl-2* gene was one of the first identified genes and is overexpressed in follicular lymphoma. *Bcl-2* is antiapoptotic, and therefore cells that overexpress it have a proliferative advantage. The *p53* protein may also be considered an apoptosis gene. It favors apoptosis in cases of severe genetic damage, and loss of this property is important in the development of cancer.

DNA Repair Genes

Mutations secondary to environment and from errors in replication are common. Under normal circumstances, DNA repair genes act to correct these errors. Disorders in DNA repair predispose to the development of cancer. One example of this is the inherited disease *xeroderma pigmentosum*. Patients lack one of several genes involved in DNA repair and are at increased risk of skin cancer caused by light exposure. Mutations in mismatch repair genes are also responsible for the increased risk of colon cancer in hereditary nonpolyposis colon carcinoma syndrome.

Additional Interactions

- Interactions with other cells, as well as the **extracellular matrix,** are important for the growth and proliferation of normal cells. Malignant cells often have alterations in these interactions, which allow them to escape contact inhibition and to escape the apoptosis normally induced when cellular interactions are disrupted. For example, **integrins** are transmembrane receptors that allow interactions with other cells and with the basement membrane. This allows for the stimulation of *ras* and other downstream pathways in the right environment. Loss of the integrin interaction results in programmed cell death under normal circumstances. Cancerous cells may overcome this by overexpressing ras or other members of its pathway. Escape from normal interactions also allows cells to metastasize and invade.
- **Telomerase** is another protein that is often overexpressed in malignant cells. Cell replication is normally accompanied by progressive shortening in the telomeres, which are repeat DNA sequences that are present at the ends of chromosomes. Shortening of the telomeres to the point that they can no longer protect cellular DNA provides a "biologic clock" that limits the lifespan of a cell and its progeny. Germ cell lines produce telomerase, which protects the telomeres and immortalizes

the cells. Normal somatic cells do not express telomerase, but many malignant cells express this protein, allowing continued replication of the cells.

- **Angiogenesis** is another process important in malignancy, particularly in distant spread of tumor cells. Tumors induce angiogenesis through a variety of mechanisms. One way is to stimulate neovascularization by the production of proangiogenic factors. Tumors may also induce neighboring macrophage and fibroblasts to elaborate angiogenic growth factors. Angiogenesis provides a way for tumors to obtain the nutrients they need to further proliferate. It is also necessary for distant spread.
- Tumors also often elaborate **proteases** and other destructive enzymes, which allow them to break down extracellular materials and to invade. They must have the ability to migrate and to hone to tissues that will permit their growth.

Tumor Progression

The development of cancer is a multistep process requiring mutations in different pathways. Each cancer likely has its own unique progression of mutations, leading to the malignant phenotype. As tumors develop, they tend to continue to acquire mutations that lead to increasing malignant potential. Within a tumor, there is variability in invasive potential, growth potential, and other attributes. Ultimately, subclones within a tumor are selected if they have attributes that allow them to be more "fit" than other subclones. Development of **colon cancer,** for example, is a relatively well-understood process. The lesions progress from adenomas to dysplasia to frank malignancy, and the genetic changes are well characterized. Mutations in the APC tumor suppressor gene initiate the process, leading to hyperproliferative cells. DNA hypomethylation also occurs, which alters gene expression, and is seen in early adenomas. Activation of ras may be the next step, leading to a more advanced adenoma with further clonal expansion. Loss of the DCC tumor suppressor gene leads to a late adenoma, and loss of p53 precedes the development of carcinoma. Further mutations occur, leading to more aggressive clones and metastasis. It is believed that many tumors have similar mechanisms that are as yet undefined. The exact involved genes and the sequence of mutation likely varies for each particular tumor type.

Future Directions

Any of the previously described mechanisms that occur in the creation of a malignant cell may be potentially manipulated in hopes of treating a tumor. Investigation into the exact roles of oncogenes, tumor suppressor genes, angiogenesis factors, and the other mechanisms described earlier may hopefully translate to treatments or cures for malignancy. The future of medical oncology likely lies in the manipulation of these "growth and death" pathways as treatment.

GENETIC CANCER SYNDROMES

The vast majority of cancers are not inherited diseases, but studies involving inherited syndromes have allowed further understanding of the biology of cancer. The following are some of the more well described (but not necessarily common) ones.

Familial Retinoblastoma

Retinoblastomas are small-cell, undifferentiated tumors of the retina. Approximately 40% of cases are familial, and they are usually bilateral and occur at an early age. The genetic change responsible is loss or alteration of the *Rb* gene. Loss of one allele occurs in the germline, and an additional somatic mutation is need for retinoblastoma to develop. The *Rb* gene product, as discussed earlier, is a negative growth regulator. Inactivation of the *Rb* gene is also seen in osteosarcoma, small-cell lung cancer, breast cancer, and leukemia.

Li-Fraumeni Syndrome

Li-Fraumeni syndrome is characterized by loss of the tumor suppressor gene, *p53*. Patients are predisposed to carcinoma, sarcoma, brain cancer, and leukemia. The p53 protein is involved in a cell cycle checkpoint induced by DNA damage and in apoptosis. Mutations in p53 are seen in all types of malignancy.

Wilms' Tumor

Nephroblastoma—Wilms' tumor—is a childhood malignancy. The *WT1* gene is responsible for this phenotype. It encodes a DNA-binding protein that belongs to a family of transcription regulators important in cell growth.

Neurofibromatosis Type I

Neurofibromatosis type I is a relatively common disorder, occurring in approximately 1 in 3000. There is a predisposition to neurofibrosarcoma and glioma in affected individuals. The NF1 gene product has been found to have homology to proteins involved in the regulation of ras. NF1 protein is believed to inactivate *ras*, and, therefore, loss of NF1 leads to unregulated growth.

Familial Adenomatous Polyposis

Familial adenomatous polyposis is characterized by loss of the APC gene and multiple polyps in the colon and rectum. Colon cancers result at an early age. The APC gene is a member of the tumor suppressor family of genes. Inactivation leads to upregulation of growth-promoting factors such as *myc* and cyclins.

Multiple Endocrine Neoplasia

Multiple endocrine neoplasia II is a dominant disorder due to gain of function mutations in the *ret* gene. Patients are predisposed to pituitary adenoma, medullary thyroid cancer, and pheochromocytoma.

Hereditary Nonpolyposis Colon Cancer

Patients with hereditary nonpolyposis colon cancer have a family history of colon cancer before the age of 50. Most of this disease is due to mutations in DNA mismatch repair genes. This confers genetic instability and an increased likelihood of mutations that result in unregulated growth.

KEY POINTS TO REMEMBER

- The genesis of a malignant tumor is a multistep process that involves derangement of multiple genes that involve the normal function of cells.
- Most malignancies do not have a clear hereditary genetic basis. Rather, acquired genetic alterations along with inherited susceptibilities and environmental factors likely lead to the genetic changes responsible for malignancy.

REFERENCES AND SUGGESTED READINGS

DeVita VT, Rosenberg SA, Hellman S, eds. *Cancer: principles and practice of oncology*, 6th ed. Philadelphia: Lippincott Williams & Wilkins, 2000.

Fauci AS, et al. *Harrison's principles of internal medicine*, 14th ed. New York: McGraw-Hill, 1998.

Friend SH, Dryja TP, Weinberg RA. Oncogenes and tumor-suppressing genes. *N Engl J Med* 1988;318:618–622.

Hahn WC, Weinberg RA. Mechanisms of disease: rules for making human tumor cells. *N Engl J Med* 2002;347:1593–1603.

Hanahan D, Weinberg RA. The hallmarks of cancer. *Cell* 2000;100(1):57–70.

Vogelstein B, Fearon ER, Hamilton SR, et al. Genetic alterations during colorectal-tumor development. *N Engl J Med* 1988;319(9):525–532.

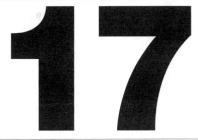

Chemotherapy

Giancarlo Pillot and
Kristan Augustin

INTRODUCTION

Medical therapy of malignancy with chemotherapy is the specific specialty of the medical oncologist, although most cancers are often treated with multiple therapies, including surgery, radiation, and chemotherapy. As a modality, it is potentially very serious in both side effects and potential for harm and should only be prescribed by physicians specifically trained and experienced in their administration. Its administration should also only be done by those specificially trained to do so. The intention of this chapter is a brief overview of the various types of chemotherapy and mechanisms of action, as well as common side effects. Table 17-1 contains a list of selected chemotherapeutic agents, their mechanism, and most common side effects.

Please see Chap. 35, Supportive Care in Oncology, for nonchemotherapeutic medication and treatment of the cancer patient.

GENERAL PRINCIPLES

Most forms of chemotherapy are agents that are toxic to cells of the human body. The justification for using substances that are toxic to normal cells is that malignant cells are preferentially sensitive to the effects of chemotherapy. In this way, a balance is intended to be struck between toxicity to malignant cells that are intended to be killed and benign, normal tissues that are intended to be spared but are often harmed as "innocent bystanders." This concept is the **therapeutic index,** which is the ratio of toxicity to tumor cells to that of normal cells. The therapeutic index is quite narrow for many antineoplastic agents. Traditional chemotherapeutic agents are in a number of classes of agents that *interfere with normal cell processes*, typically DNA synthesis or repair. However, it should be appreciated that these agents may act in methods other than simple cell killing (e.g., as initiators of apoptosis or maturation agents). Several newer agents are being developed that depart from the traditional concept of cell killing as their primary action. These agents are *targeted to specific receptors in the cancer cell*, often in pathways specifically dealing with maturation. As the understanding of the molecular basis of malignancy matures, these agents will become a larger part of our armamentarium.

Cell Cycle

The growth and division of cells can be conceptualized by the **cell cycle.** There are several phases to the life cycle of the dividing cell, including **g**rowth (G) phases, **s**ynthesis (S) phase, and a **m**itosis (M) phase. There also is a "rest" phase, or G0, in which cells are not actively participating in the cell cycle. Cells can then undergo terminal differentiation or reenter the cell cycle. Not all cells are actively in the proliferative portion of the cell cycle. Many chemotherapeutic agents are **cell cycle–specific** (i.e., they only have activity in certain parts of the cell cycle). Those that are **non–cell cycle–specific** may cause damage to a cell in any part of the cell cycle.

TABLE 17-1. SELECTED CHEMOTHERAPEUTIC AGENTS, CLASSIFICATION, AND SELECTED SIDE EFFECTS

Chemotherapy agent	Classification	Selected side effects
Fluorouracil (Adrucil, Efudex, Fluoroplex)	Antimetabolite (fluoropyrimidine)	Stomatitis, palmar-plantar erythrodysthesia, diarrhea, myelosuppression
Capecitabine (Xeloda)	Antimetabolite (fluoropyrimidine)	Stomatitis, palmar-plantar erythrodysthesia, diarrhea
Cytarabine (Cytosar-U, Tarabine PFS)	Antimetabolite (pyrimidine antagonist)	Myelosuppression, neurotoxicity, mucositis, nausea and vomiting, conjunctivitis, diarrhea
Gemcitabine (Gemzar)	Antimetabolite (pyrimidine antagonist)	Myelosuppression
Mercaptopurine (Purinethol)	Antimetabolite (purine antagonist)	Myelosuppression
Thioguanine	Antimetabolite (purine antagonist)	Myelosuppression
Pentostatin (Nipent)	Antimetabolite (purine antagonist)	Myelosuppression
Fludarabine (Fludara)	Antimetabolite (purine antagonist)	Myelosuppression, reduced immune function
Cladribine (Leustatin)	Antimetabolite (purine antagonist)	Myelosuppression Reduced immune function
Methotrexate (Abitrexate, Folex, Mexate, Rheumatrex)	Antimetabolite (folate antagonist)	Myelosuppression, nausea and vomiting, mucositis
Hydroxyurea (Hydrea)	Miscellaneous	Myelosuppression
L-Asparaginase (Elspar, Ervinar)	Miscellaneous	Anaphylaxis, nausea and vomiting, fever, malaise, acute pancreatitis, hypofibrinogenemia, hepatotoxicity, hyperglycemia
Vinblastine (Velban, Alkaban AQ, Velsar)	Tubulin interactive agents (vinca alkaloids)	Myelosuppression
Vincristine (Oncovin, Vincasar PFS, Vincaxome)	Tubulin interactive agents (vinca alkaloids)	Neuropathy, constipation, paralytic ileus
Vinorelbine (Navelbine)	Tubulin interactive agents (vinca alkaloids)	Myelosuppression, mucositis, nausea and vomiting, neurotoxicity
Paclitaxel (Taxol)	Tubulin interactive agents (taxanes)	Myelosuppression, peripheral neuropathy, hypersensitivity reaction, alopecia
Docetaxel (Taxotere)	Tubulin interactive agents (taxanes)	Myelosuppression, peripheral neuropathy, fluid retention, alopecia

(*continued*)

TABLE 17-1. CONTINUED

Chemotherapy agent	Classification	Selected side effects
Irinotecan (Camptosar)	Topoisomerase I inhibitor	Myelosuppression, diarrhea
Topotecan (Hycamtin)	Topoisomerase I inhibitor	Myelosuppression, nausea and vomiting, diarrhea
Etoposide (VePesid)	Topoisomerase II inhibitor (nonintercalator)	Myelosuppression, mucositis
Teniposide (Vumon)	Topoisomerase II inhibitor (nonintercalator)	Myelosuppression, mucositis
Cyclophosphamide (Cytoxan, Neosar)	Alkylating agent (oxazaphosphorine)	Myelosuppression, nausea and vomiting, hemorrhagic cystitis, cardiomyopathy
Ifosfamide (Ifex)	Alkylating agent (oxazaphosphorine)	Myelosuppression, nausea and vomiting, hemorrhagic cystitis, neurotoxicity
Mechlorethamine (Mustargen)	Alkylating agent (nitrogen mustard)	Nausea and vomiting, myelosuppression
Chlorambucil (Leukeran)	Alkylating agent (nitrogen mustard)	Myelosuppression, pulmonary fibrosis
Melphalan (Alkeran)	Alkylating agent (nitrogen mustard)	Myelosuppression
Busulfan (Busulfex, Myleran)	Alkylating agent (alkyl sulfonate)	Myelosuppression, hepatotoxicity, pulmonary fibrosis, seizures
Carmustine (BiCNU, Gliadel Wafers)	Alkylating agent (nitrosourea)	Myelosuppression, nausea and vomiting, mucositis
Lomustine (CeeNU, CCNU)	Alkylating agent (nitrosourea)	Myelosuppression
Streptozocin (Zanosar)	Alkylating agent (nitrosourea)	Nephrotoxicity, nausea and vomiting
Cisplatin (Platinol, Platinol-AQ)	Alkylating agent (platinum)	Myelosuppression, nausea and vomiting, peripheral neuropathies, nephrotoxicity, ototoxicity
Carboplatin (Paraplatin)	Alkylating agent (platinum)	Thrombocytopenia, nausea and vomiting, peripheral neuropathies, nephrotoxicity
Oxaliplatin (Eloxatin)	Alkylating agent (platinum)	Peripheral neuropathies, nausea and vomiting, diarrhea
Thiotepa (Thioplex)	Alkylating agent (ethylenimine)	Cystitis (intravesical), myelosuppression (IV)
Dacarbazine (DTIC-Dome)	Alkylating agent (miscellaneous)	Myelosuppression, nausea and vomiting
Temozolomide (Temodar)	Alkylating agent (miscellaneous)	Myelosuppression, nausea and vomiting

(continued)

TABLE 17-1. CONTINUED

Chemotherapy agent	Classification	Selected side effects
Bleomycin (Blenoxane)	Antitumor antibiotic	Pulmonary toxicity, acute febrile reactions
Mitomycin C (Mutamycin)	Antitumor antibiotic	Myelosuppression
Daunorubicin (Cerubidine)	Topoisomerase II inhibitor (intercalator/anthracycline)	Myelosuppression, mucositis, cardiotoxicity
Doxorubicin (Adriamycin)	Topoisomerase II inhibitor (intercalator/anthracycline)	Myelosuppression, mucositis, cardiotoxicity
Idarubicin (Idamycin)	Topoisomerase II inhibitor (intercalator/anthracycline)	Myelosuppression, mucositis, cardiotoxicity
Mitoxantrone (Novantrone)	Topoisomerase II inhibitor (intercalator/anthracenedione)	Myelosuppression, mucositis, cardiotoxicity
Epirubicin (Ellence)	Topoisomerase II inhibitor (intercalator/anthracycline)	Myelosuppression, mucositis, cardiotoxicity
Imatinib (Gleevec)	Miscellaneous	Nausea
Trastuzumab (Herceptin)	Monoclonal antibody	Cardiotoxicity, infusion reaction
Gemtuzumab (Mylotarg)	Monoclonal antibody	Myelosuppression, infusion reaction
Rituximab (Rituxan)	Monoclonal antibody	Myelosuppression, infusion reaction
Alemtuzumab (Campath)	Monoclonal antibody	Myelosuppression, nausea, infusion reaction, viral and *Pneumocystis carinii* pneumonia complications

ANTIMETABOLITES

Antimetabolites attempt to interfere with the normal synthesis pathways of the tumor cell. They are often involved in inhibiting DNA or RNA synthesis. They mostly act in the S phase of the cell cycle, and, therefore, the major toxicities are given to actively replicating normal tissues such as in the GI tract and marrow.

Pyrimidine Antagonists

- **Fluorouracil (5-FU) (Efudex, Fluoroplex)** inhibits thymidylate synthase. It must be metabolized in the cell before being incorporated into DNA. Most common toxicities of continuous infusion (e.g., in head and neck cancer therapy) include GI toxicity and mucositis. There can be bone marrow suppression at bolus doses such as when used in colon cancer therapy.
- **Ara-C (cytarabine) (Cytosar-U)** has side effects that include myelosuppression and gastroenteritis. Cytarabine can cause severe mucositis in the oral cavity. High-dose regimens are toxic to the cerebellum, and this side effect needs to be monitored (having the patient sign his or her name daily is one way to assess for this). In addition, high-dose regimens cause conjunctivitis, which is prophylaxed with steroid drops.
- **Gemcitabine (Gemzar)** is another antimetabolite that has myelosuppression as a toxicity.

Purine Antagonists

- **Mercaptopurine (6-MP) (Purinethol, Puri-Nethol)** requires conversion by intracellular enzymes before activation. Elimination is by xanthine oxidase, which is inhibited by allopurinol, so the combination should be avoided. It is often used in the therapy of leukemia.
- **Fludarabine (Fludara)** is another antimetabolite that causes neurotoxicity.

Folate Antagonist

Methotrexate (Folex, Rheumatrex, Trexall) inhibits dihydrofolate reductase, which is required for thymidylate synthesis and purine metabolism. Leucovorin can inhibit the actions of this drug. Its dose is limited by toxicity to the GI tract (mucositis) and bone marrow.

MICROTUBLE AGENTS

- **Vinca alkaloids** consist of vinblastine (Velban, Velbe) and vincristine (Oncovin, Vincasar PFS). They are isolated from the periwinkle plant. They bind to tubulin and inhibit cell division by inhibiting assembly into microtubles necessary for cell mitosis and are active in the M phase. Vincristine frequently causes neurotoxicity, whereas vinblastine causes marrow suppression.
- The **taxanes—paclitaxel (Taxol)** and **docetaxel (Taxotere)**—are isolated from the Pacific and European yew (which is more widely available), respectively. They also bind to microtubules, but they inhibit their disassembly, which also inhibits cell division. They are used in ovarian, lung, and breast cancers. Their toxicities are chiefly marrow suppression, neurotoxicity, and alopecia.

TOPOISOMERASE INHIBITORS

Topoisomerase inhibitors act on the topoisomerase enzymes, which are active in the winding (topoisomerase II) and unwinding (topoisomerase I) of DNA. This results in strand breaks and inhibits replication and translocation. These agents primarily act in the S phase of the cell cycle.

Topoisomerase I Inhibitors

- **Irinotecan** is often used in metastatic carcinoma of the colon or rectum. Its common toxicities include alopecia, diarrhea (both an early and late form), and myelosuppression.
- **Topotecan** is often used in the treatment of metastatic carcinoma of the ovary and of small-cell lung cancer. Its major toxicity is myelosuppression.

Topoisomerase II Inhibitors

- **Etoposide (VP-16) (Etopophos, Toposar, VePesid)** is used in some leukemias and lymphomas, as well as sarcomas.
- **Doxorubicin (Adriamycin, Doxil, Rubex), daunorubicin (Cerubidine), and idarubicin (Idamycin)** also produce free radicals and intercalating adjacent DNA base pairs in addition to inhibiting topoisomerase II. They are GI toxic and also decrease WBC counts. They cause severe skin damage when they extravasate. A major problem is cumulative cardiotoxicity, which is irreversible and has a cumulative effect. This occurs in approximately 2% of patients who receive cumulative doses of 550 mg/m^2. If the patient has received mediastinal radiation, the dose ceiling is 450 mg/m^2 for doxorubicin or 400 mg/m^2 for daunorubicin. Typically, an evaluation of heart function is necessary before initiation of these agents.

ANTITUMOR ANTIBIOTIC

Antitumor antibiotics are products of microbes that have activity against malignancies. They cause their effect by intercalating adjacent DNA base pairs, stopping transcription and DNA damage. They are relatively nonspecific in the cell cycle. **Bleomycin (Blenoxane)** is used in many combination regimens. It is not very myelotoxic but causes pulmonary fibrosis.

ALKYLATING AGENTS

This group of agents includes some of the first used chemotherapeutic agents. They directly bind to DNA and initiate cross-linking and strand breaks, causing toxicity and cell death. A comparatively high incidence of secondary malignancies is related to their use, and they can cause sterility.

- **Cyclophosphamide (Cytoxan, Neosar)** is used in a wide variety of malignancies. It can cause direct bladder toxicity when its metabolite is excreted in the urine. This can be prevented by MESNA and brisk hydration. If a course of cyclophosphamide is interrupted, the MESNA should typically be continued, because it is a protective agent, not the toxic agent. It can also cause myelosuppression and myocarditis.
- **Ifosfamide (Ifex)** is a similar chemical to cyclophosphamide. It is also typically administered with MESNA, as it has an even higher incidence of cystitis. It also can be neurotoxic.
- **Melphalan (Alkeran)** is a PO agent used in multiple myeloma. Its major toxicity is pulmonary fibrosis.
- **Busulfan** is profoundly marrow toxic and is used in many preparative regimens for bone marrow transplant.
- **Carmustine (BCNU, BiCNU)** therapy is complicated by delayed myelosuppression. It is lipid soluble and thus penetrates the CNS well. Renal insufficiency may also occur with its use.
- **Platinum** is a precious metal also used as a chemotherapy agent. **Cisplatin** (Platinol, Platinol-AQ) and **carboplatin** (Paraplatin) are the most commonly used forms. Cisplatin is toxic to kidneys and complicated by *severe* nausea and vomiting, which can occur in acute and delayed forms. This should be anticipated and treated *before* it occurs. Carboplatin is more neurotoxic and causes more thrombocytopenia but has less kidney toxicity.

OTHER AGENTS

- **Leucovorin (Wellcovorin)** acts as a folate analog. This medication is often used as an "antidote" to antifolate drugs such as methotrexate. It can be also given with 5-FU to enhance its binding to thymidylate synthase, enhancing its toxicity.
- **Hydroxyurea (Droxia, Hydrea)** inhibits ribonucleotide reductase. There is usually mild toxicity leading to leukopenia, which is typically easily reversible on discontinuation. It is useful for treatment of chronic myelogenous leukemia (CML).
- **L-Asparaginase (Elspar)** is an enzyme that, when infused, depletes the available pool of circulating asparagine. It can cause an anaphylactic reaction.

NOVEL AGENTS

There are several therapies for malignant disease that do not necessarily have effect by causing direct toxicity but are targeted therapies to specific signaling pathways.

Hormonal Therapy

Endocrine-related tumors are often affected by hormone therapy (e.g., antiestrogens in breast cancer, thyroid hormone to suppress thyroid cancer, and antiandrogens to inhibit prostate cancer). These are not discussed here, and the reader is referred to

Chap. 19, Breast Cancer, and Chap. 27, Urologic and Male Genital Malignancies, regarding those tumors.

Cell Marker Antibodies

Many tumor cells have specific cell-surface markers at various stages of their development. The most widely used examples are leukemias and lymphomas, which express different markers at different stages of maturity. Rituxan is a specific antibody to CD-20 (i.e., a B-cell marker) that is used in the treatment of certain B-cell lymphomas.

Signaling Pathways

Often, malignant transformation results from discrete gene rearrangements, causing loss of function, overexpression, or loss of regulation of function. Bcr-abl is a constitutively expressed tyrosine kinase found in some GI stromal tumors and CML. Imatinib mesylate (Gleevec) is a selective inhibitor of this gene product and has had dramatic success in treatment of CML. **ATRA** (all-*trans*-retinoic acid) is similar to retinoic acid and binds to the gene products of acute promyelocytic leukemia, causing differentiation of these cells.

KEY POINTS TO REMEMBER

* Cytotoxic chemotherapeutic agents typically have a narrow therapeutic index.
* Chemotherapeutic agents should typically only be ordered by clinicians experienced in their use.
* The use of chemotherapeutic agents requires close and careful monitoring.

REFERENCES AND SUGGESTED READINGS

Bast RC Jr, ed. *Cancer medicine: an official publication of the American Cancer Society*. New York: B.C. Decker, 2000.

Canal P, Chatelut E, Guichard S. Practical treatment guide for dose individualisation in cancer chemotherapy. *Drugs* 1998;56(6):1019–1038.

Chernecky C, Sarna L. Pulmonary toxicities of cancer therapy. *Crit Care Nurs Clin North Am* 2000;12(3):281–295.

DeVita VT, Rosenberg SA, Hellman S, eds. *Cancer: principles and practice of oncology*, 6th ed. Philadelphia: Lippincott Williams & Wilkins, 2000.

Fauci AS, et al. *Harrison's principles of internal medicine*, 14th ed. New York: McGraw-Hill, 1998.

Sonis ST, Fey EG. Oral complications of cancer therapy. *Oncology (Huntingt)* 2002;16(5):680–686.

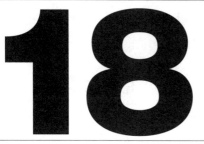

Introduction to Radiation Oncology

Parag J. Parikh and
Imran Zoberi

INTRODUCTION

Radiation oncology unifies the study of cancer with the therapeutic use of radiation. The radiation oncologist is the medical specialist who decides when and how to best use radiation. Under the supervision of the radiation oncologist, an array of nonmedical specialists, including physicists, dosimetrists, and technicians, assist in the planning and delivering of radiation to patients. This chapter introduces some of the basic principles of radiation oncology, some common treatment strategies, and an overview of the common toxicities that may be encountered in the inpatient setting. For a more complete description of these issues, the reader is referred to one of the textbooks listed at the end of this chapter [1–3].

PHYSICAL AND BIOLOGIC PRINCIPLES

- **Ionizing radiation** is energy that causes the ejection of an orbital electron and may be either electromagnetic (photons, gamma rays) or particulate (electrons, protons, or other atomic particles). In the majority of the world, photons and electrons are used. The energy of photons that can be generated in the clinic has increased over the years, which allows more doses to be delivered to internal malignancies, while respecting the tolerance of the skin to radiation. **Radiation dose** is measured in energy per unit mass, where 1 J/kg is 1 gray (Gy). The previously used term, **rad**, is equal to 1 centigray (cGy).
- Radiation causes DNA damage in both normal tissues and tumor cells. In general, *cells are most susceptible in G1, G2, and M phases of the cell cycle*. Susceptible cells may enter apoptotic cell death by a variety of mechanisms or undergo necrosis. Hypoxic cells are thought to be less susceptible to radiation than well-oxygenated cells, owing to preferential free radical formation. Fractionated radiotherapy (radiation given in multiple small doses over a given period instead of a single large dose) allows normal tissue to repair sublethal damage and repopulate while the tumor cells resort themselves in the cell cycle and become better oxygenated. A great deal of current research involves the cell cycle–signaling pathways involved in each aspect of the damage, repair, and reoxygenation pathways.

RADIATION TREATMENT GOALS AND METHODS

- Radiation can be given by directing x-rays from a treatment machine to the patient (**external beam radiotherapy**) or by placing a radioactive source in close proximity to the patient (**brachytherapy**). Brachytherapy is most often used in gynecologic cancers, prostate cancer, and head and neck cancer. Sometimes both techniques will be used to provide optimal dose distribution.
- Radiation can be given for **curative** or **palliative** intent and commonly is the definitive treatment. Often, it is combined with chemotherapy and surgery in the complete cancer care of the patient. It can be given before (neoadjuvant) or after

(adjuvant) the definitive therapy. Many solid tumors are treated with radiation and chemotherapy at the same time (concurrent chemoradiation).

- Accurate tumor **localization** is essential for optimum delivery of radiation. This can be done clinically (e.g., in palliative cases and gynecologic cancers) or using radiographic studies. Clinical localizations are done on whole brain patients and for some patients with bone metastases. These are quick and allow the patient to start treatment immediately but do not allow for conformal delivery of radiation. To plan most radiotherapy, the patient needs to have a **simulation** ("sim") in which he or she is brought to the radiation oncology department to make a treatment plan. This plan will aid in delivering the maximal dose of radiation to tumor tissue while attempting to avoid healthy tissue. Either two-dimensional (2D) (fluoroscopy, plain x-rays) or three-dimensional (3D) (CT scanners) methods can be used to generate images for treatment planning. These are sometimes merged with other radiologic modalities such as MRI, U/S, angiography, or PET scanning to better delineate tumor localization. Often, specialized **immobilization devices** are constructed for the patient during simulation to reduce intertreatment variation in patient position. After the simulation, the radiation oncologist develops a **treatment plan.** The time between initial consultation and the first treatment can often be 2–3 wks. **Patients are best served by early consultation of the radiation oncology team.**

- In general, for external beam radiotherapy, a patient will be placed on a flat, mobile, treatment table each day during the course of radiation therapy. Marks on the patient's skin and any immobilization devices are used to obtain accurate and precise patient positioning. Each treatment may last 10–30 mins. The total course of radiation therapy can vary from 1 day (prostate brachytherapy) to several weeks (fractionated external beam radiotherapy). Most fractionated treatment is given once/day, 5 days/wk, although some treatments are given more frequently.

INDICATIONS FOR URGENT RADIATION THERAPY

Urgent radiation therapy is useful in certain oncologic emergencies. Spinal cord compression is the only true radiation oncology emergency and is described further in Chap. 35, Oncologic Emergencies. It is imperative that radiation oncology and surgical services are consulted early and that an MRI of the entire spine is obtained as soon as possible. Brain metastases can be treated with radiation therapy, with timing depending on symptoms and patient's performance status. Uncontrolled bleeding of tumors (breast, gynecologic, lung, colon, or bladder are common sites) often responds well to radiation therapy. Superior vena cava (SVC) syndrome, the compression of the SVC by tumor (most often small-cell lung cancer), can be palliated by radiation. Resolution of SVC syndrome takes weeks with radiation therapy. Although SVC syndrome by itself is rarely fatal, these tumors can often encase other critical structures of the mediastinum.

LATE EFFECTS AND TISSUE TOLERANCE

Radiation therapy balances side effects to normal tissue with delivering adequate doses to the tumor. Side effects are divided into **late** (months to years after completion of radiation therapy) vs **acute** (during radiation therapy). The tolerance of normal tissue varies from patient to patient and depends on the dose of radiation, the fractionation scheme, and the volume of the organ exposed. The most common fractionation scheme is 1.8–2 Gy/day. Based on animal experiments and best available human data, the concept of the $TD_{x/y}$ was developed, which is the $x\%$ cumulative incidence of a certain complication in y years. Table 18-1 shows the doses with which one can expect 5% of patients to develop a late complication in 5 yrs as a function of volume of organ treated. These data represent general parameters and may not apply to an individual clinical situation. A radiation oncologist may elect to exceed these dose levels or be more conservative in individual cases.

TABLE 18-1. NORMAL TISSUE TOLERANCE TO THERAPEUTIC IRRADIATION: DOSE (GY) THAT TYPICALLY CAUSES A 5% INCIDENCE OF LATE COMPLICATIONS IN 5 YRS (TDS/S)

	Fraction of organ irradiated			
	$^1/_3$	$^2/_3$	$^3/_3$	End point
Kidney	50	30	23	Clinical nephritis
Brain	60	50	45	Necrosis/infarction
Lung	45	30	17.5	Pneumonitis
Heart	60	45	40	Pericarditis
Esophagus	60	58	55	Clinical stricture/perforation
Stomach	60	55	50	Ulceration/perforation
Small intestine	50	unk	40	Obstruction/perforation/fistula
Colon	55	unk	45	Obstruction/perforation/fistula/ulceration
Rectum	75	65	60	Severe proctitis/necrosis/fistula
Liver	50	35	30	Liver failure
Spinal cord	5 cm[a]	10 cm[a]	20 cm[a]	
	50	50	47	Myelitis/necrosis

unk, unknown.

[a]As the spinal cord is an organ in a series, doses of radiation to spinal cord are for lengths of the spinal cord and not for fraction of organ irradiated. These doses are those required to cause toxicity to the stated length of spinal cord.

Adapted from Emami B, Lyman J, Brown A, et al. Tolerance of normal tissue to therapeutic irradiation. *Int J Radiat Oncol Biol Phys* 1991;21:109–122; and Chao KS, Perez C, Brady L. *Radiation oncology: management decisions*. Philadelphia: Lippincott–Raven, 1999:24.

COMMON TREATMENT GUIDELINES AND ASSOCIATED ACUTE EFFECTS

The following is a brief description of current "off-protocol" treatment regimens. It must be emphasized that many patients are treated according to research protocols, which vary considerably. Acute toxicities of radiation therapy are typically related to direct toxicity to tissue in the path of the radiation. Most radiation-alone acute effects can be managed on an outpatient basis. With concurrent chemoradiation, acute effects have increased substantially and may require inpatient management. This is especially seen with head and neck, lung, and GI cancers.

Palliative Therapy

Brain metastases, bone metastases, and other palliative treatments are often given 20–40 Gy over 1–3 wks. This is a larger fraction size than used in most curative treatments, because there is less concern for late effects and a greater interest in minimizing treatment time for patient convenience.

Bone Metastases

Bone metastases can be treated with 6–8 Gy single doses to 42 Gy at 200 cGy/day depending on the number, location, and the patient's life expectancy. For patients with multiple bone metastases, radioactive strontium, samarium, or yttrium can be used to decrease pain.

Lung Cancer

Medically inoperable stage I and II lung cancer and stage III non–small-cell lung cancer are often treated with definitive radiotherapy, typically to a dose of 60–70 Gy. In many patients, the mediastinum is irradiated, which can result in the acute toxicity of esophagitis. The resultant odynophagia can lead to dehydration or significant weight loss, which may require inpatient management. Shortly after the completion of radiotherapy, a radiation pneumonitis or, very rarely, a radiation pericarditis may occur. Antiinflammatory steroid therapy is the mainstay of treatment for both of these conditions. 3D conformal radiation therapy, involving treatment planning based on CT scans, is being investigated as a method to increase dose to tumor while avoiding normal lung. Radiation therapy is used as adjuvant treatment in select cases of locally advanced non–small-cell lung cancer treated with definitive surgery. Both chemotherapy and radiation therapy play a central role in the definitive management of limited-stage small-cell lung cancer.

Esophageal Cancer

Radiation therapy with concurrent chemotherapy is used either as definitive treatment for esophageal/gastroesophageal junction tumors or as neoadjuvant treatment. As for the lung, esophagitis is the major acute toxicity.

CNS

After maximal safe surgical resection, *primary brain tumors* may be treated to 50–60 Gy depending on the area of the brain involved. *Brain metastases* are normally treated to 20–30 Gy. Radiosurgery, either by linear accelerator or by gamma knife, can be used on patients with few metastatic lesions—<4 cm. Radiosurgery involves a single day of treatment. Mild mental deterioration is seen in developing children and the elderly. Hospital admission is generally secondary to neurologic changes from tumor progression and, rarely, from treatment toxicity.

Head and Neck

In general, early-stage head and neck cancers are equally well treated with surgery or radiation. Advanced head and neck cancers require surgery and postop radiation, radiotherapy alone, or chemoradiation. Doses are typically 60–70 Gy. Multiple treatments per day (hyperfractionation) are often used. Side effects include xerostomia, odynophagia, dysphagia, and hoarseness. The acute toxicity often results in dehydration, which may require administration of IV fluids or placement of a gastric tube for nutritional support. Chemotherapy has been shown to improve outcome in the definitive radiotherapy of advanced head and neck cancers at the cost of 1–3% treatment-associated mortality and 20–30% risk of hospitalization for esophagitis. Treatment-associated deaths are rare with radiotherapy alone, and the frequency of hospitalization for acute toxicity is generally ≤10%.

Breast

Radiation is used in breast conservation therapy as well as postmastectomy in certain patients with large initial tumors, positive lymph nodes, or positive resection margins. The dose to the breast is normally 54–60 Gy. Acute side effects are most often limited to skin reactions, but pneumonitis, lymphoedema, and carditis can occur as late reactions. Hospitalization is a distinctly rare event for any acute radiotherapy effect in the breast.

Prostate

Prostate cancer can be treated either with external beam radiation therapy or prostate brachytherapy ("seeds"). External beam radiation is anywhere from 60–80 Gy. The most common side effects are urethritis and cystitis, which are managed as an outpatient in the vast majority of patients. *Rates of impotence and cure* are similar among external radiation therapy, brachytherapy, and radical prostatectomy.

Colon/Rectal

Radiation is not often used in most colon cancers, except in those that are locally advanced (often fixed or perforated) and need preop radiation therapy. The confines of the pelvis make surgical resection of rectal cancer more of a challenge vs colon cancer. Preop radiation therapy is used in most cases to facilitate surgical resection, for sphincter preservation, and to treat the poorly accessible presacral lymph nodes. Rectal cancer doses are 20–50 Gy, depending on the size of the lesion and whether it is preop or postop. Radiation therapy–induced proctitis is generally quite mild unless concurrent chemotherapy (generally 5-fluorouracil) is administered. In this case, proctitis can be severe enough to cause dehydration leading to hospitalization. Patients often develop and may need nutritional support. Patients also can develop diarrhea.

Anal

Most anal malignancies can be managed with definitive radiotherapy plus adjuvant chemotherapy with surgery reserved for salvage. Although generally of squamous histology, anal cancers respond well to low doses of radiotherapy. Typical curative doses are 30–54 Gy, classically given with concurrent mitomycin-C and 5-fluorouracil. Acute toxicities are mainly myelosuppression from mitomycin-C, proctitis, cystitis, hemorrhoid exacerbation, and skin reaction in the perineum.

Pediatrics

Radiation is used in many pediatric tumors. Total body irradiation and irradiation of sanctuary sites are used in leukemia, and many lymphoma protocols involve local irradiation. Many sarcomas are treated with radiation after or instead of surgery. Most CNS tumors are treated in part with radiation as well. Treatment varies per site, and long-term effects on development limit dose.

Lymphoma/Total Body Irradiation

Lymphomas are very radioresponsive, and doses from 20–45 Gy are used, depending on the type of lymphoma and chemotherapy regimen. Treatment is normally very well tolerated, with some cytopenia and fatigue with larger fields and some nausea/vomiting when the abdomen is treated. **Total body irradiation** is used as part of the preparative scheme for peripheral blood stem cell transplant protocols. The occurrence of 550 cGy in a single fraction is very common, although fractionated total body irradiation is also used in certain protocols. This is normally well tolerated, except for self-limiting parotitis and nausea and vomiting.

Gynecologic

Cervical and uterine corpus cancers are often treated with radiation therapy. Most advanced cervical cancers are treated with definitive radiotherapy, and numerous phase III trials have demonstrated equivalent survival outcome between radical hysterectomy and radiotherapy for early cervical cancer. Radiation is generally used as adjuvant therapy in uterine corpus tumors. Radiotherapy for most gynecologic malignancies uses **brachytherapy**, because it better delivers the dose to the at-risk tissues, while sparing the bladder and rectum. Doses are anywhere from 50–85 Gy. Patients can develop proctitis, enteritis, and urethritis/cystitis, depending on the dose and tumor location. As with other sites, with the advent of concurrent chemoradiation (CDDP) in cervical cancer, the frequency of admission for acute toxicity has increased.

KEY POINTS TO REMEMBER

- Consult radiation oncology before starting therapeutic chemotherapy or surgery to allow for optimum multidisciplinary management of the malignancy. Evaluating the patient in his or her presenting state is of inordinate value to the radiation oncologist.
- When radiation toxicity is in the differential, consult a radiation oncologist. He or she can help with diagnosis and treatment.
- The only true radiation oncology emergency is spinal cord compression, although there are other "urgent" indications for radiation therapy.
- Consider urgent radiation oncology consults when faced with SVC syndrome, new brain metastases, or uncontrolled bleeding.

REFERENCES

1. Perez C, Brady L, eds. *Principles and practices of radiation oncology*, 3rd ed. Philadelphia: Lippincott–Raven, 1997.
2. Rubin P, ed. *Clinical oncology for medical students and physicians: a multidisciplinary approach*, 7th ed. Philadelphia: W.B. Saunders, 1993.
3. Gunderson L, Tepper J, eds. *Clinical radiation oncology*. Philadelphia: Churchill Livingstone, 2000.

19

Breast Cancer

Marcia L. Chantler

INTRODUCTION

Breast cancer is the most commonly diagnosed malignancy in women (other than skin cancer) and follows lung cancer as the leading cause of cancer deaths among women. Breast cancer mortality rates have been remarkably stable over the past 60 yrs. However, in the 1980s, the mortality rate began to decline slightly. It is likely that at least some of the decline is due to screening, although medical therapy also may have contributed some. Identifiable risk factors for breast cancer include age, early menarche, late menopause, nulliparity, personal or family history of breast cancer, and exogenous estrogens, as well as environmental factors. Primarily thought of as a disease of women, men actually make up 1% of new breast cancer diagnoses each year.

Epidemiology

- In 2002, an estimated 203,500 new breast cancers will be diagnosed in the United States, and 39,600 deaths will occur from the disease. A woman has a 12% lifetime risk of developing breast cancer and a 3.5% chance of dying from it.
- The majority of women diagnosed with breast cancer have no known **risk factors.** Fewer than 10% of all breast cancers are hereditary. The known risk factors for breast cancer include age, early menarche, late menopause, nulliparity, history of breast cancer, or benign breast disease, as well as other familial and environmental factors.
- The **median age** for the diagnosis of breast cancer is 60–65 yrs. In addition, the incidence and risk of developing breast cancer increases with age. 80% of cases occur in postmenopausal women. Breast cancer is extremely rare in women in their teens or early 20s and uncommon in women under 35. After age 35 yrs, the risk of breast cancer begins to increase, rising sharply after menopause.
- **Estrogen** plays an integral role in the growth and development of breast cancer cells. This is reflected in the increased risk of developing breast cancer associated with longer exposure to endogenous estrogens, such as early menarche (before age 12), late menopause (after age 55 yrs), and first pregnancy after age 30 yrs or nulliparity. The risk of exogenous estrogens, including oral contraceptives and estrogen replacement therapy (ERT), and the association with breast cancer has been studied extensively. The Women's Contraceptive and Reproductive Experiences (CARE) study showed no increased risk of breast cancer linked with oral contraceptive use, regardless of length, timing, or age at use. However, ERT is associated with an increase in the incidence of breast cancer. Data from the Women's Health Initiative showed a 26% increased risk of breast cancer in women taking estrogen plus progestin compared to those taking placebo after an average of 5.2 yrs. In women taking estrogen alone, there is no evidence of an increased risk for breast cancer. The increased risk of breast cancer appears to be reduced after stopping ERT.
- Proliferative breast lesions with or without atypical hyperplasia are associated with up to a fivefold increase in the risk of the development of breast cancer. **Lobular carcinoma *in situ* (LCIS)** is associated with the highest risk for development of an invasive malignancy, 8–11 times that of the general population. Nonproliferative breast lesions, such as cysts, fibroadenomas, or ductal ectasia, are not associated with an increased risk for breast cancer. Women with a history of a previous breast

cancer have a three- to fourfold increase in risk of a second breast cancer. Whereas the risk of a second breast cancer persists for up to 30 yrs after the original diagnosis, the median time interval to development is 4 yrs.

- The **BRCA1** and **BRCA2 genes** have been identified and linked with inherited breast cancer. Women with mutations in the BRCA1 or BRCA2 gene have an estimated 40–85% lifetime risk of developing breast cancer. The BRCA1 gene is located on the long arm of chromosome 17 and is associated with a concomitant increase in ovarian malignancies. BRCA2 is located on the long arm of chromosome 13 and is associated with male breast and prostate cancer. Other familial syndromes associated with a genetic inheritance of breast cancer risk include Li-Fraumeni and Cowden syndrome.
- Women exposed to chest wall radiation during childhood (ages 10–19 yrs) for Hodgkin's disease have been shown to be at an increased risk for developing breast cancer throughout their lives. Other environmental factors, such as alcohol, dietary fat, or cholesterol intake, have not been shown conclusively to be associated with an increased risk of breast cancer.

Staging

The American Joint Committee on Cancer (AJCC) staging system provides a strategy for grouping breast cancer patients based on primary tumor size, nodal involvement, and the presence of metastatic disease (TNM classification is in Table 19-1). The most important prognostic factor in women with breast cancer is *axillary nodal status*, followed by *hormonal receptor status* and *HER2/neu overexpression*. However, only axillary nodal status is included in the current tumor staging criteria. The determination of the primary tumor and axillary nodal stage is from pathologic specimens at the time of surgery. Radiology testing should not preclude the surgical staging of the axillary lymph nodes with the exception of grossly metastatic disease. Any woman who presents with palpable lymphadenopathy or has positive lymph nodes diagnosed at surgery should have radiology testing performed to look for distant sites of disease.

CAUSES

Pathophysiology

- Most invasive breast cancers are adenocarcinomas, which can be quite heterogeneous in histologic appearance. **Infiltrating (invasive) ductal carcinoma** accounts for approximately 80% of all breast cancers and originates from the cells lining the ducts of the breast. Infiltrating ductal carcinomas metastasize predominately to the bones, liver, lungs, and brain. **Lobular carcinomas** make up 10% of malignant breast cancers and originate from the terminal ductules of the breast lobules. Lobular carcinomas are associated with bilateral tumors in up to 20% of cases and also tend to be associated with multicentric (≥ 2 tumors in separate quadrants of the breast) disease within the same breast. Lobular carcinomas have a predilection to metastasize to the meninges, serosal surfaces, and mediastinal and retroperitoneal lymph nodes.
- Less common types of breast carcinomas include medullary, tubular, mucinous, and papillary. These variants carry a relatively favorable prognosis. **Paget's disease** of the nipple is a specialized form of ductal carcinoma that arises from the main excretory ducts in the breasts and involves the skin of the nipple and areola. Inflammatory carcinomas involve the lymphatic structures in the dermis and infiltrate widely throughout the breast tissue. **Inflammatory carcinomas** are not a special morphologic pattern but are clinically diagnosed based on swelling, erythema, and tenderness in the involved breast and are associated with more aggressive disease.
- The **estrogen receptor (ER) and progesterone receptor (PR)** belong to a class of nuclear receptor proteins that, when activated by the hormone-receptor complex, results in gene activation, mRNA transcription, and cell proliferation. ER and PR can be used as both predictive and prognostic factors in women with breast cancer and should be assessed on all patients with breast cancer. One-third of all premenopausal and two-thirds of all postmenopausal breast cancers are ER-positive. Patients with tumors that express either ER or PR have an improved prognosis and are more likely

TABLE 19-1. TNM CLASSIFICATION AND AJCC STAGING FOR BREAST CANCER

Primary tumor (T)

Tis	Carcinoma *in situ*
T1	Tumor ≤ 2 cm in greatest dimension
T2	Tumor >2 cm but not >5 cm in greatest dimension
T3	Tumor >5 cm in greatest dimension
T4	Tumor of any size with chest wall involvement, *peau d'orange*, skin ulceration, satellite skin nodules, or inflammatory carcinoma

Axillary nodal status (N)

N0	No axillary nodal involvement
N1	Ipsilateral axillary nodal involvement
N2	Ipsilateral, fixed, or matted axillary nodal involvement
N3	Ipsilateral internal mammary nodal involvement

Distant metastatic disease (M)

M0	No distant sites of disease detected
M1	Distant sites of disease detected, including ipsilateral supraclavicular lymph node involvement

AJCC stage

Stage 1	**T1**	**N0**	**M0**
Stage 2A	**T1**	**N1**	**M0**
	T2	**N0**	**M0**
Stage 2B	**T2**	**N1**	**M0**
	T3	**N0**	**M0**
Stage 3A	**T1–2**	**N2**	**M0**
	T3	**N1–2**	**M0**
Stage 3B	**T4**	**Any N**	**M0**
	Any T	**N3**	**M0**
Stage 4	**Any T**	**Any N**	**M1**

Adapted from American Joint Committee on Cancer. *AJCC cancer staging manual*, 5th ed. Philadelphia: Lippincott–Raven, 1997.

to benefit from hormonal therapy. Although ER and PR are associated together, PR does not provide useful clinical information independent of the ER status.
* All breast cancers should also be tested for HER2/neu overexpression for complete risk stratification and to identify the potential use of a monoclonal antibody, trastuzumab (Herceptin), directed at the **HER2/neu receptor.** The HER2/neu protein (also known as *c-erb-2*) is a transmembrane tyrosine kinase receptor that is overexpressed in approximately 30% of invasive breast cancers. Overexpression of HER2/neu is associated with ER-negative disease and high-grade histology and is an overall poor prognostic factor. Immunohistochemical testing is commonly used to identify HER2/neu overexpression, but there is little standardization of reporting HER2/neu expression on breast cancer cells. Fluorescent *in situ* hybridization can be used to measure HER2/neu gene amplification to confirm overexpression in patients with weakly positive (1+ or 2+) immunohistochemical staining.

MALE BREAST CANCER

Male breast cancer (MBC) makes up approximately 1% of all breast cancers, and there has not been a recent increase in incidence as has been seen in female breast cancer

(FBC). This is likely due to the recent onset of aggressive screening in women. Similar to FBC, tumor size and the presence and number of positive lymph nodes are the most important prognostic factors. In addition, survival is also comparable to FBC when matched for stage and grade. MBC in some instances is due to hormonal alterations in estrogen and androgen balance; those with Klinefelter syndrome, testicular pathology (e.g., cryptorchidism, testicular injury, orchitis), and infertility have an increased risk. Treatment is similar to that of FBC. Although MBC is relatively rare, the diagnosis should always be considered in any male patient with a breast mass.

SCREENING

- Monthly breast self-exam is frequently advocated as a screening tool for breast cancer, but there is little evidence for showing its effectiveness in reducing mortality rates in breast cancer. The breast self-exam is most useful in conjunction with a clinical breast exam (CBE) by an experienced physician and mammography. Only 15% of all breast cancers are detected on a CBE. The American Cancer Society recommends a CBE be performed q3yrs in women ages 20–39 yrs, and yearly in women >40 yrs.
- The current **mammography** screening recommendations for **average-risk patients** is q1–2yrs beginning at age 40 yrs. There are currently no data to support the role of a "baseline" mammogram between the ages of 35–40 yrs. For women ≥ 50 yrs, yearly screening mammography should be performed. In women >50, screening mammography is associated with a 30% reduction in breast cancer mortality from early detection. This same benefit has not been seen with in woman <50 yrs and is the basis for controversy on the role of screening mammography in this age group.
- In women with a **strong family history** of breast cancer, annual mammography should begin 5–10 yrs earlier than the age at which a family member was diagnosed with breast cancer. **Ductal lavage** is a new investigational technique that is being evaluated as a new screening tool for the early detection of breast cancer. Ductal lavage uses a thin, flexible catheter to introduce a saline solution into the mammary ducts located on the nipple. The fluid collected from the ducts is then analyzed for malignancy. Currently, ductal lavage should not be used for screening purposes outside the role of a clinical trial.

PRESENTATION

History

A woman who presents with a new breast mass should have a complete history and physical exam. Symptoms related to a new mass, including duration, tenderness, relationship to menstrual cycle, and nipple discharge, should be elicited. Nipple discharge is a common complaint in women. There is an increased concern of malignancy if the discharge is unilateral, spontaneous, or bloody, especially in a postmenopausal woman. A *negative family history* does not exclude malignancy, given that most women who develop breast cancer do not have a family history of the disease. A personal history of prior malignancies, such as colon or ovarian, places a woman at greater risk for breast cancer through the association with the BRCA1 gene. Other risk factors should be assessed in the history, including menstrual history, history of breast pathology, and a complete medication history, especially recent or current use of ERT.

Physical Exam

- The physical characteristics of a breast mass can be helpful in determining a diagnosis. A thorough breast exam should begin with the patient disrobed to the waist and sitting in the upright position. One should begin with a careful inspection for breast symmetry, contours, and retraction of the skin. Other changes in the skin can include erythema, thickening, or peau d'orange appearance. Close inspection of the nipple can reveal rashes, ulceration, thickening, or discharge that may help identify an underlying malignancy or Paget's disease of the breast.
- To palpate the breast during the CBE, the patient should be supine with her arms raised above head. The normal adult breast often has an uneven texture and feels nodular or lumpy, termed **physiologic nodularity.** It is often bilateral, and may be evident

throughout the entire breast or only in parts of it. Nodularity may increase premenstrually and during pregnancy. Note the characteristics of any nodules including location, size, shape, consistency, demarcation, tenderness, and mobility. The axilla should be examined with the patient in a sitting position. A complete exam for lymphadenopathy includes evaluation for supra- and infraclavicular lymph nodes in addition to the axilla.
- The final element of the breast exam should include compressing the areola to try to elucidate any nipple discharge. A nonmilky or bloody unilateral nipple discharge suggests underlying breast pathology and should be evaluated further. The most common source of nipple discharge is an intraductal papilloma, which is a benign lesion.

Differential Diagnosis

The individual risk of a primary breast cancer can be characterized as high or low based on the patient's age, presenting symptoms, history of breast pathology, and family history. For example, a new breast mass in a woman >50 yrs should be considered malignant until proved otherwise, whereas, in women <35 yrs with a similar lesion, cancer is possible but uncommon. The differential diagnosis of a breast mass can be broad, including malignancies such as primary breast cancer, lymphoma, or sarcoma, or benign breast lesions such as cysts, fibroadenomas, and fat necrosis. Skin conditions, such as sebaceous cysts, abscesses, or thrombophlebitis, may present with a palpable mass. The history and physical exam will help aid in the differential diagnosis, but ultimately a biopsy is confirmatory.

WORKUP

Lab Evaluation

- Lab tests do not directly aid in the staging of breast cancer but can allow the clinician to focus on possible metastatic sights of disease. A CBC can detect abnormalities in blood cell lines that may suggest bone marrow infiltration. The spread of breast cancer to the liver or bones may cause abnormalities in blood chemistries, such as calcium, serum glutamic-oxaloacetic transaminase (aspartate aminotransferase), serum glutamic-pyruvic transaminase (alanine aminotransferase), and alkaline phosphatase. Abnormal blood tests can give the physician an objective marker to assess for clinical response after therapy in patients without identifiable measurable disease.
- **Tumor markers** (CEA 19-9, CA 15-5, or CA 27-29) have been evaluated for the ability to diagnose, monitor therapy, and predict recurrence of breast cancer. Tumor markers are not accurate to be used for screening or diagnosis. However, in patients with advanced disease and no other measurable disease, tumor markers can assist in the monitoring of response to therapy.

Diagnostic Evaluation

- A solid mass is best evaluated with **diagnostic mammography.** Mammography allows the physician to assess the radiologic characteristics of the mass and the remainder of breast tissue in the ipsilateral and contralateral breast. U/S can be useful to determine whether a lesion is cystic or solid. Aspiration of a cystic mass may be helpful. **Cytology** may reveal malignant cells, but the absence of malignant cells does not rule out a malignant lesion.
- After radiologic evaluation to determine location and characteristics of the mass, a biopsy can be obtained using several different methods. **Fine-needle aspiration** (FNA) is a simple method for obtaining material for cytologic exam that can be performed in the clinician's office. False-negative rates for FNA can be as high as 10% even among the most experienced technicians. If a negative result is obtained from FNA, **a core (needle) or excisional biopsy** should be done to obtain appropriate tissue for pathologic review. The majority of these biopsies can also be performed in the outpatient setting. A core biopsy that confirms a benign lesion does not need further evaluation. If the biopsy reveals only normal breast tissue, further surgical biopsy is recommended if the lesion is suspicious for cancer. Needle localization or stereotactic biopsies are helpful in this situation. Both methods use specialized radiology localiza-

tion to aid the surgeon in obtaining the appropriate tumor specimen. For less suspicious breast lesions, a 6-mo follow-up mammogram is recommended.

MANAGEMENT

Treatment

The treatment of breast cancer uses a multidisciplinary approach, including surgery, hormonal or chemotherapy, and radiation therapy. Treatment strategies are characterized based on the AJCC staging and menopausal and hormone receptor status. HER2/neu overexpression is also advancing as a key element in the treatment strategies of breast cancer. Currently, outside of a clinical trial, treatment decisions based on HER2/neu overexpression are limited to metastatic disease.

Carcinoma In Situ

- **Ductal carcinoma** *in situ* (DCIS) (also known as **intraductal carcinoma**) is the noninvasive form of breast cancer that is being encountered more frequently with the increased use of screening mammography. These lesions are most often identified on mammography as clustered microcalcifications with or without a palpable mass. Surgical treatments for DCIS range from local excision to total mastectomy.
- Patients with small foci of microcalcifications isolated in one quadrant of the breast may be a candidate for **lumpectomy and irradiation.** Local chest wall irradiation after lumpectomy reduces the rates of ipsilateral breast tumor recurrences by >50% compared to lumpectomy alone. Mastectomy is an alternate surgical option for patients with DCIS. Routine axillary nodal dissection is not recommended based on a low (<5%) incidence of axillary nodal metastases in patients with DCIS. Tamoxifen given after surgery and radiation therapy has also been demonstrated to reduce the rate of all breast cancer events (noninvasive or invasive ipsilateral tumors and new contralateral tumors) by up to 40%.
- **LCIS** is not detected on physical exam and is always an incidental finding on breast biopsies performed for another reason. The terminology of LCIS is a misleading one. LCIS is not a premalignant lesion. It is a marker that identifies women at an increased risk—8–11 times that of the general population—for the development of an invasive breast cancer in either breast. Of interest, the majority of subsequent cancers are infiltrating ductal rather than lobular carcinomas.
- LCIS can be managed by **observation** alone after biopsy. There is no evidence that reexcision after the initial biopsy to obtain histologically negative surgical margins is required. The increased risk of breast cancer persists beyond 20 yrs, so careful observation and mammography should be performed indefinitely in these women. Bilateral prophylactic mastectomies are an alternate option for women who are unwilling to accept the increased risk of bilateral breast cancers. Radiation therapy has no role in the management of LCIS. Tamoxifen (Nolvadex D, Emblon, Fentamox, Soltamox, Tamofen) (20 mg daily) is associated with a 56% decrease in the risk of all breast cancer events in women with LCIS when taken for 5 yrs.

Early-Stage Breast Cancer

- Surgical options for the management of breast cancer include **breast-conserving therapy (BCT)** followed by radiation therapy, **mastectomy with breast reconstruction,** or **modified radical mastectomy** alone. The presence of metastases to the axillary lymph nodes remains the most important prognostic factor in patients with breast cancer. Therefore, **axillary lymph node dissection** remains an important part of the surgical approach in breast cancer patients. Randomized clinical trials prove that overall survival is equivalent between BCT followed by radiation therapy and mastectomy in women with breast cancer. The selection of a surgical approach depends on the location and size of the lesion, other abnormalities present on the mammogram, breast size, and the patient's attitude toward breast preservation. Multicentric disease (≥ 2 primary tumors in separate quadrants), extensive malignant-appearing microcalcifications on mammogram, pregnancy, and previous breast or mantle irradiation are absolute contraindications for BCT. A history of collagen vascular disease is a relative contraindication to BCT. Patients with a history of collagen vascular disease may develop marked soft tissue fibrosis and bone necrosis after adjuvant radiation, resulting in a poor cosmetic and potentially deforming surgical outcome.

- In an effort to decrease the occurrence of **lymphedema** and **pain** associated with axillary lymph node dissection while maintaining accurate staging, surgeons are using **sentinel lymph node (SLN) biopsy** in women with breast cancer. The SLN is defined as the first node in the lymphatic chain that receives lymphatic flow from the entire breast, being at the highest risk for harboring occult metastatic disease in breast cancer patients. Vital blue dye and/or technetium-labeled sulfur are injected in and around the tumor or biopsy site. The surgeon can map the dye and radioactive compound drainage to the axilla and identify the SLN, which is then biopsied. The SLN can be identified in >90% of patients with breast cancer, with false-negative rates ranging from 0–10%. No further axillary node dissection is necessary if the SLN biopsy is negative. If the SLN is positive for malignancy, further treatment options include a full axillary node dissection, axillary radiation, or no further surgery and adjuvant chemotherapy. SLN biopsies are only being performed on women without palpable axillary lymph nodes on physical exam.

- **Neoadjuvant therapy** with the use of hormonal or chemotherapeutic agents has been shown to be effective in downsizing the dimensions of the primary tumor stage, thus allowing for BCT. Chemotherapy regimens that result in high response rates include cyclophosphamide, doxorubicin, and 5-fluorouracil (CAF); doxorubicin and cyclophosphamide (AC); and cyclophosphamide, methotrexate, and 5-fluorouracil (CMF), with the anthracycline-based regimens used most commonly. Newer neoadjuvant regimens with an anthracycline-based regimen followed by a taxane are also effective. Chemotherapy is given preop for a total of four cycles or to a maximum tumor response. In a postmenopausal, hormone-receptor-positive patient, the use of hormonal agents (tamoxifen or an aromatase inhibitor) can be used to shrink the primary tumor size. 10–15% of women receiving neoadjuvant therapy have been shown to have no residual tumor at the time of surgery. In women with residual malignancy found at the time of surgery, additional hormonal or chemotherapy is recommended.

- **Radiation therapy** to the intact breast after BCT is standard treatment based on several randomized trials that have shown higher local recurrence rates with BCT alone compared to BCT with radiation therapy. Radiation treatments are administered daily to the intact breast over a 5- to 6-wk period. A radiation boost to the tumor bed is often administered, although its necessity is currently controversial. Patients with positive axillary nodes may benefit from regional nodal irradiation in addition to irradiation of the intact breast. For patients with negative axillary nodes, regional nodal irradiation is not recommended.

- In postmastectomy patients with positive surgical margins, primary tumors >4.5 cm or involvement of ≥ 4 lymph nodes, the risk of local recurrence is significantly high enough to consider adjuvant chest wall and axillary radiation therapy. Radiation therapy can decrease the rates of local recurrence in addition to adjuvant chemotherapy. Anthracycline chemotherapy has radiation-sensitizing effects and should not be given concurrently for the risk of higher radiation–associated toxicities. Therefore, radiation therapy is typically given after completion of adjuvant chemotherapy, within the first 6 mos after mastectomy.

- **Adjuvant systemic therapy** with either chemotherapeutic or hormonal agents has demonstrated significant improvement in disease-free and overall survival in both premenopausal and postmenopausal women, with or without lymph node metastases. Candidates for adjuvant therapy are chosen based on the risk of recurrence, including primary tumor size >1 cm, axillary lymph node involvement, and ER-negative disease. Currently, there are no convincing data to support the use of any known biologic factor other than hormone receptor status in selecting which breast cancer patients should receive adjuvant therapy. Current studies are underway to determine whether HER2/neu overexpression or other biologic markers are related to prognosis and should subsequently influence the choice of adjuvant therapy regimens.

- The decision to recommend **adjuvant hormonal therapy** with **tamoxifen** should be based on the presence of hormone receptors in the primary tumor, regardless of age, menopausal status, involvement of axillary lymph nodes, or tumor size. Adjuvant hormonal therapy should not be recommended in patients whose breast cancers are ER-negative or PR-negative, because clinical trials have not shown any benefit on disease-free or overall survival. Tamoxifen (20 mg daily) reduces recurrence rates by 47% and mortality by almost 26%. This benefit appeared to be irrespective of age or menopausal status. Other clinical trials have favorably demonstrated a 50% reduction in contralateral breast recurrences as well. The current recommendation is to continue tamoxifen for 5 yrs. Switching to another hormonal agent [raloxifene (Evista) or an aromatase inhibitor] after 5 yrs of tamoxifen use is not currently recommended but is the focus of ongoing clinical trials. In patients receiving chemotherapy, tamoxifen can be initiated either during or at the completion of the chemotherapy.
- Clinical trials are also currently underway to look at the effectiveness of the **aromatase inhibitors** in combination with tamoxifen or alone in the adjuvant setting in postmenopausal women. Preliminary results from the Arimidex and Tamoxifen Alone and in Combination trial show that anastrozole (Arimidex) has better results for preventing disease recurrence than tamoxifen after 2.5 yrs of follow-up in the study. However, anastrozole is also associated with a higher rate of bone fractures, as aromatase inhibitors are not beneficial to bone preservation when compared with tamoxifen. Present recommendations are that tamoxifen remains the standard adjuvant hormonal therapy until further data from this trial can mature and be reported. This study does provide the clinician with an alternative option for the use of aromatase inhibitors if the patient is a poor candidate for tamoxifen (high clotting risk, high endometrial cancer risk) in the adjuvant setting.
- For **premenopausal ER-positive women,** alternative strategies of hormonal therapy include ovarian ablation through surgery or radiation therapy to the ovaries, and chemical suppression of ovarian function with **luteinizing hormone–releasing hormone (LHRH) agonists** such as goserelin. Aromatase inhibitors are contraindicated in premenopausal women with functioning ovaries due to the insufficient blockade of ovarian estrogens. New clinical trials are evaluating the use of LHRH agonists plus aromatase inhibitors in premenopausal patients.
- **Chemotherapy** in the adjuvant setting has demonstrated reductions in the risk of recurrence and mortality rates of 25% and 15%, respectively, regardless of age, menopausal or hormonal status, or axillary lymph node involvement. Current literature now supports that four to six courses of treatment (3–6 mos) provide optimal benefit. Additional courses of chemotherapy add to treatment-related toxicity with no substantial improvement in overall outcome. Current chemotherapy regimens are given in an outpatient setting on an every 21- to 28-day schedule (Table 19-2). The use of anthracycline-containing regimens over non–anthracycline-containing regimens is preferred based on statistically significant survival advantages. However, there is also a higher incidence of hospitalizations for febrile neutropenia in patients treated with anthracycline-based chemotherapy. Several ongoing trials are attempting to define the value of taxanes in the treatment of early-stage breast cancer. The current standard of practice is to initiate adjuvant chemotherapy 4–6 wks after surgery before the initiation of radiation. Existing comorbid conditions should

TABLE 19-2. COMMON BREAST CANCER ADJUVANT CHEMOTHERAPY REGIMENS

Cyclophosphamide/methotrexate/5-fluorouracil (CMF) × 6 cycles

5-Fluorouracil/doxorubicin/cyclophosphamide (FAC) × 6 cycles

5-Fuorouraucil/epirubicin/cyclophosphamide (FEC) × 6 cycles

Doxorubicin/cyclophosphamide (AC) × 4 cycles

AC × 4 cycles followed by single-agent paclitaxel × 4 cycles (AC + T)

be considered in the decision to offer adjuvant chemotherapy, as adverse effects related to chemotherapy drugs may influence the overall benefits.

Treatment of Advanced and Metastatic Breast Cancer

- **Advanced breast cancer** includes those subsets of patients with tumors >5 cm in size, inflammatory breast tumors, and any tumor with fixed or matted axillary lymphadenopathy or internal mammary lymph node involvement. Surgery is typically limited to a biopsy to confirm the diagnosis and identify receptor status. Neoadjuvant chemotherapy is effective in this patient population and may allow for tumor shrinkage to adequately allow for surgical resection with clear margins. Advanced breast cancer is associated with a poor prognosis and a high rate of local and distant recurrences, leading to a similar treatment approach as that for metastatic disease.
- **Metastatic breast cancer (MBC)** remains an incurable disease with a median survival of 18–24 mos. The primary goal of treatment for patients with metastatic disease is to prolong survival and palliate symptoms related to the disease rather than curing patients. The management of MBC depends on the site and extent of metastases, hormone receptor status, and HER2/neu overexpression. Patients with MBC can be divided into two groups for treatment decisions: low and high risk. Patients in the low-risk group include those patients with a long disease-free interval; hormone receptor–positive tumors; and bone, soft tissue, or limited visceral organ involvement. High-risk patients include those with rapidly progressive disease or extensive visceral involvement, as well as those patients whose disease becomes refractory to hormonal therapy. See Fig. 19-1 for an example of a treatment pathway for MBC.
- In low-risk patients with advanced or MBC and ER-positive disease, **hormonal therapy** can achieve initial response rates as high as 60–70%. ER-negative tumors exhibit no clinical benefit from first-line hormonal therapy. In postmenopausal women, first-line hormonal therapy consists of either **tamoxifen** or the **newer aromatase inhibitors.** Present data show that the aromatase inhibitors [anastrozole (Arimidex), letrozole (Femara), and exemestane (Aromasin)] produce higher

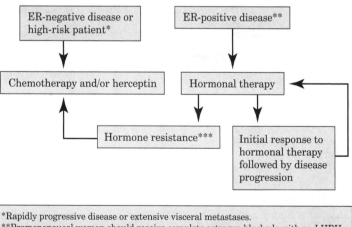

FIG. 19-1. Treatment pathway for advanced and metastatic breast cancer. ER, estrogen receptor.

response rates and longer remissions than tamoxifen and are currently preferred as first-line agents. The current treatment recommendation in premenopausal ER-positive women with locally advanced or MBC is the combination of an LHRH agonist and tamoxifen. This combination has demonstrated an improvement in time to disease progression and survival compared with an LHRH agonist alone. An important phenomenon related to hormone therapy is the **"flare" response,** defined as a temporary worsening of signs and symptoms of the disease within the first few weeks to months of treatment. Clinicians should be aware of this phenomenon to avoid premature discontinuation of a potentially beneficial treatment. The onset of action for hormonal therapy is slow—on the order of months—and is important to consider before labeling a patient resistant to hormonal therapy.

- **Fulvestrant** (Faslodex) is an ER antagonist that binds to the ER in a competitive manner with affinity comparable to that of estradiol. In addition to competitive binding to the ER, fulvestrant downregulates the ER protein in human breast cancer cells. Fulvestrant has been approved for the treatment of ER-positive MBC in postmenopausal women whose disease has progressed after receiving tamoxifen or an aromatase inhibitor. Fulvestrant is given as a once-a-month IM injection.

- Patients who have a clinical response after initiation of a hormonal therapy may benefit from **second- and third-line hormonal therapies** when the cancer begins to progress. Other hormonal therapies in addition to tamoxifen and the aromatase inhibitors include fulvestrant, megestrol acetate, fluoxymesterone (Halotestin), and diethylstilbestrol (DES). Subsequent response rates with second- and third-line agents become lower but remain as high as 20–40%. With each subsequent hormonal therapy, the duration of a clinical response becomes shorter, and, ultimately, the disease will become refractory to hormone treatment. Second- and third-line hormonal therapy should be chosen based on the adverse side effect profile of each drug. Systemic chemotherapy can be recommended in patients whose disease becomes refractory to multiple lines of hormonal therapy.

- **Tamoxifen** is extremely well tolerated by most patients, with <5% of patients discontinuing therapy due to related toxicities. The most common side effects from tamoxifen include **hot flashes** and vaginal discharge or irritation. Clonidine (Catapres) or the newer antidepressants (SSRIs) can lessen the severity of hot flashes. The development of **endometrial cancer** in women on tamoxifen occurs at a rate 2–7 times more than in women not on the drug. The endometrial cancers are typically of lower grade and stage and treated with hysterectomy. Women on tamoxifen should have yearly pelvic exams, and any abnormal vaginal discharge or bleeding should be evaluated promptly. However, the routine use of endometrial biopsy, hysteroscopy, and transvaginal U/S as screening tools for endometrial cancer in asymptomatic women on tamoxifen has not proved effective. **Thromboembolic events** also occur at a higher rate in patients on tamoxifen, and the use of tamoxifen should be avoided in women at high risk of developing blood clots. Tamoxifen assists in the preservation of bone mineral density in postmenopausal women but is associated with a decrease in bone mineral density in premenopausal women.

- **Aromatase inhibitors** are also well tolerated in women with breast cancer. The main side effects of these drugs include hot flashes and vaginal dryness at rates similar to tamoxifen. Other side effects include **myalgias,** headache, nausea, and peripheral edema. Aromatase inhibitors are associated with fewer thromboembolic events and endometrial malignancies when compared with tamoxifen. The potential long-term endocrinologic effects on bone, lipid metabolism, and cardiovascular risk from aromatase inhibitors are not yet known.

- **High-risk patients** with rapidly progressive disease, extensive visceral involvement, or disease that becomes refractory to hormonal therapy may benefit from chemotherapy. Many chemotherapeutic agents are active against advanced-stage breast cancer, including anthracycline-based combinations, such as CAF, and newer combinations with taxanes are gaining favor in MBC. Many single-agent drugs also have activity in MBC, such as doxorubicin (Adriamycin, Doxil, Rubex), capecitabine (Xeloda), vinorelbine (Navelbine), and gemcitabine (Gemzar). All chemotherapy regimens have similar overall response rates in MBC, and individual chemotherapy regimens are offered based on the toxicity profile and patient's performance status. Once a patient develops progressive disease on one regimen, subsequent agents may be offered if the patient desires further treatment. At some point in the clinical course, the disease burden from MBC may interfere with the patient's ability to tolerate further treatment options, and supportive or palliative care should be offered to the patient and family.

- Among patients with MBC, **HER2/neu overexpression** occurs in 25–30% of cases. HER2/neu overexpression is associated with relative resistance to treatment with anthracycline- or taxane-based chemotherapy. **Trastuzumab** is a humanized monoclonal antibody targeted to the HER2/neu protein. The drug is approved for use in combination chemotherapy as first-line therapy and as a single-agent drug in second- and third-line therapy in MBC. In the original trials with trastuzumab as a single agent in first-line therapy, trastuzumab achieved response rates of 20–25%. The combination of chemotherapy with trastuzumab is the only treatment for MBC that shows a statistically significant improvement in overall survival. Trastuzumab is overall well tolerated, with minimal side effects as compared with standard chemotherapy. The use of trastuzumab in combination with anthracyclines has been associated with severe cardiac toxicity in up to 15% of patients and should not be used in combination with this drug class.

- Although patients with bone-only metastatic disease have a better prognosis than those with visceral metastases, **bone metastases** are a catastrophic complication of breast cancer that lead to pain, fractures, spinal cord compression, and hypercalcemia. Traditionally, treatment of symptomatic bone metastases has been with analgesics, localized radiation, or surgery. Although improvements in pain and quality of life have been obtained from the use of these therapeutic options, their use for the prevention of progression of bone lytic metastases has been ineffective. Several studies have evaluated the use of **bisphosphonates**, either alone or in addition to chemotherapy, and have shown a reduction in bone pain and the progression of lytic bone metastases. IV pamidronate (Aredia) infusion (90 mg IV over 2 hrs) was the first bisphosphonate to demonstrate this benefit. Zoledronate (Zometa) is an alternate IV bisphosphonate that is 1,000 times more potent than pamidronate and has a much shorter infusion time (4 mg IV over 15 mins). All patients with bone metastases should be maintained on an IV bisphosphonate q3–4wks for the duration of their treatment.

Follow-Up Recommendations

- Follow-up exams should be individualized either to reflect the patient's risk of recurrence or to monitor treatment or disease progression. The **overall prognosis** for a patient with breast cancer is based on the clinical stage. See Table 19-3 for estimated survival rates. The role of routine lab testing and imaging studies to detect metastatic disease when it is asymptomatic is controversial. No randomized trials have demonstrated a benefit based on routine lab or radiology testing compared to a careful history and physical exam. The clinical role of tumor markers (CEA, CA 15-3, CA 27-29) is also unproven.

TABLE 19-3. BREAST CANCER STAGE AND 5-YR SURVIVAL RATES

Stage	5-yr survival rates (%)
1	87
2A	78
2B	68
3A	51
3B	42
4	13

- Current recommendations for **follow-up office visits** with an accompanying history and physical exam are q3–4mos for the first 2 yrs after diagnosis, then q4–6mos for the subsequent 3–5 yrs after diagnosis. Particular attention on the physical exam should be placed on areas of metastasis, including bilateral breast exam, lymph nodes, liver, chest wall, and bones. A chest x-ray, routine lab data, and mammography should be performed yearly. A mammogram of the radiated breast is typically recommended q6mos for the first 1–2 yrs. The routine use of CT scans or bone scans has been shown to be of no benefit and can be performed as indicated by the patient's symptoms. Patients with advanced breast cancer or MBC may be followed more closely based on treatment schedules, response to treatment, and overall symptoms and performance status.

KEY POINTS TO REMEMBER

- Breast cancer is the most commonly diagnosed malignancy in women and follows lung cancer as the leading cause of cancer deaths among women. Early detection and treatment are the only chance for improved survival.
- Identifiable risk factors for breast cancer include age, early menarche, late menopause, nulliparity, history of breast cancer or benign breast disease, and exogenous estrogens, as well as other familial and environmental factors.
- Male breast cancer makes up 1% of new breast cancer diagnoses and in some cases may be related to a disruption in the androgen to estrogen ratio.
- One-third of all premenopausal and two-thirds of all postmenopausal breast cancers are ER-positive. ER-positive disease is associated with an improved prognosis over ER-negative disease.
- The biologic marker HER2/neu protein is seen in approximately 30% of invasive breast cancers and is associated with ER-negative disease, high-grade histology, chemotherapy resistance, and an overall poor prognosis.
- The most important prognostic factor in women with breast cancer is axillary nodal status, followed by hormonal receptor status.
- BCT with radiation therapy and mastectomy both demonstrate equivalent survival rates.
- SLN biopsy is useful to provide accurate surgical staging of the axilla and is associated with less lymphedema.
- Radiation is a standard adjuvant therapy after BCT. In postmastectomy patients, reasons to consider adjuvant radiation include positive surgical margins, large primary tumors, and axillary lymph node involvement.
- Adjuvant hormonal and/or chemotherapy are recommended in all breast cancer patients with primary tumors >1 cm, positive axillary or SLN involvement, and ER-negative disease.
- MBC remains an incurable disease, but hormonal therapy in ER-positive patients can lead to longer time to disease progression and improved survival.
- The combination of chemotherapy and trastuzumab shows a statistically significant improvement in overall survival in the treatment for MBC.
- Bisphosphonates reduce bone pain and the progression of lytic bone metastases in breast cancer patients.

REFERENCES AND SUGGESTED READINGS

American Joint Committee on Cancer. *Manual for staging of cancer*, 5th ed. Philadelphia: JB Lippincott, 1997:171–180.

Early Breast Cancer Trialists' Collaborative Group. Effects of radiotherapy and surgery in early breast cancer: an overview of randomized trials. *N Engl J Med* 1995;333:1444.

Early Breast Cancer Trialists' Collaborative Group. Polychemotherapy for early breast cancer: overview of the randomized trials. *Lancet* 1998;352:930.

Fisher B, Constantino J, Fisher B, et al. Pathologic findings from the National Surgical Adjuvant Breast Project (NSABP) Protocol B-17. Intraductal carcinoma (ductal carcinoma in situ): the National Surgical Adjuvant Breast and Bowel Project Collaborating Investigators. *Cancer* 1995;75:1310.

Fisher B, Constantino JP, Wickerham DL, et al. Tamoxifen for prevention of breast cancer: report of the National Surgical Adjuvant Breast and Bowel Project P-1 Study. *J Natl Cancer Inst* 1998;90:1371.

Fisher ER, Anderson S, Tan-Chiu E, et al. Fifteen-year prognostic discriminants for invasive breast carcinoma: National Surgical Adjuvant Breast and Bowel Project Protocol-06. *Cancer* 2001;91(8 Suppl):1679.

Hortobagyi GN, Theriault RL, Lipton A, et al. Long-term prevention of skeletal complications of metastatic breast cancer with pamidronate. Protocol 19 Aredia Breast Cancer Study Group. *J Clin Oncol* 1998;16:2038.

Krag D, Weaver D, Ashikaga T, et al. The sentinel node in breast cancer. A multicenter validation trial. *N Engl J Med* 1998;337:941.

Nabholtz JM, Buzdar A, Pollack M, et al. Anastrozole is superior to tamoxifen as first-line therapy for advanced breast cancer in postmenopausal women: results of a North American multicenter randomized trial. *J Clin Oncol* 2000;18:3758.

NIH Consensus Statement 2000. For which patients should adjuvant chemotherapy be recommended: adjuvant therapy for breast cancer. *NIH Consens Statement* 2000;17:1.

Slamon DJ, Godolphin W, Jones La, et al. Studies of the HER2/neu proto-oncogene in human breast and ovarian cancer. *Science* 1989;8:2127.

Slamon DL, Leyland-Jones B, Shak S, et al. Use of chemotherapy plus a monoclonal antibody against HER2 for metastatic breast cancer that overexpresses HER2. *N Engl J Med* 2001;344:78.

Thomas DB. Breast cancer in men. *Epidemiol Rev* 1993;15:220.

Thomas DB, Jimenez LM, McTiernan A, et al. Breast cancer in men: risk factors with hormonal implications. *Am J Epidemiol* 1992;135:734.

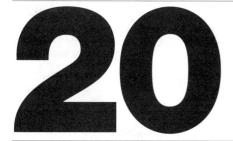

Lung Cancer

Amanda F. Cashen

INTRODUCTION

Lung cancer is the leading cause of cancer mortality in men and women in the United States. The overall incidence of lung cancer had been increasing for decades but has recently reached a plateau. However, the incidence continues to increase in women due to a lag in the smoking pattern. A major public health goal in reducing total mortality from lung cancer remains reducing the prevalence of smoking. This chapter reviews the physiology of lung cancer, as well as staging and a brief overview of treatment. Lung cancer is first divided into two broad groups: small-cell lung cancer (SCLC) and non–small-cell lung cancer (NSCLC), based on histology. Their clinical behavior and management are different and, therefore, discussed separately. Also reviewed in this chapter is the general workup of a solitary lung nodule.

EPIDEMIOLOGY AND RISK FACTORS

The incidence of lung cancer is approximately 70 cases/100,000 men and 35 cases/ 100,000 women. In the United States, there are >150,000 deaths from lung cancer each year. There is a clear, dose-dependent relationship between **tobacco** use and lung cancer. Squamous cell and SCLCs in particular are associated with tobacco smoking. Other exposures have also been associated with lung cancer, including asbestos, radon, bis(chloromethyl)ether, polycyclic aromatic hydrocarbons, chromium, nickel, and arsenic compounds. There are well-identified familial clusters of lung cancers, although no specific gene has been identified as predisposing to lung cancer.

NON–SMALL-CELL LUNG CANCER

NSCLC comprises four pathologic subtypes:

- **Squamous cell lung cancer** usually arises in proximal bronchi and can cause obstruction of the larger airways.
- **Adenocarcinoma** is the most common subtype, representing 40% of lung cancers in North America. It usually arises in the lung periphery.
- **Bronchoalveolar carcinoma** is a subtype of adenocarcinoma that grows along alveolar septa. It can present as a single nodule or multiple nodules or as a rapidly progressive multilobar disease that radiographically resembles pneumonia. It is not associated with tobacco smoking.
- **Large-cell carcinoma** is the least common subtype.

Clinical Features

- Presenting signs and symptoms of lung cancer depend on the size, location, and degree of spread of the tumor. Lung cancer can present as an asymptomatic lung nodule found incidentally on chest x-ray. **Local symptoms** can include cough, wheeze, hemoptysis, dyspnea, postobstructive pneumonia (due to tumors that occlude major bronchi), pain (particularly with pleural or chest wall involvement), dysphagia (due to esophageal compression by tumor or lymphadenopathy), and hoarseness (caused by laryngeal nerve involvement). Apical tumors that invade the lower brachial plexus can present with *Pancoast's syndrome,* which is a brachial plexopathy, Horner's syndrome, and shoulder pain. Mediastinal lymphadenopathy that compresses the superior vena cava (SVC) can cause *SVC syndrome,* which most commonly presents with dyspnea and facial swelling. **Systemic symptoms** usually accompany more advanced disease and can include weight loss, fatigue, and loss of appetite. Metastatic disease also may cause symptoms specific to the involved organs. For example, patients may have pain from bony metastases, dyspnea from pericardial or pleural effusions, or headache and neurologic deficits from brain metastases. Although adrenal and liver metastases are common, they are usually asymptomatic.

- NSCLC has been associated with numerous **paraneoplastic syndromes.** *Clubbing* results from proliferation of connective tissue at the ends of the digits and usually improves with treatment of the tumor. *Hypercalcemia* is due to ectopic parathyroid hormone production by the tumor. *Pulmonary hypertrophic osteoarthropathy* is a syndrome consisting of bone and joint pain, clubbing, and increased alkaline phosphatase. It can be diagnosed by plain films (which show periosteal inflammation) or bone scan (which shows increased uptake symmetrically in long bones).

Diagnostic Workup and Staging

A simplified version of the current staging system for NSCLC is described in Table 20-1. (The full staging system further divides tumors into A and B stages based on size and node status.) The goal of the initial workup is to establish the diagnosis of malignancy and to determine accurately the clinical stage of the cancer, so that candidates for potentially curable surgical resection are identified. Strategies for obtaining a pathologic diagnosis of a lung mass include **sputum cytology** (optimally from three early morning sputum collections), biopsy by **percutaneous fine-needle aspiration,** and **bronchoscopy with biopsy.** Once the diagnosis of NSCLC has been confirmed, recommended imaging studies include a **chest x-ray and a chest CT scan,** which can reveal the size of the tumor, extent of invasion of local structures, and presence of regional lymph node metastases. **PET scan** is also useful, as it has high accuracy in detecting disease metastatic to lymph nodes and distant sites, and it can aid in the differentiation of benign and malignant lung nodules. *Potential lymph node metastases* identified on imaging studies should be confirmed with direct biopsy. Mediastinoscopy is the most accurate means of staging mediastinal lymph nodes and should be performed when nodal involvement cannot be defined with chest CT. *Pleural effusions* should always be examined by thoracentesis, as a tumor associated with a malignant effusion is inoperable. The best way to identify the presence of distant metastases is with a thorough history and physical exam. Further imaging exams (i.e., head CT, abdominal CT, bone scan) should be directed by the patient's symptoms and are not required in asymptomatic patients who have early-stage tumors.

Treatment Modalities

- **Surgery,** either pneumonectomy or lobectomy, is the best chance for cure for patients with stages I and II disease. Patients with malignant pleural effusion (stage IIIB) and those with distant metastases (stage IV) are treated with chemotherapy only. There is no role for palliative surgery in the management of lung cancer.
  - **Preop workup** includes spirometry, arterial blood gases, and ·V/·Q scan to establish both that FEV_1 will be >1.2 L postresection and that the patient does not have hypercapnia or cor pulmonale.
- **Radiation therapy (XRT)** is used for cure in unresectable disease, for adjuvant therapy after surgery, or for palliation of locally advanced or metastatic disease. *Toxicities of XRT* include pneumonitis (shortness of breath, tachypnea, tachycardia, fever, nonproductive cough, infiltrate on chext x-ray 1–3 mos after XRT), pulmonary fibrosis, acute esophagitis, pericarditis, and Lhermitte's syndrome.
- In locally advanced disease, **chemotherapy** can be combined with surgery and/or XRT with curative intent. In stage IIIB and stage IV disease, chemotherapy is usu-

ally the single-treatment modality with the goal of prolongation of survival and palliation of symptoms.

Prognosis

Prognosis correlates with stage (Tables 20-1 and 20-2). Poor prognostic factors are age >60 yrs, male gender, and mucin production in the tumor. Histologic type does not affect prognosis. In advanced disease (stages III and IV), good performance status and absence of weight loss confer better prognosis.

TABLE 20-1. TNM STAGING SYSTEM FOR NON–SMALL-CELL LUNG CANCER

Tumor (T)	
T0	No tumor
Tx	Tumor by cytology but no lesion found
Tis	Carcinoma *in situ*
T1	<3 cm
T2	>3 cm or involves the main bronchus or 2 cm or more distal to the carina or invades the visceral pleura or with atelectasis extending to the hilum
T3	Extends to chest wall, diaphragm, pericardium, or mediastinal pleura or main bronchus tumor <2 cm from carina, or causes total atelectasis of the lung
T4	Invades mediastinal structures, trachea, vertebra, or carina or malignant effusion present
Node (N)	
NX	Cannot assess regional nodes
N0	No regional lymph nodes
N1	Metastasis to ipsilateral peribronchial and/or ipsilateral hilar lymph nodes and intrapulmonary nodes (even if directly invaded by primary tumor)
N2	Metastasis to ipsilateral mediastinal and/or subcarinal lymph nodes
N3	Metastasis to contralateral mediastinal or hilar nodes, ipsilateral or contralateral scalene or supraclavicular lymph nodes
Metastases (M)	
M0	No metastases
M1	Distant metastases
Staging	
I	T1–2, N0, M0
II	T1–2, N1, M0
	T3, N0, M0
IIIA	T3, N1, M0
	T1–3, N2, M0
IIIB	Any T4, any N3, M0
IV	Any M1

Adapted from Mountain CF. Revisions in the International System for Staging Lung Cancer. *Chest* 1997;17(Suppl):S3–S10.

TABLE 20-2. LONG-TERM SURVIVAL IN NON–SMALL-CELL LUNG CANCER

Stage	5-Yr survival (%)
I	40–60
II	25–35
III	5–15
IV	1

Management

Stages I and II

Stage I and II tumors are considered resectable, as they have extended no further than adjacent resectable structures or first-level lymph nodes. The optimal treatment is surgical resection with lobectomy or pneumonectomy. Patients who are not candidates for surgery because of poor lung function or comorbid conditions should be considered for XRT administered with curative intent. Postoperative XRT decreases local recurrence in stage II disease but does not confer any improvement in survival. There is no role for adjuvant chemotherapy outside the context of clinical trials in patients with resected stages I or II NSCLC.

Stage III

For unresectable stage IIIA and all stage IIIB disease, combined modality therapy is the basic approach to care. Several large prospective studies have shown that addition of chemotherapy to radiation improves long-term survival over radiation alone in patients with stage III NSCLC. Surgery alone is not curative for patients with stage IIIA disease. These patients are often treated with combined-modality therapy with chemotherapy and radiation. Whether addition of surgery to chemoradiation would improve survival in patients with stage IIIA disease is being studied in clinical trials. Patients with stage IIIB disease (invasion of mediastinal organs or contralateral lymph node involvement) are not candidates for surgery and are treated with chemotherapy and radiation. Patients who are classified as stage IIIB disease because of malignant pleural effusion are treated with chemotherapy only.

Stage IV

Chemotherapy provides modest improvement in survival. There has been a three- to fourfold improvement in 1-yr survival with combination chemotherapy over best supportive care. Several new agents have now become available for the management of metastatic NSCLC. They include vinorelbine (Navelbine), gemcitabine (Gemzar), paclitaxel (Taxol), docetaxel (Taxotere), and irinotecan (Camptosar). It has been shown that gefitinib (Iressa), a specific inhibitor of epidermal growth factor receptor tyrosine kinase, has been shown to cause disease stabilization lasting several months in nearly 30–50% of patients who recur after initial therapy.

Palliative Care

For patients who have poor performance status and do not benefit from chemotherapy, treatment may focus on palliation of symptoms. A brief palliative course of XRT may reduce disease bulk, relieving dyspnea, pain, or other symptoms. Targeted XRT may also treat pain and complications from bony or brain metastases.

Follow-Up

There is no general consensus on the appropriate follow-up for a patient who has had complete resection of NSCLC. Recurrences may be local or distant and will occur in up to 30% of patients with stage I disease and 50% of patients with stage II disease over the subsequent 5 yrs. After resection, careful history and physical exam and a CXR should be obtained at intervals of 3–4 mos, with the frequency of follow-up visits decreasing over time. Further studies (chest, abdomen, or head CT scan; bone scan; PET scan) should be obtained if signs or symptoms suggest recurrent disease. Blood tests and sputum cytology do not have a role in routine follow-up. Unfortunately, even with close follow-up, it is unlikely that recurrent disease will be resectable and curable.

SMALL-CELL LUNG CANCER

Clinical Features

- SCLC accounts for 13% of lung cancers in the United States. As opposed to NSCLC, SCLC tends to grow more rapidly, be more often associated with diverse paraneoplastic syndromes, and be more (initially) chemosensitive. The presenting signs and symptoms of SCLC are similar to those of NSCLC. Although SCLCs can present as asymptomatic lung nodules found on imaging studies, most patients with this type of lung cancer present with symptoms, especially cough, dyspnea, and chest pain. Because SCLCs are often centrally located, they can cause hemoptysis, postobstructive pneumonia, and wheezing. 10% of patients have SVC syndrome at presentation.
- **Paraneoplastic syndromes** associated with SCLC include the following:
  - **SIADH:** antidiuretic hormone production by the tumor leads to hyponatremia.
  - **Cushing's syndrome:** Ectopic ACTH production leads to symptoms of adrenal excess.
  - **Neurologic paraneoplastic syndromes,** including peripheral neuropathy and encephalomyelitis, are thought to be due to the production of autoantibodies.
  - **Lambert-Eaton syndrome** is caused by an autoantibody that impairs acetylcholine release at the neuromuscular junction, leading to proximal muscle weakness and hyporeflexia. It is diagnosed with electromyography.

Diagnostic Workup and Staging

A TNM (tumor, node, metastases) staging system is not used to classify SCLC. Instead, SCLC is described either as **limited stage,** with disease confined to one hemithorax that is encompassed in a radiation field, or as **extensive stage,** which describes all other patterns of disease. Initial workup should include comprehensive history and physical exam; screening lab work, including CBC, liver function tests, alkaline phosphatase, and lactate dehydrogenase; and chest x-ray. A **CT scan** is useful for defining the extent of intrathoracic disease and for detecting abdominal metastases. Further workup can include a head CT and bone scan. **Bone marrow biopsy no longer has a role in the workup of SCLC.** Once disease has been found outside of the thorax, workup for additional sites of metastasis is not necessary, except if metastasis requiring immediate intervention (e.g., to weight-bearing bone or CNS) is suspected.

Treatment

Chemotherapy is the primary modality used in the treatment of SCLC, and inferior results are obtained when surgery or XRT are used alone.

Limited Stage
Surgery does not play a role in the management of patients with SCLC. For patients with limited-stage disease, combined modality treatment with chemotherapy and XRT to the chest is standard.

Extensive Stage
Extensive disease is treated with chemotherapy alone. The commonly used standard chemotherapy regimens for SCLC include combinations of carboplatin (Paraplatin) or cisplatin (Platinol) with etoposide (Etopophos, Toposar, VePesid). It has recently been shown that irinotecan in combination with cisplatin may produce superior results compared with cisplatin and etoposide. Overall response rate to chemotherapy is 60–80%, but nearly all patients eventually relapse.

Palliative Care

Patients with poor performance status or significant comorbidities may not be able to tolerate aggressive chemotherapy. These patients may receive only XRT or attenuated schedules of chemotherapy, with the goal of relieving symptoms.

Prognosis

Stage (limited vs extensive), performance status, and serum lactate dehydrogenase are the factors that most reliably correlate with outcome. The median survival of limited-stage disease treated with chemotherapy and XRT is 15–26 mos. However, nearly **30% of patients with limited-stage SCLC could potentially be cured with chemoradia-tion.** The median survival of extensive-stage disease treated with chemotherapy is 7–12 mos. Only 5% of patients with extensive disease survive to 2 yrs.

Follow-Up

Most patients treated for SCLC will relapse, usually in the first 2 yrs after diagnosis. Therefore, they should have close follow-up with a medical oncologist for the identification of symptoms, physical exam findings, or lab and chest x-ray abnormalities that suggest recurrent disease.

OTHER TUMORS OF THE LUNG

A small percentage of lung malignancies are **carcinoid tumors,** which are derived from neuroendocrine cells and arise in the bronchi. Carcinoids can produce a variety of systemically active substances that cause the carcinoid syndrome: flushing, diarrhea, and wheezing. They can also cause bronchial obstruction. In the lung, carcinoids tend to grow slowly and are associated with a 5-yr survival of 77–87%. Please see Chap. 26, Endocrine Malignancies, for further information. Other malignant tumors of the lung are very uncommon, including adenoid cystic carcinoma and mucoepidermoid tumors, arising from bronchial salivary glands, and sarcomas and other soft tissue tumors.

SOLITARY LUNG NODULE

- A solitary lung nodule is a single lesion completely surrounded by lung parenchyma that is <3 cm in diameter. Lung nodules may be malignant or benign. Benign etiologies include infectious granulomas (most common benign lesions), hamartomas, noninfectious granulomas, and adenomas. Lesions >3 cm, termed **masses,** are almost always malignant and should be managed as lung cancer.
- The first goal of the **workup** of a solitary lung nodule is to assess the probability that the nodule is malignant. Patient characteristics that increase the likelihood of malignancy include age, smoking history, presence of hemoptysis, and personal history of malignancy. Chest x-ray and chest CT should be performed to provide information about the nodule's size and appearance. Nodules with a spiculated appearance are more likely to be malignant; calcified nodules and nodules that have not increased in size over time are more likely to be benign. Previous x-rays or scans, if available, can provide critical information regarding the evolution of the nodule. After the initial assessment, the nodule can be classified as benign, malignant, or indeterminate. *Benign nodules* should be followed with serial chest x-ray or chest CT every 3–6 mos for 2 yrs. Nodules that have a high probability of *malignancy* may be pursued with open biopsy and subsequent possible resection for cure. Indeterminate nodules will require further testing. **Percutaneous fine-needle aspiration** is useful for biopsy of peripheral nodules; larger, central lesions can be biopsied with **bronchoscopy. Video-assisted thoracoscopic surgery** with resection of the nodule is the definitive diagnostic procedure; it can be considered in patients with low surgical risk. **PET scanning** is sensitive and specific for the differentiation of benign and malignant lesion, and it has the advantage of providing

staging information if occult nodal or distant metastases are identified. A nodule that appears benign on PET scan should be followed by serial chest x-rays or CT scans to ensure that it does not change over time.

KEY POINTS TO REMEMBER

- Adenocarcinoma is the most common type of lung cancer.
- Paraneoplastic syndromes associated with NSCLC include clubbing, hypercalcemia, and pulmonary hypertrophic osteoarthropathy. Paraneoplastic syndromes associated with SCLC include SIADH, Cushing's syndrome, and various neurologic syndromes.
- The staging workup of NSCLC focuses on identifying tumors that can be resected and thereby potentially cured.
- The staging workup of SCLC focuses on identifying local vs advanced disease.
- Most SCLCs are symptomatic and metastatic at the time of presentation. Chemotherapy with or without radiation is the primary treatment modality.
- NSCLCs that cannot be resected or that recur after resection have a poor prognosis.
- Limited-stage SCLC is a curable disease in approximately 30% of patients treated by chemoradiation.

REFERENCES AND SUGGESTED READINGS

Deslauriers J, Gregoire J. Clinical and surgical staging of non-small cell lung cancer. *Chest* 2000;117(4 Suppl):96S–103S.

Ginsberg RJ, et al. Non-small cell lung cancer. In: DeVita VT Jr, Hellman S, Rosenberg SA, eds. *Cancer: principles and practice of oncology*, 6th ed. Philadelphia: Lippincott Williams & Wilkins, 2001:925–983.

Mountain CF. Revisions in the international system for staging lung cancer. *Chest* 1997;17(suppl):S3–S10.

Murren J, et al. Small cell lung cancer. In: DeVita VT Jr, Hellman S, Rosenberg SA, eds. *Cancer: principles and practice of oncology*, 6th ed. Philadelphia: Lippincott Williams & Wilkins, 2001:983–1018.

Ost D, Fein A. Evaluation and management of the solitary lung nodule. *Am J Respir Crit Care Med* 2000;162:782–787.

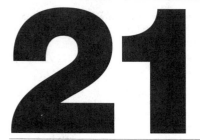

Colorectal Cancer

Ron Bose

INTRODUCTION

Tumors of the lower GI tract are one of the most common cancers diagnosed in the United States and a leading cause of cancer death. They often have a prolonged asymptomatic phase before becoming clinically apparent. However, when detected early, they can be surgically cured in a high percentage of cases. This chapter gives an overview of the presentation of colon cancers, pathophysiology, staging, and general principles of treatment.

EPIDEMIOLOGY

Colorectal cancer (CRC) is the third most common cancer after prostate and lung in men and breast and lung in women and accounts for approximately 15% of all cancers diagnosed in the United States. In the United States, there were approximately 94,000 new cases of colon cancer and 37,000 new cases of rectal cancer in 2000. CRC also ranks third in mortality with approximately 48,000 deaths from colon cancer and 8,600 deaths from rectal cancer in 2000. The overall incidence of CRC in the United States has been declining since 1985 for unclear reasons. The incidence of CRC increases with age, with approximately 90% of cases diagnosed in those >50 yrs. The median age of newly diagnosed patients is 70 for men and 73 for women. Peak incidence occurs in the eighth decade of life. The lifetime risk for CRC is 6% in average-risk persons living in the United States.

PATHOPHYSIOLOGY

Most CRCs are thought to develop from **adenomatous polyps** that arise from the colonic mucosa. Studies have shown that adenomatous polyps can become malignant over a period of 5–20 yrs. The common histologies of a polyp are tubular, tubulovillous, or villous. Villous adenomas are most likely to become malignant. Other characteristics of a higher propensity for malignancy are size >1 cm in diameter or a high grade of dysplasia. Adenomatous polyps are found in approximately 35% of persons in autopsy studies. Up to 5% of polyps are believed to become malignant over time. >95% of CRCs are **adenocarcinomas.** Of these, >80% are moderately differentiated. Other histologic types seen are undifferentiated, squamous, carcinoid, leiomyosarcomas, and hematopoietic and lymphoid neoplasias. *Poor prognosis* is associated with colloid and signet ring subtypes of adenocarcinoma, which together represent approximately 20% of tumors.

Risk Factors

- Persons with a **first-degree relative** with a history of CRC have an increased risk for CRC, especially if the relative has had CRC before the age of 45. Another strong risk factor is a **personal history** of CRC. Persons with a history of other malignancies, such as breast cancer, are also at increased risk of CRC. A history of radiation therapy to the abdomen or pelvis, such as in the case of endometrial cancer, increases the CRC risk. **Increasing age,** especially >50, is associated with an increased incidence of CRC. Those patients <40 represent <3% of cases, whereas those >50 represent >85% of cases. The seventh and eighth decades are the most affected.

- There are several CRC syndromes. **Familial adenomatous polyposis** (FAP) is an autosomal dominant disease caused by a defect in the APC gene that leads to colon cancer in 100% of patients by the age of 40 if they are left untreated. Persons affected will have up to thousands of adenomatous polyps in their bowel that have malignant potential. Persons with FAP should have a prophylactic subtotal colectomy by age 30. Aggressive screening for the development of cancer is also indicated before colectomy. Other cancers are also associated with this syndrome, and screening and treatment recommendations for their prevention are still in development. **Hereditary nonpolyposis colorectal cancer** (HNPCC) is inherited in an autosomal dominant manner and often leads to malignancies in the right side of the colon with a mucinous histology. Often, these tumors may arise without going through a polyp phase and, therefore, are seen as flat adenomas. HNPCC is also associated with cancers of the endometrium, ovary, stomach, and hepatobiliary system. Persons with this disease are also recommended to have a prophylactic subtotal colectomy. **Other inherited syndromes** associated with an increased risk of CRC include Gardner's syndrome, Turcot syndrome, Muir-Torre's syndrome, and Peutz-Jeghers syndrome.
- There are also several other risk factors that are associated with a clear increase in CRCs and therefore should be monitored carefully. These include persons with a history of **ureterosigmoidostomies.** Persons with **inflammatory bowel disease,** especially ulcerative colitis but also Crohn's disease, are at increased risk.
- The role of **diet** in CRC is somewhat controversial. Dietary factors that have been associated with CRC include a low-fiber and high-fat diet. Other dietary factors with a speculated role in CRC are calcium, vitamin D, folate, and alcohol. Increased intake of calcium, vitamin D, and folate have been associated with a decreased relative risk, whereas alcohol in some studies is associated with an increased risk. Unlike most malignancies, smoking cigarettes does not seem to be associated with an increased risk for CRC. There may also be an inverse association with ASA or other NSAID use.

Screening

- Screening methods used to detect CRC include **fecal occult blood testing (FOBT), endoscopy,** and **barium enema.** CRC is suitable for screening, because early detection is associated with improved survival due to detection of more curable lesions, and its incidence is high enough that screening can be cost-effective with acceptable positive predictive values. Available screening tests have acceptable sensitivity and specificity, but different tests are variably effective in early detection. The tests also have various risks and practical acceptability for patient and physician. It should be noted that these guidelines for screening tests are only appropriate for the *asymptomatic* patient. Anyone with warning signs of CRC requires more aggressive investigations, typically colonoscopy.
  - **FOBT** is the least expensive and most widely used screening test for the detection of CRC. There are problems with its sensitivity, which has been reported to be 18–93% with a specificity of >90%. Sensitivity will be affected by the size of the polyp and continuous bleeding from the polyp. Specificity is affected by NSAID use, other sources of GI bleeding, consumption of red meat, and certain vegetables in the diet. Hydration of samples before testing them is not recommended, as this worsens specificity of the test.
  - **Flexible sigmoidoscopy** examines up to 60 cm of the rectum and distal colon and can detect approximately 50% of CRC cases. Its advantages are that it can be performed in the primary care physician's office and that it has a specificity of nearly 100%. However, it has the advantage of not assessing the entire colon, and biopsies cannot be obtained during the procedures. Abnormalities found necessitate a follow-up colonoscopy for biopsy.
  - **Double-contrast barium enema** is a radiologic method for detection of CRC and is the safest of the visualization methods. It does require a bowel preparation. It also has the disadvantage like FOBT of requiring subsequent endoscopy for biopsy of identified lesions.

- **Colonoscopy** is considered the gold standard for detection of CRC but is associated with a higher complication rate and a higher cost than the other methods. It also involves more extensive preparation before the procedure and sedation during it.
- Most groups concerned with prevention recommend annual FOBT after age 50 yrs, combined with flexible sigmoidoscopy q5yrs, or colonoscopy q10yrs. They also recommend screening at an earlier age if risk factors, such as a history of inflammatory bowel disease, or genetic risk, such as family members with CRC or a known defect such as HNPCC or FAP are present. A ground rule of thumb is to begin screening 10 yrs before the age of cancer diagnosis of the family member affected in those with a family history. It should be noted that it is not completely clear which approach is best for colon cancer screening at this time.

PRESENTATION

- CRC presents because of symptoms or because of a positive screening test for the disease. It is relatively asymptomatic until the tumor is large in size. Most of the symptoms with which patients present are nonspecific and are found commonly in patients without CRC. Symptoms associated with CRC are often related to the **location of the tumor** within the bowel; therefore, *right-sided lesions* more often present with symptoms of anemia and occasionally of melena. *Left-sided lesions* more commonly cause obstruction, tenesmus, constipation, bright-red blood per rectum, and other changes in bowel habits. Other symptoms on presentation include fatigue, anorexia, failure to thrive, and right upper quadrant pain associated with liver metastasis.
- The most common presenting **symptoms,** although, are those associated with anemia. Because the bleeding is insidious, patients often have an iron-deficiency anemia and may have symptoms of pica. Because CRC is a cause of anemia, it is important to evaluate any person who presents with an unexplained anemia for CRC, especially men and postmenopausal women.
- Signs found on **physical exam** of CRC include those of anemia such as pallor in the conjunctivae and the nail beds. Rarely, a palpable mass will be present in the abdomen or the rectum. Patients may also have gross blood or melanotic stool in the rectal vault. If liver metastases are present, patients my have hepatomegaly and tenderness to palpation in the right upper quadrant. On barium enema, an "apple core" lesion may be seen, which suggests colon cancer. *Streptococcus bovis* bacteremia and/or endocarditis is also a sign of CRC, and persons diagnosed with this should be evaluated for colon cancer.

Diagnosis

Diagnosis is by detection on routine screening or workup due to a suspicion of CRC. History and physical exam can be revealing. CRC should be suspected with unexplained anemia in men and postmenopausal women, in those with GI bleeding, unexplained changes in bowel habits, and as a search for an unknown primary tumor. Colonoscopy is the diagnostic procedure of choice, as it will detect tumors, collect biopsies, and potentially cure benign polyps and carcinoma *in situ*. Other modes less often used to diagnose colon cancer include barium enema and sigmoidoscopy. CT or MRI scans are generally not useful in making a diagnosis.

MANAGEMENT

Initial Evaluation of the Colon Cancer Patient

- A **history and physical** are, of course, the first step in colon cancer evaluation.
- A **CBC** will give information about an iron-deficiency anemia that may be associated. CRC most often metastasizes to the liver, lung, adrenals, ovaries, and bone. **Liver function tests** may be elevated in a person with metastatic disease to the liver. An elevation in the alkaline phosphatase can be seen in association with liver and bone metastases. A **carcinoembryonic antigen (CEA)** is often obtained for follow-up after treatment, as a rise in CEA after treatment may be seen with recurrence. A chest x-

TABLE 21-1. AMERICAN JOINT COMMITTEE ON CANCER TNM (TUMOR, NODE, METASTASES) SYSTEM FOR COLORECTAL CANCER STAGING

T

Tis	Carcinoma *in situ*: intraepithelial or invasion of the lamina propria
T1	Invasion of the submucosa
T2	Invasion into the muscularis mucosa
T3	Invasion through the muscularis mucosa into the subserosa
T4	Invasion through visceral peritoneum or invasion into adjacent organs

N

N0	No lymph node metastases
N1	Metastases in one to three lymph nodes
N2	Metastases in four or more lymph nodes

M

M0	No distant metastases
M1	Distant metastases present

Adapted from American Joint Committee on Cancer. AJCC cancer staging manual, 5th ed. Philadelphia: Lippincott–Raven, 1997.

ray may be used to rule out pulmonary metastasis. Many would advocate an abdominal CT scan to evaluate the liver and other abdominal organs for metastatic disease.
- **All patients should have the remainder of their bowels evaluated by colonoscopy** or barium enema to rule out synchronous lesions. Up to 3–5% of patients have another focus of CRC in their bowels. Patients should also have a tissue biopsy before therapy to confirm the diagnosis.

Surgical Staging

- Surgery is important for accurate staging of CRC. The preferred staging system for CRC is the American Joint Committee on Cancer (AJCC) TNM (tumor, node, metastases) system (Table 21-1).
- Pathologic stages are delineated in Table 21-1. It uses the degree of tumor invasion, the presence of positive lymph nodes, and the presence of distant metastasis to classify the disease in one of four stages. Although the AJCC TNM staging system is the preferred staging system today, the Duke staging system with the Astler-Coller modification is often referred to in older literature (Table 21-2).

TABLE 21-2. STAGING OF COLORECTAL CANCER BY AMERICAN JOINT COMMITTEE ON CANCER TNM (TUMOR, NODE, METASTASES) SYSTEM (AND DUKE STAGE EQUIVALENTS)

Stage	T	N	M	Duke Stage
0	Tis	N0	M0	N/A
I	T1 or T2	N0	M0	A, B1
II	T3 or T4	N0	M0	B2
III	Any T	N1 or N2	M0	C
IV	Any T	Any N	M1	D

N/A, not applicable.

TABLE 21-3. TREATMENT FOR VARIOUS STAGES OF COLON CANCER

Stage	Treatment
0	Polypectomy/surgical resection
I	Surgery alone
II	Surgery ± chemotherapy
III	Surgery + chemotherapy
IV	Palliative chemotherapy, metastasis resection (limited cases)

Treatment

As with all tumors, the goals of therapy need to be clearly delineated from the beginning and reevaluated throughout the patient's course. **Colon cancer is a surgically curable disease**, with the best chance for cure at the earliest stages of disease. Chemotherapy can be added to improve cure rates in higher-stage tumors or as palliation in incurable tumors (Table 21-3).

Surgery

Surgery is undertaken with an intent to cure in 75% of those with colon cancer. Many of the remainder will also require surgery to prevent obstruction, perforation, or bleeding.

- **Wide excision** of the tumor with a distal margin of approximately 5 cm is recommended for curative surgery. The length of colon and mesentery resected is determined by the vascular anatomy. If the tumor is adherent to or invades another organ, an en bloc excision must also be done. This excision prevents seeding and allows the possibility of cure. If the surgical intent is palliation instead of cure, a simple resection or diversion is used to lessen morbidity from the procedure. In stage IV cancer, some patients may benefit from resection of metastases. Modest 5-yr survivals have been obtained in those with limited liver metastases that have been resected.
- **Prophylactic total abdominal colectomy** for high-risk individuals without current colon cancer is a controversial topic among colorectal surgeons. Although most recommend this for those with FAP, others also believe that a total colectomy should be offered to patients with HNPCC, and those who present with a colon cancer before the age of 40. Prophylactic oophorectomy has been advocated for some women with CRC, but this also remains controversial.

Chemotherapy

- **Adjuvant chemotherapy** is administered to prevent relapse, which occurs mainly at distant sites with colon cancer. Overall, 50% of those with macroscopic clearance of their disease through surgery will recur. 5-Fluorouracil (5-FU) (Efudex, Fluoroplex) and leucovorin is now the standard of therapy for stage III colon cancer. 5-FU works by inhibiting the synthesis of thymidine, which can be incorporated into DNA and RNA. Leucovorin (folinic acid) increases binding of 5-FU to thymidylate synthase, which increases its antimetabolite role. This leads to apoptosis in rapidly dividing cells. 5-FU is only cytotoxic in those cells undergoing DNA synthesis and cell division. See Chap. 16, Chemotherapy, for more details.
- The mortality rate is higher with **stage III disease,** and it is clear that **adjuvant chemotherapy improves outcome.** Controversy remains, although, over adjuvant chemotherapy for stage II disease. Because the 5-yr survival rate is 75–80% in stage II colon cancer, the relative reduction in deaths is predicted to be small. Because there seems to be only a small benefit to treating stage II disease, the current focus is on finding subgroups within the stage II colon cancer population that will be more likely to benefit from treatment. Chemotherapy is typically only indicated currently as part of a clinical trial in **stage II colon cancer,** although some high-

risk groups may receive chemotherapy. Some examples of high-risk groups include those patients who present with a total obstruction or a perforated tumor.

- Also ongoing are trials that compare survival using irinotecan (Camptosar), a topoisomerase-I inhibitor, with 5-FU and leucovorin vs 5-FU and leucovorin alone. Additional trials are also looking at the role of oxaliplatin (Eloxatin), a newer platinum analog in the adjuvant setting. These agents have clear established use in the treatment of metastatic colon cancer. Additional experimental agents are being investigated that interfere with angiogenesis (new vessel formation) or inhibit certain cellular-signaling pathways thought to be altered in malignant cells. Interested patients with stage IV disease should be referred for clinical trials when possible.

Prognosis

The four stages have great significance in the prognosis and treatment of the disease. In the United States between 1973 and 1997, overall 5-yr survival with CRC was 61%. Stage I was associated with >95% 5-yr survival. Stage II had an 87% 5-yr survival. Stage III had a 55% 5-yr survival, and stage IV was associated with a <5% 5-yr survival and a median survival of around 11 mos. 5-yr survival correlates well with cure of the disease. Other prognostic factors include the number of lymph nodes positive. Increasing N stage is associated with decreased survival. Tumor invasiveness is also associated with poorer outcomes. Those with invasion through the bowel wall into adjacent organs or into veins tend to do worse than those with the same stage without invasion.

Rectal Cancer

- **Surgery** is used in rectal cancer also to cure the disease and plays a role in palliative therapy. The rectum is the distal 15 cm of the large bowel and resides within the bony pelvis. The most important feature of the rectum is the lack of a serosa for these tumors. Because of this anatomy, local recurrence for rectal cancer is high, and adjuvant therapy may be needed to make a tumor resectable. Even with these difficulties, 50% of those who have surgery will be cured. Surgery in the pelvis can be technically demanding because there is a decreased area in which to work. Accordingly, surgery is used in conjunction with radiation or chemoradiation, and this multimodality approach has been associated with decreased recurrence. Approaches aimed at sphincter preservation, obviating the need for colostomy, can often be performed if a 2-cm margin can be obtained.
- Compared to colon cancer, rectal cancer is much more likely to **recur locally** rather than distally. Only approximately 25% of patients have distant metastases. Therapy is therefore tailored to prevent local recurrence in stages II and III cancers. Currently, surgery along with 5-FU and radiation is used to treat rectal cancer, leading to significant improvements in overall survival as compared to treatment with surgery alone. Areas of study involve the comparisons of preop and postop combined modality therapy and timing and use of chemotherapy. Most American centers are adopting preop radiation therapy as a standard, especially for low-lying tumors.

Complications

Tumor Related

Complications that can result from CRC often produce the symptoms with which patients present. These include **bowel obstruction, anemia,** and **abdominal pain.** More serious complications can include peritonitis after perforation, fistula formation, and malnutrition. Complications can also result from sites of metastatic disease. Liver metastases can lead to hyperbilirubinemia and coagulopathies, and pulmonary metastases, when advanced, may result in cough or shortness of breath. Patients may also develop pain at sites of metastases.

Treatment Related

Complications of treatment are commonly related to surgery and chemotherapy but can also occur with radiation therapy. Postop mortality rates are 1–5%. Major morbidity includes bowel and bladder dysfunction, sexual dysfunction, anastomotic leaks, and bowel obstruction. The need for a permanent colostomy can be psychologically upsetting.

Follow-Up

With the risk of recurrent CRC being nearly 50% for stage III colon cancer patients, studies are ongoing to address how closely and extensively patients should be followed to detect recurrence. One controversial area remains the measurement of CEA levels. Because all patients with CRC are in a high-risk group for new primary CRCs, colonoscopy is widely recommended 1 yr after surgery and then q3yrs to detect new primary lesions. Routine chest x-ray and CT scans have also been examined in detections of recurrence and improving survival but are not routinely recommended now.

ANAL CANCER

Epidemiology

Anal cancer accounts for approximately 1% of all CRCs in the United States. It is now more common in men than women, although in the past, the number of cases in women has been five times that in men. Its incidence generally increases with age, with peak incidence in the sixth and seventh decades of life. The incidence is increasing in men <40 yrs. Histologically, 63% of anal cancers are squamous cell carcinomas. Basaloid transitional cell carcinomas (cloacogenic) make up 23% of cases. More rare types are adenocarcinoma, basal cell, and melanoma.

Risk Factors

The risk factor most commonly associated with anal cancer is **human papilloma virus** (HPV) infection. HPV 16 and 18 have been linked to the disease. This is seen in both men and women. In women, increased anal cancers are seen with HPV-associated cervical cancer. In men, anal cancer is more frequently associated with receptive anal intercourse and HPV. As many as 70% of anal cancers are positive for HPV.

Other risk factors include immunosuppression such as that seen after renal transplant. Immunosuppression with AIDS also seems to be associated with an increased incidence. Current cigarette smoking is also a risk factor for anal cancer with a relative risk of seven- to ninefold for smokers.

Presentation and Diagnosis

Anal cancers present with **bleeding** 50% of the time. Other symptoms include pain, mass, constipation, diarrhea, and pruritus. Often the symptoms are ascribed to hemorrhoids, and delays in diagnosis occur. Approximately 25% of people are asymptomatic when the cancer is discovered. **Physical exam findings** include an **anal mass** and **lymphadenopathy.** On palpation, an anal mass will often be firm and indurated. Notes should be made of the location of the mass, including its position relative to the dentate line. Anal cancers are divided into those of the anal margin and those of the anal canal. The line of demarcation is a zone approximately halfway between the dentate line and the anal verge. Anoscopy, proctoscopy, and transrectal U/S are used to visualize the mass. Diagnosis is made by incisional biopsy of the mass and any inguinal lymphadenopathy.

Staging

Staging is based on the TNM system (Table 21-4).

Treatment

Very small tumors at the anal margin may be treated with wide local excision, but combined chemotherapy and radiation therapy has been the preferred treatment for locore-

TABLE 21-4. STAGING OF ANAL CANCER

T		
	Tis	Carcinoma *in situ*
	T1	Tumor is ≤2 cm in diameter
	T2	Tumor is between 2 and 5 cm in diameter
	T3	Tumor is >5 cm
	T4	Tumor of any size that invades adjacent organs such as the vagina, urethra, or bladder
N		
	N0	No regional lymph nodes involved
	N1	Metastases in unilateral internal iliac or inguinal lymph node
	N3	Metastases in perirectal and one inguinal lymph node and/or bilateral internal iliac or inguinal lymph nodes
M		
	M0	No distant metastases present
	M1	Distant metastases present
	Stage I	T1, N0, M0
	Stage II	T2, 3; N0; M0
	Stage IIIA	T1–3, N1, M0 or T4, N0, M0
	Stage IIIB	T4, N1, M0 or any T, N2–3, M0
	Stage IV	Any T, any N, M1

gional disease. Treatment is with mitomycin C (Mutamycin) and 5-FU with concurrent radiation. In several trials, 5-yr survival varied between 64–83% with combined modality therapy. After treatment, close medical follow-up is needed to screen for recurrence.

Prognosis

Prognosis is based on staging. T1 and T2 tumors have >80% 5-yr survival, whereas T3 and T4 tumors have 5-yr survivals of <20%. Inguinal lymphadenopathy and male gender are also related to a poorer prognosis. Tumors in the anal margin have a more favorable prognosis than those in the canal.

KEY POINTS TO REMEMBER

- CRC must be suspected in unexplained anemia in men and postmenopausal women.
- The main risk factors for colon cancer include personal and family history of colon cancer and age.
- CRC screening strategies only apply when screening asymptomatic patients.
- CRC is a surgically curable disease, with later stages yielding poorer long-term survival rates.
- Chemotherapy for CRC is useful in higher-stage disease.
- Rectal cancer typically has a more difficult operative approach.
- Rectal cancers have a high rate of local recurrence and are, therefore, treated with combined modality treatment in stages II and III disease.
- The preferred approach of screening for CRC is not yet certain, but most groups concerned with prevention recommend annual FOBT after age 50 combined with flexible sigmoidoscopy every 5 yrs or colonoscopy every 10 yrs.
- Anal cancer is associated with HPV infection.

REFERENCES AND SUGGESTED READINGS

Janne PA, Mayer RJ. Chemoprevention of colorectal cancer. *N Engl J Med* 2000;342:1960–1966.

Midgley R, Kerr D. Colorectal cancer. *Lancet* 1999;353:391–399.

Peeters M, Haller DG. Therapy for early stage colorectal cancer. *Oncology (Huntingt)* 1999;13:307–315; discussion, 315–317, 320–321. [Review.]

Petrelli N, Herrera L, Rustum Y, et al. A prospective randomized trial of 5-fluorouracil versus 5-fluorouracil and high dose leucovorin versus 5-fluorouracil and methotrexate in previously untreated patients with advanced colorectal carcinoma. *J Clin Oncol* 1987;5:1559–1565.

Poon MA, O'Connell MJ, Moertel CG, et al. Biochemical modulation of fluorouracil: evidence of significant improvement of survival and quality of life in patients with advanced colorectal carcinoma. *J Clin Oncol* 1989;7:1407–1417.

Saltz LB, Cox JV, Blanke C, et al. Irinotecan plus fluorouracil and leucovorin for metastatic colorectal cancer. *N Engl J Med* 2000;343:905–914.

Schatzkin A, Lanza E, Corle D, et al. Lack of effect of a low-fat, high fiber diet on the recurrence of colorectal adenomas. *N Engl J Med* 2000;342:1149–1155.

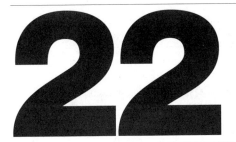

Other Gastrointestinal Malignancies

Ron Bose

This chapter deals with upper GI tumors and tumors of the pancreas, liver, and biliary tract. Tumors of the GI tract outside the colon are much more rare than colorectal cancer. However, some of these tumor types have been increasing in incidence over the last several years. In this chapter, the upper GI tumors (stomach and esophageal cancer) have been grouped together, whereas pancreatic, hepatic, and biliary tumors are discussed separately. Carcinoid tumors also often involve the GI tract but are discussed in Chap. 26, Endocrine Malignancies.

ESOPHAGEAL AND GASTRIC CANCER

Epidemiology

The incidence of *esophageal cancer* in the United States has been rising since the 1990s, and now approximately 8.8 new cases/100,000 population are diagnosed each year. There have also been changes in the locations and histology of esophageal cancers, with the adenocarcinomas of the distal esophagus now being the most common type diagnosed. There is believed to be an association with the presence of Barrett's esophagitis, and there may be an increased risk by simply having symptoms of gastroesophageal reflux disease. *Gastric cancer* is relatively rare in the United States, with approximately 23,000 new cases diagnosed per year. However, in contrast to esophageal cancer, its incidence has decreased dramatically during the 20th century. Risk factors include history of atrophic gastritis, cigarette smoking, *Helicobacter pylori* infection, and Barrett's esophagitis. There is a striking variation in the worldwide incidence of these tumors, however, with esophageal and stomach cancer being leading causes of cancer deaths in certain parts of the world, especially parts of Asia (especially China and Singapore), Central and South America (especially Costa Rica and Brazil), and Africa and the Middle East (especially Iran). The care provider should remember to carefully screen patients from these high-risk populations.

History and Physical Exam

Initial symptoms of **esophageal cancer** may include dysphagia and weight loss, and progressive dysphagia to solid or liquid foods is a classic history. Extraesophageal spread can cause pain, hoarseness (secondary to recurrent laryngeal nerve involvement), aspiration, tracheal narrowing, or tracheoesophageal fistula. **Gastric cancer** may present with pain, weight loss, vomiting, early satiety, or upper GI bleed. Signs of spread to the liver, such as hepatomegaly or ascites; to pleura, such as malignant effusion; or to lymph nodes may be present.

Diagnosis

Upper endoscopy with biopsy is the gold standard for diagnosis of upper GI tract tumors. **Barium studies** may also be used for diagnosis but are less sensitive and do not allow for biopsy of suspicious lesions. Given that approximately 3% of gastric ulcers are found to be malignant, many **gastric ulcers found on upper endoscopy should be considered for biopsy**. Repeat endoscopy is also often done to document resolution of ulcer disease.

TABLE 22-1. TUMOR, NODE, METASTASIS (TNM) SYSTEM FOR ESOPHAGEAL AND STOMACH CANCER

Tis	Carcinoma *in situ*		Mx	Cannot assess
T1	Invades submucosa		M0	No metastases
T2	Invades muscularis propria		M1	Metastases present
T3	Invades adventitia			
T4	Invades adjacent structures			
For esophageal cancer			**For stomach cancer**	
Nx	Cannot assess		Nx	Cannot assess
N0	No regional nodes involved		N0	No regional nodes involved
N1	Unilateral, mobile nodes		N1	<7 Regional nodes
N2	Bilateral, mobile nodes		N2	7–15 Regional nodes
N3	Nonmobile nodes		N3	>15 Regional nodes

Staging and Prognosis

Staging workup includes a thorough history and physical, basic labs (CBC, liver functions, basic metabolic panel), and imaging via chest x-ray and CT of chest and/or abdomen. Other potentially useful tests include endoscopic U/S, which can help gauge depth and length of tumor or guide biopsy of paraesophageal lymph nodes. In some cases, laparoscopy can be used to rule out peritoneal involvement. In addition, mediastinoscopy is being studied to see whether better staging can guide therapeutic choices. In addition, laparoscopy can be useful to allow insertion of a gastric feeding tube or a jejunostomy tube to ensure adequate nutrition during neoadjuvant therapy. Bone scans may be performed to diagnose bony involvement. Bronchoscopy is indicated in patients with symptoms of tracheal involvement or with tumors of the upper or middle one-third of the esophagus. Tables 22-1, 22-2, and 22-3 show a simplified version of the TNM staging system for stomach and esophageal cancer. Prognosis is primarily based on a patient's TNM staging as is seen in Table 22-2.

Treatment Options

Esophageal Cancer

- **Esophagectomy** can be performed for potentially resectable lesions with the goal of surgical cure and negative margins. It is more readily accomplished with

TABLE 22-2. STAGING, TREATMENT, AND SURVIVAL FOR ESOPHAGEAL CANCER

Stage	TNM	Standard treatment	5-yr survival
0	Tis, N0, M0	Surgery, XRT	>90%
I	T1, N0, M0	Surgery CMT	>50%
IIa	T2, 3; N0; M0	Surgery CMT	15–30%
IIb	T1, 2; N1; M0	Surgery CMT	10–30%
III	T3, N1, M0 or T4, any N, M0	CMT ± palliative surgery	<10%
IV	Any T, N, M1	RT ± chemotherapy	Rare

CMT, combined-modality therapy; RT, radiation; XRT, radiation therapy.

TABLE 22-3. STAGING, TREATMENT, AND SURVIVAL FOR STOMACH CANCER

Stage	TNM	Standard treatment	5-yr survival (%)
0	Tis, N0, M0	Surgery	>90
Ia	T1, N0, M0	Surgery	60–80
Ib	T1, N1, M0 or T2, N0, M0	Surgery ± CMT	50–60
II	T1, N2, M0 or T2, N1, M0	Surgery ± CMT	30–40
IIIa	T2, N2, M0 or T3, N1, M0 or T4, N0, M0	Surgery ± CMT	20
IIIb	T3, N2, M0	Palliative chemo, RT or surgery	10
IV	T4; N1, 2; M0 or any T, N3, M0 or any T, N, M1	Same as IIIb	<5

CMT, combined-modality therapy; RT, radiation; TNM, tumor, node, metastases.

midesophageal and distal lesions. When resection for cure is impossible, palliative approaches can include laser therapy, stenting, and feeding gastrostomy tube.

• **Radiation therapy** can be used preop, postop, or in the palliative setting. It is often offered with chemotherapy [combined-modality treatment (CMT)]. CMT can be a primary treatment for poor surgical candidates. Some recent studies suggest that survival rates for patients with esophageal cancer are similar with the use of surgery or the use of radiation therapy and chemotherapy. Radiation therapy alone is not equivalent to surgery or CMT and should be used when palliation alone is the goal. 5-Fluorouracil (5-FU) (Efudex, Fluoroplex), cisplatin (Platinol, Platinol-AQ), and mitomycin C (Mutamycin) are frequently used agents. Additional modalities include brachytherapy, which is the placement of an isotope-producing substance into the tumor mass.

Gastric Cancer

Resection of the primary tumor and lymph nodes is the only modality for a cure of gastric cancer. Surgical resection depends on the site and extent of the tumor, and surgical exploration should be undertaken in the absence of known tumor spread. **Subtotal gastrectomy** is often preferred when an adequate margin of tissue is possible, as it has lower morbidity with comparable survival rates to complete gastrectomy. However, it may not be possible in patients with more proximal or large lesions. **Radiation therapy** has a limited role in gastric cancer but may be used in the adjuvant (postop) setting in conjunction with chemotherapy. A recent large trial has confirmed that radiation therapy and 5-FU–based chemotherapy should be given postresection in the adjuvant setting. This randomized trial showed minimal morbidity and superior cure rates with this approach. **Chemotherapy** regimens often include 5-FU or cisplatin. Other agents, such as doxorubicin (Adriamycin), mitomycin C, etoposide (Etopophos, Toposar, VePesid), taxanes, and others, have also been considered. In general, gastric tumors are very responsive to chemotherapy, but such responses are short. Because of the high response rate, many patients have been using chemotherapy neoadjuvantly, but this approach remains investigational.

Complications

Tumor growth can cause significant **dysphagia.** It can range from difficulty with solid foods or liquids to oral secretions. Palliative therapy to allow swallowing of secretions or feeding tubes may be considered. Surgical complications of therapy include anastomotic leak, stricture, and bleeding. Tracheoesophageal fistulae may occur, which predisposes patients to aspiration pneumonia. These fistulae generally require surgical intervention. Vitamin B_{12} deficiency occurs in long-term survivors (5–10 yrs) in all cases of total gastrectomies and in 20% of subtotal resections.

Follow-Up

Follow-up should appreciate the **field effect,** in that patients with esophageal cancers are typically at risk for all aerodigestive tract tumors due to shared risk factors. Patients should be followed for screening of head and neck, lung, and recurrent esophageal tumors.

Screening

Given the rarity of these tumors in the United States, there is no justification for routine screening for esophageal or stomach cancer at this time. However, in countries of high incidence (e.g., Japan), screening for stomach cancer via endoscopy or upper GI imaging is standard for those >50 yrs.

PANCREATIC CANCER

Pancreatic cancer is the fifth leading cause of cancer death in the United States. It has an annual incidence of approximately 12.3/100,000. It is a rarely curable disease because of the advanced stage at presentation in the majority of patients and the poor response to therapy of unresectable or recurrent tumors.

Clinical Features

Initial **symptoms** at presentation can include abdominal or back pain, weight loss, nausea, vomiting, painless jaundice, fatigue, and depression. The presenting symptom of new-onset depression or diabetes can be striking. **Physical findings** such as palpable abdominal mass, jaundice, ascites, Courvoisier's sign (painless palpable gallbladder), Virchow's node (left supraclavicular), and Sister Mary Joseph's node (periumbilical) may be occasionally found. Paraneoplastic syndromes, such as Trousseau's syndrome (migratory superficial phlebitis), idiopathic deep venous thrombosis, myositis syndromes, and Cushing's syndrome, may rarely be presenting symptoms. Many pancreatic tumors are *asymptomatic* until they are well advanced, especially those located in the tail of the pancreas.

Diagnostic Evaluation

In addition to a thorough history and physical and basic labs, imaging modalities such as **U/S or CT scan** may be performed. CT is typically preferred, and high-resolution views of the pancreas should be obtained. Tissue diagnosis may be obtained by percutaneous needle biopsy, laparoscopy, endoscopic retrograde cholangiopancreatography, or ascitic fluid cytology. Ca19-9 levels may be obtained as a baseline and followed for response/recurrence. Staging is by the TNM system and is reviewed in simplified form in Table 22-4.

Management
Surgery
An experienced surgeon is needed to determine resectability, but patients with positive liver, peritoneal, or distant metastases or Virchow's or Sister Mary Joseph's nodes are typically unresectable. The standard procedure is a pancreaticoduodenectomy with choledochojejunostomy, cholecystectomy, and gastrojejunostomy (Whipple procedure). This is a major surgery, which entails considerable morbidity. Palliative procedures, such as biliary bypass or endoscopic stent, may also be undertaken.

TABLE 22-4. TNM SYSTEM FOR PANCREATIC CANCER

Tx	Cannot assess	Nx	Cannot assess
T0	No evidence of primary tumor	N0	No regional nodes
Tis	Carcinoma *in situ*	N1	Positive regional nodes
T1	<2 cm in greatest dimension	Mx	Cannot asses metastasis
T2	>2 cm	M0	No metastases
T3	Extension into duodenum, bile duct, peri-pancreatic tissue	M1	Metastases present
T4	Extension to stomach, spleen colon, or large blood vessel		

Stage

0	Tis, N0, M0
I	T1, 2; N0; M0
II	T3, N0, M0
III	T1–3, N1, M0
IVa	T4, any N, M0
IVb	Any T, any N, M1

Radiation

Radiation with concurrent chemotherapy is frequently used both in the postop and palliative settings.

Chemotherapy

5-FU is often used in CMT, whereas gemcitabine (Gemzar) is the standard agent for metastatic disease. Metastatic disease treated with gemcitabine has shown to improve the survival and the quality of life for these patients. Given the poor prognosis of these cancers and the evidence that many have specific genetic/signaling defects, a number of experimental agents are being developed to treat them.

Prognosis

T1 and T2 lesions without distant spread are potentially resectable and are associated with 5–35% 5-yr survival rates. Median survival for unresectable disease has been as short as 6 mos, but many trials are now reporting median survivals of treated patients closer to 12 mos.

Complications

Pain management is paramount in pancreatic cancer patients. In addition to standard analgesics, celiac plexus block may be an option in selected patients. Biliary obstruction and subsequent cholangitis should be relieved by stenting or draining procedures.

HEPATOBILIARY CANCER

Hepatocellular Carcinoma

- Hepatocellular cancer is a rare cancer in the United States, with an annual incidence of approximately 2.4/100,000, but is a very common tumor type in some areas of the world, such as Southeast Asia and Africa. The **incidence** in the United States has risen strikingly over the last few decades, subsequent to a *rise in incidence of hepatitis B and C.* **Risk factors** for hepatic cancer include hepatitis B, hepatitis C, and cirrhosis of any cause. Cirrhotic patients have a roughly 3% yearly incidence of hepatocellular carcinoma.

- Patients on **presentation** may have nonspecific complaints of abdominal pain, malaise, weight loss, or fever. Imaging via U/S or CT scan is typically the first step to diagnosis, and biopsy is usually by percutaneous needle biopsy. Alpha-fetoprotein is elevated in 85% of cases but can be nonspecific.

- **Staging and prognosis** depend on number, size, and presence of vascular invasion by the tumor. Prognosis ranges from 5–55% 5-yr survival, depending on ability to undergo surgical resection. Only approximately 10% of hepatocellular carcinomas are resectable at time of diagnosis.

- These tumors are highly vascular. **Staging workup** includes CT scan or MRI to define anatomic relationships and vascular anatomy, but angiography may be needed to completely reveal the anatomy. **Multifocal disease** is common, especially in patients with a history of cirrhosis. There is a TNM staging system for these tumors, and the interested reader is referred to the most recent American Joint Committee on Cancer staging manual.

- Stages can be roughly split into **localized resectable, localized unresectable,** and **advanced cancers.** Localized resectable lesions are single masses that may be completely resected with a margin of normal liver for an attempt at cure. Localized unresectable lesions are those that are confined to a localized area of the liver but are not amenable to resection with a tissue margin owing to proximity of vascular structures, amount of tissue resection required, or poor health of the patient. Given that many patients with these tumors are cirrhotic, many cannot tolerate more than a small wedge resection. Advanced liver cancers are metastatic lesions to nodes or other tissues or those that affect both lobes of the liver. The most important prognostic indicators are size of the tumor mass and degree of hepatic impairment, with cirrhosis conferring a poor outcome.

- **Surgery** is the primary curative modality of treatment for localized resectable lesions. As mentioned earlier, few patients are candidates because of advanced disease at presentation. Overall health status is an important consideration on deciding to which patients to offer resection, and worse outcome is associated with poorer Child's functional status. Recurrent local disease may also be treated surgically, with potential for cure.

- Given the hypervascularity of these tumors, **chemoembolization** has been attempted via the hepatic artery and may provide a survival benefit. Infusion of lipiodol after resection for cure may increase survival. Arterial infusion of Gelfoam or other embolization agents may have a role in unresectable disease. Other local therapies include **intralesional injection of ethanol** for unresectable localized lesions. Radiation therapy may be used in unresectable disease as well. Radiofrequency ablation and cryosurgery are other potentially promising modalities for unresectable disease.

- **Chemotherapy** has been used in unresectable localized disease. Adriamycin is the most commonly used agent, and this may be infused systemically or by hepatic artery infusion.

- Given the frequent association with cirrhosis, **liver transplant** has been investigated as treatment of both the primary tumor and concomitant cirrhosis. Liver transplant has been used successfully in trials for the treatment of hepatocellular carcinoma, despite the use of immunosuppression postop. In one trial, patients with fewer than 3 lesions smaller than 3 cm or a single lesion smaller than 5 cm had a 4-yr survival rate of approximately 85%.

- **Prevention** of these tumors may be achieved by decreasing the burden of cirrhosis or chronic liver inflammation. Hepatitis B vaccination is very effective at protecting against the virus, and vaccination in a high-incidence country has been shown to decrease the subsequent incidence of hepatocellular carcinoma. Hepatitis C is now adequately screened for in the blood supply. Treatment of hepatitis C with interferon may decrease the subsequent risk of hepatocellular carcinoma. Patients with hepatitis C should be screened with annual alpha-fetoprotein levels and liver U/S.

Cholangiocarcinoma

Cholangiocarcinoma and gallbladder cancer are rare cancers of the biliary system, with approximately 7,000 cases diagnosed per year. Gallbladder polyps and calcification are risk factors for gallbladder cancer, as well as is a history of gallstones (although the rarity of gallbladder cancer **does not warrant screening** in those with a history of gallstones). Cholangiocarcinoma is more common in patients with a history of primary sclerosing cholangitis, with lifetime risk ranging from 10–20%. These tumors may present with symptoms of acute or chronic cholecystitis, although jaundice and weight loss are more common. U/S or abdominal CT can be used for imaging, although **endoscopic retrograde cholangiopancreatography** is often needed for tissue diagnosis and demonstration of extent of tumor. Treatment is surgical, but few patients are resectable at time of presentation. Unresectable tumors are those with bilateral intrahepatic duct involvement, portal vein entrapment, or bilateral invasion of hepatic artery branches. Biliary stenting or cholecystostomy tubes may be used for palliation of biliary obstruction.

KEY POINTS TO REMEMBER

- Progressive dysphagia is a classic presentation of esophageal cancer.
- The incidence of esophageal cancer has been increasing in the United States, with a predominance of adenocarcinoma as the histologic type. More intensive screening is appropriate for first-generation patients from high-risk countries (Japan, China, Singapore, Costa Rica, Brazil).
- Upper endoscopy is the diagnostic test of choice in the evaluation of esophageal or stomach cancer.
- Patients with upper digestive tract tumors are at high risk for subsequent aerodigestive tract tumors owing to shared risk factors.
- Surgical intervention is the approach for cure of stomach and esophageal cancers, but chemoradiation may have a role alone for esophageal tumors.
- Pancreatic cancer is typically advanced at time of presentation.
- Hepatocellular cancer is increasing in incidence, likely owing to the burden of hepatitis B and C and alcoholic cirrhosis in this country.
- Patients with hepatitis C should be screened with annual alpha-fetoprotein levels and liver U/S.

REFERENCES AND SUGGESTED READINGS

Chang M-H, Chen C-J, Lai M-S, et al. Universal hepatitis B vaccination in Taiwan and the incidence of hepatocellular carcinoma in children. *N Engl J Med* 1997;336:1855–1859.

de Groen PC, Gores GJ, LaRusso NF, et al. Medical progress: biliary tract cancers. *N Engl J Med* 1999;341:1368–1378.

El-Serag HB, Mason AC. Rising incidence of hepatocellular carcinoma in the United States. *N Engl J Med* 1999;340:745–750.

Fuchs CS, Mayer RJ. Medical progress: gastric carcinoma. *N Engl J Med* 1995;333:32–41.

Lagergren J, Bergström R, Lindgren A, et al. Symptomatic gastroesophageal reflux as a risk factor for esophageal adenocarcinoma. *N Engl J Med* 1999;340:825–831.

Mazzaferro V, Regalia E, Doci R, et al. Liver transplantation for the treatment of small hepatocellular carcinomas in patients with cirrhosis. *N Engl J Med* 1996;334:693–699.

U.S. Cancer Statistics Working Group. *United States cancer statistics: 1999 incidence*. Atlanta: Department of Health and Human Services, Centers for Disease Control and Prevention and National Cancer Institute, 2002.

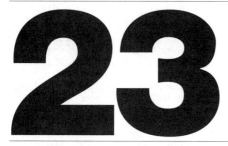

Malignant Melanoma

Amanda F. Cashen

INTRODUCTION

Malignant melanoma is the sixth most common cancer in American men and the seventh most common in American women. It occurs on the most readily visible organ of the body, and the cure rate is excellent when lesions are excised when still superficial. Unfortunately, metastatic melanoma is rarely curable. There is some evidence that sunscreen application may decrease squamous cell carcinomas, although the data is conflicting regarding all types of skin cancers. It is possible that use of sunscreen is associated with patients who then pursue more sun exposure, and some studies therefore suggest an *increased* incidence. However, evidence strongly correlates sun (and other UV) exposure with development of skin cancers, and avoidance of peak sun exposure (midday sun) when possible is prudent. A sunscreen with an SPF of at least 15 should be liberally applied, especially when peak sun exposure occurs between 10 AM and 4 PM and reapplied appropriately. Protective clothing, hats, and sunglasses with UVA and UVB protection may also be helpful. Tanning booths should be avoided. The USPTF has not recommended for or against routine screening for skin cancer in patients without a prior history. However, a whole-body skin exam (most easily done by referral to a dermatologist) may be prudent yearly for select high-risk patients. Public education about sun avoidance, sunscreen use, identification of suspicious lesions, and careful self-screening exams are the patient's best tools for reducing the incidence and mortality of melanoma.

Epidemiology and Risk Factors

The incidence of melanoma has been steadily increasing (3–7%/yr in people of European dsscent) over the past decades, with a current incidence of 14–15/100,000. Prevalence is highest in white individuals of European descent, and a white American's lifetime risk of developing melanoma is 1 in 85. **Known risk factors** include sun exposure, presence of large congenital nevi, dysplastic nevi, or multiple nevi; family or personal history of melanoma; sunburns during childhood; fair complexion; and blue eye color.

CAUSES

Clinical Features and Natural History

The **ABCDE** mnemonic describes common characteristics of melanomas: *A*symmetry, *B*order irregularity, *C*olor variegation, *D*iameter >5 mm, *E*nlargement, or *E*levation. Bleeding and ulceration can occur and are associated with worse prognosis. Melanomas have historically been categorized by morphologic appearance. Superficial spreading melanomas are the most common morphologic type. They may have years of radial growth before vertical growth and metastasis occur. Other morphologic types include nodular melanoma, which has early vertical growth; lentigo maligna melanoma, which typically presents on the face of older persons; and acral lentiginous melanoma, which occurs on the palms, soles, and under the nails and is the most common presentation of melanoma in black individuals. Melanoma also rarely occurs in the eye or on mucosal surfaces.

EVALUATION

Diagnosis

Screening for potentially malignant skin lesions should be part of a comprehensive physical exam. In addition, patients at risk for melanoma should be encouraged to examine themselves regularly for new or changing skin lesions. Suspicious lesions should be examined by **excisional biopsy,** as other biopsy techniques (such as punch biopsy) may not provide crucial information about lesion thickness.

Staging

Staging is based on the **thickness of tumor** and the presence of **nodal or distant metastases.** It also incorporates presence or absence of **ulceration,** number of nodes involved, and the site of distant metastasis. (See reference 1 for the complete staging system.) A general simplification of the staging system is as follows:

* Stage I melanoma is a localized lesion <1 mm in thickness or a 1- to 2-mm-thick melanoma without ulceration.
* Stage II is localized and >2 mm in thickness or >1 mm thick with ulceration.
* In stage III melanoma, spread to regional lymph nodes has occurred.
* In stage IV disease, distant metastases are present.

MANAGEMENT

Localized Disease (Stages I and II)

Wide local excision is the standard treatment for stages I and II melanomas. Excision recommendations are 1-cm margins for lesions <1 mm in depth and 2-cm margins for lesions >1 mm in depth. **Sentinel lymph node biopsy** frequently is performed before wide local excision of lesions ≥ 1 mm to rule out subclinical lymph node metastases. After excision of stage I lesions, no further treatment is recommended. Patients with stage II lesions, especially those with lesions >4 mm, can be treated with **adjuvant chemotherapy** similar to that used for stage III disease.

Regional Disease (Stage III)

Patients with stage III melanoma can present with a positive sentinel lymph node biopsy, clinically palpable lymph nodes, or in-transit metastasis (i.e., melanoma in the skin or subcutaneous tissue sharing lymphatic drainage with the primary tumor). Preop workup for patients with regional disease includes chext x-ray, lactate dehydrogenase (LDH), and CT scans as clinically indicated. Treatment usually involves **lymph node dissection,** both for regional control of disease and for prognostic information, as the number of positive lymph nodes is predictive of survival. In-transit disease can be treated with **isolated limb perfusion** with melphalan. **Interferon-alpha** is the best-studied adjuvant therapy for stage III melanoma. Most studies have found improved relapse-free and/or overall survival in high-risk patients treated with adjuvant interferon-alpha for 1 yr after resection of the primary tumor and regional lymph nodes. Adjuvant therapy with vaccines derived from melanoma cells shows promise and is currently under study.

Distant Metastatic Disease (Stage IV)

The most common sites of **metastatic melanoma** are (in descending order of frequency) skin and lymph nodes, lung, liver, brain, bone, and intestine. Presence of visceral metastases (except those to lung) and presence of high LDH are associated with worse prognosis than metastases limited to skin, lymph nodes, or lung. Workup of patients with metastatic disease includes brain MRI, chest/abdomen/pelvis CT or PET scan, CBC, liver function tests, and LDH. **Chemotherapy has little impact on metastatic melanoma,** and survival in patients with distant metastases is poor. Resection of solitary skin, lung, or brain metastases can be considered. No chemotherapy regimen has consistently proved superior to single-agent dacarbazine (DTIC-Dome), which has a response rate of 14–20%, although many regimens, including immunotherapy with interleukin-2 and interferon, are under study. Of note, a small percentage of patients with metastatic melanoma have a dramatic response to interleukin-2, with durable complete remission of disease.

FOLLOW-UP

Patients with tumors <1 mm in depth should have follow-up with a dermatologist to screen for new or recurrent melanoma. Patients with tumors 1–4 mm in depth should have annual chest x-ray and LDH and dermatology follow-up. Patients with stage III melanoma should follow up with a medical oncologist and dermatologist and have semiannual chest x-ray, LDH, and CBC. Patients with metastatic disease will need close follow-up with a medical oncologist.

PROGNOSIS

Overall 5-yr survival for patients with melanoma is 90%, but survival falls off dramatically with increasing stage. Tumor thickness and presence or absence of ulceration are the most important prognostic factors in localized cutaneous melanoma. Lesions <1 mm in thickness without ulceration are associated with a 10-yr survival of almost 90%, whereas lesions >4 mm are associated with a 5-yr survival <60%. The prognosis of regional disease correlates with the number of positive lymph nodes, with median survival of 90 mos for one positive node and 15 mos for more than four positive nodes. The overall 5-yr survival for stage III disease is approximately 40%. Stage IV melanoma is associated with a median survival of 6–9 mos. Elevated LDH correlates with the presence of metastatic disease and confers a worse prognosis.

KEY POINTS TO REMEMBER

- Worldwide over the last 50 yrs, the incidence of melanoma has been increasing (currently 3–7%/yr in people of European descent.
- Skin lesions suspicious for melanoma should be removed by excisional biopsy to allow measurement of lesion depth.
- Prognosis of localized disease depends on the depth of the lesion. Most patients with stage I disease are cured with excision of the melanoma.
- Metastatic melanoma is poorly responsive to chemotherapy and rarely curable, although a few patients have a dramatic response to immunotherapy.

SUGGESTED READING

Arndt KA, et al. Melanoma. In: Koh HK, Barnhill RL, Rogers GS, eds. *Cutaneous medicine and surgery*. Philadelphia: WB Saunders, 1996;1576.

Green A, et al. Daily sunscreen application and betacarotene supplementation in prevention of basal-cell and squamous-cell carcinomas of the skin: a randomised controlled trial. *Lancet* 1999;354:723–729.

Kirkwood JM, Strawderman MH, Ernstoff MS, et al. Interferon alfa-2b adjuvant therapy of high-risk resected cutaneous melanoma: the Eastern Cooperative Oncology Group Trial EST 1684. *J Clin Oncol* 1996;14:7.

Lotze MT, et al. Melanoma. In: DeVita VT Jr, Hellman S, Rosenberg SA, eds. *Cancer: principles and practice of oncology*, 6th ed. Philadelphia: Lippincott Williams & Wilkins, 2001:2012–2069.

Up To Date. Primary prevention of melanoma. Available at: http://www.uptodateonline.com/application/topic.asp?file-skin_can/2052&type-A&selectedTitle-4~52. Accessed August 2003.

US Preventative Task Force Web Site. Skin cancer screening document. Available at: http://www.ahrg.gov/clinic/ajpmsupp/skcarr.htm. Accessed August 2003.

REFERENCE

1. Balch CM, Buzaid AC, Soong SJ, et al. Final version of the American Joint Committee on Cancer staging system for cutaneous melanoma. *J Clin Oncol* 2001;19:3635–3648.

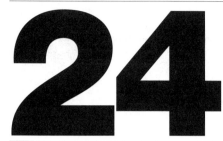

Head and Neck Cancer

Geoffrey L. Uy

Head and neck cancers are a diverse group of malignancies accounting for approximately 5% of newly diagnosed invasive malignancies per year. Because of the location of these tumors, these patients face unique problems with symptoms of the malignancy and in its treatment. Of these malignancies, 90% of non–salivary gland tumors arise from squamous epithelium. For this reason, salivary gland tumors are discussed separately.

SQUAMOUS HEAD AND NECK CANCERS

Epidemiology and Risk Factors

Head and neck cancers have a significant **male predominance** in terms of both mortality and incidence, with a >2:1 male to female predominance in new cases and deaths per yr. These tumors are estimated to account for approximately 40,000 new cases/yr, with an estimated 11,000 deaths/yr. The main **risk factors** for development of these malignancies are tobacco in any form and alcohol use. Tobacco and alcohol use increase the risk of cancer in a dose-dependent fashion and are synergistic in their effects. Sun exposure has been associated with an increased risk of carcinoma of the lip. **Nasopharyngeal carcinoma,** although rare in the United States, is endemic in the Far and Middle East and in Africa, accounting for 18% of newly diagnosed malignancies in Southeast China. In these areas, nasopharyngeal cancer is associated with Epstein-Barr virus infection in genetically predisposed individuals.

Pathophysiology

Malignancies of the head and neck are classified by their anatomic location, which is divided into (a) lip and oral cavity; (b) pharynx, which is subdivided into the nasopharynx, oropharynx, and hypopharynx; (c) larynx; (d) nasal cavity and sinuses; and (e) salivary glands. With the exception of salivary gland tumors, squamous cell carcinoma accounts for >90% of head and neck tumors.

Clinical Presentation

Most head and neck cancers are moderately advanced at the time of diagnosis, including tumors of the oral cavity that are easily accessible to inspection and exam by the patient and physician. The clinical presentation of these malignancies varies on the anatomic location of the tumor. **Cancers of the nasal cavity** can present with epistaxis, nonhealing ulcer, or obstruction. **Nasopharyngeal cancer** can present with a neck mass but may also have serous otitis media or cranial nerve involvement. **Oral cancers** usually present with a nonhealing ulcer. Leukoplakia and erythroplakia are frequently associated with dysplastic changes or invasive carcinoma. **Laryngeal cancers** can present with sore throat, odynophagia, referred ear pain, hoarseness, or enlarged neck nodes. The **Plummer-Vinson** syndrome, characterized by iron-deficiency anemia, mucosal atrophy, and esophageal webs, is frequently associated with carcinoma of the oral cavity and pharynx.

Initial Evaluation and Staging

- The **initial workup** of suspected head and neck cancers includes a careful inspection of the oral mucosa, including palpation of the floor of the mouth, tongue, and neck. Suspicious lesions are biopsied for histologic confirmation and grading. **Imaging studies** should include a chest radiograph, Panorex x-ray, and CT or MRI of the head and neck to help further delineate disease extent at presentation. **Panendoscopy,** including esophagoscopy with direct laryngoscopy, helps characterize the primary lesion and evaluates for possible second tumors, as there is a 10–15% incidence of synchronous primary tumors. Bronchoscopy may be useful but is not required in the evaluation for a second primary tumor.
- Staging for head and neck cancer is according to the American Joint Committee on Cancer TNM system, with different staging for oropharyngeal and laryngeal cancers.
- Occasionally, patients present with cervical lymphadenopathy **without an identifiable primary tumor.** In these cases, if fine-needle aspiration of the lymph node histology is consistent with squamous cell carcinoma, evaluation for an occult head and neck malignancy should be performed. See Chap. 33, Cancer of Unknown Primary Site, for further details.

Management

- Management of patients requires a **multidisciplinary** approach, including head and neck surgeons and radiation and medical oncologists. Radiation and surgery are the mainstays of treatment with head and neck cancers. Chemotherapy is reserved for patients with regionally advanced disease or as adjuvant therapy.
- **Single-modality treatment** with either surgery or definitive radiation treatment results in similar rates of disease control and survival in 40% of patients who present with **stage I or stage II** (node negative with tumor size <4 cm) disease. The choice of treatment modality depends on accessibility of the tumor and potential side effects of treatment.
- Most patients with head and neck cancers present with **locally advanced disease.** Patients with resectable disease undergo surgery followed by adjuvant radiation therapy. For patients with locally advanced, unresectable disease, treatment includes concurrent radiation and chemotherapy. Chemotherapeutic regimens usually combine cisplatin (Platinol, Platinol-AQ) with 5-fluorouracil (Efudex, Fluroplex). Research has been focused on combined modalities for patients with recurrent or metastatic disease; treatment with combined modalities is indicated for prolongation of life with palliation of symptoms.
- Treatment of **suspected or proven metastases** to cervical nodes involves a comprehensive dissection, removing all node groups. Newer, modified, radical procedures are able to remove cervical lymph node groups with selective preservation of the sternocleidomastoid, jugular vein, and spinal accessory nerves. Selective neck dissections are reserved for patients without clinical nodal disease but have a high risk of nodal disease based on the tumor size, grade, and location. Selective dissections are valuable in selecting candidates for adjuvant radiation therapy.
- A multidisciplinary approach is essential to minimize the **complications** of the malignancy and treatment. Speech pathologists are helpful, as surgical resection can lead to chronic aspiration and vocal cord dysfunction. Plastic surgeons and prosthodontists are often used to reduce cosmetic deformities of the tumor resection. Radiation treatment can result in xerostomia, mucositis, dysphagia, and odynophagia. In addition, a high incidence of hypothyroidism is seen in those who have received radiation to the entire thyroid or pituitary gland.
- Patients should have close follow-up for evaluation of local recurrence and distant metastases, as well as physical therapy and speech pathology follow-up if needed. In addition, patients should be advised on smoking and alcohol cessation.

SALIVARY GLAND TUMORS

Salivary gland tumors may arise either in major glands located in the parotid, sub-mandibular, and sublingual glands or in minor glands located in the oral mucosa, palate, uvula, floor of mouth, posterior tongue, retromolar area and peritonsillar area, pharynx, larynx, and paranasal sinuses. Salivary gland tumors account for approximately 5% of all head and neck cancers and are varied in their histologic patterns into low- or high-grade malignancies. Approximately 80% arise from the parotid gland, but of those, 80% are benign. In contrast, 95–100% of tumors arising from the sublingual gland are malignant. Treatment usually involves surgical resection of the gland. Prognosis is more favorable for low-grade tumors and those located in major glands, especially in the parotid. For aggressive or bulky tumors, resection is often combined with postoperative radiation.

KEY POINTS TO REMEMBER

- Alcohol and tobacco use in any form are the major risk factors for head and neck cancers.
- Single-modality treatment with either surgery or radiation therapy provides equivalent survival rates in early-stage (I or II) head and neck cancers.
- Salivary gland tumors most commonly arise from the parotid, of which 75–80% are benign.

REFERENCES AND SUGGESTED READINGS

Forastiere A, Koch W, Trotti A, et al. Head and neck cancer. *N Engl J Med* 2001;345:1890–1900.

Lewin F, Norell SE, Johansson H, et al. Smoking tobacco, oral snuff, and alcohol in the etiology of squamous cell carcinoma of the head and neck. *Cancer* 1998;82:1367–1375.

Mendenhall WM, Amdur RJ, Stringer SP, et al. Radiation therapy for squamous cell carcinoma of the tonsillar region: a preferred alternative to surgery? *J Clin Oncol* 2000;18:2219–2225.

Spiro RH. Salivary neoplasms: overview of a 35-year experience with 2,807 patients. *Head Neck Surg* 1986;8:177–184.

Vokes EE. Head and neck cancer. *Semin Oncol* 1994;21:279.

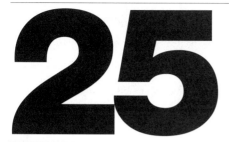

Sarcoma

Holly M. Magiera

INTRODUCTION

Sarcomas are a heterogeneous group of tumors comprised of cells of mesenchymal origin. Tumors of soft tissues include benign and malignant lesions, with benign being more common. Sarcomas are locally aggressive with variable ability to metastasize. There is a wide range of symptoms and signs associated with sarcoma, given the variable sites of origin. In general, sarcomas can be divided into soft tissue tumors and bone tumors.

SOFT TISSUE SARCOMA

Soft tissue sarcoma (STS) may arise from a variety of tissues, including muscle, fat, fibrous tissue, vessels, and peripheral nerve tissue.

Epidemiology

STS is a rare disease with approximately 5000–8000 new cases annually and an incidence of 2/100,000. They account for 1% of adult malignancies and 15% of childhood malignancies. There is an equal gender distribution. Approximately 60% of STS occurs in the extremities, with twice as many occurring in the lower extremities. 30% occur in the trunk/abdomen, and 10% occur in the head and neck. These tumors differ from carcinoma in that they do not develop *in situ* lesions and do not develop from preexisting benign lesions. Currently, *approximately 50% of patients* diagnosed with a sarcoma die of their disease. Metastatic disease is clinically present initially in only 10% of patients, but 40–60% of patients with large, deep, high-grade STS will eventually develop distant disease. Median survival once metastatic disease is diagnosed is 8–12 mos.

Pathophysiology

Most cases of STS are sporadic; however, a number of etiologic factors have been identified. **Radiation** is a risk factor, and the tumors tend to develop at least 3 yrs after treatment. Radiation-related sarcomas often are high grade, and the most frequent type is malignant fibrous histiocytoma. Certain **chemicals** have been implicated, including dioxin and thorotrast. **Genetic conditions** include syndromes such as neurofibromatosis I, Li-Fraumeni syndrome, and familial retinoblastoma. Lymphangiosarcoma has been associated with chronic edema, such as that resulting from a mastectomy. In addition, the majority of sarcomas have chromosomal aberrations, with t(x;18)(p11;q11) being common.

Clinical Presentation

Patients typically present with an **asymptomatic mass.** Patients often relate a history of trauma, but this is unlikely to have any etiologic significance. Low-grade sarcomas tend to grow slowly and may have been present for many years before presentation. High-grade sarcomas typically double q1–2mos and can become quite large over a short period. Patients may experience pain if there is entrapment of neurovascular structures or involvement of bone. Tumors in the hip girdle may present with lower-back pain, sciatica, diverticulitis, or other inflammatory processes. Retroperitoneal sarcomas presenting with abdominal mass and pain are present more often. Sarcomas may grow quite large before they are obvious on exam. **Physical exam** generally reveals a solid mass that may be deep or superficial. If a mass is >5 cm and deep, it should be presumed to be sarcoma until proven otherwise. High-grade sarcomas may have significant necrosis and can be confused with hematoma or abscess. Sarcoma may also present as extremity swelling due to compromise of venous flow, and patients may be initially diagnosed with the associated deep venous thrombosis.

Evaluation and Imaging

- Patients with masses suspicious for sarcoma should undergo **radiologic evaluation and biopsy.** The differential diagnosis includes benign soft tissue tumors as well as carcinoma, lymphoma, and melanoma. The most common benign tumors include lipoma, desmoid tumor, neurofibroma, hemangioma, and schwannoma.
- Sarcoma of the head and neck or extremities should be evaluated with **plain films** and with **MRI.** Plain films may reveal soft tissue mineralization (which is typical for synovial sarcoma) or may reveal skeletal reaction to the tumor. MRI is valuable for assessing fat and distinguishing it from surrounding tissues. This may assist in the diagnosis of the lesion and, in addition, it allows for planning of the biopsy and subsequent surgery. For retroperitoneal and abdominal sarcomas, CT is the imaging modality of choice. This also allows assessment of the liver, which is a frequent metastatic site for these tumors.
- In addition to evaluating the primary lesion with imaging, **distant metastatic disease** may also be assessed. STS spreads *hematogenously*, and the lung is the most common site of metastasis. Chest x-ray may be sufficient for small, low-grade lesions, but chest CT should be used for all others.

Biopsy

An accurate **biopsy** diagnosis is essential for STS. Any lesion >5 cm or a rapidly growing lesion should be biopsied. The placement of the biopsy tract is also critical, as it will be seeded with tumor and must be excised at the time of resection. Generally, the preferred technique is open incisional biopsy performed by a surgeon with experience in resection of STS. Hemostasis is also very important, as a hematoma may require enlarging radiation fields or may interfere with planned resection.

Pathology

Histologic evaluation should be performed at an experienced center, as **grade is critically important** to the prognosis. STSs are named for their tissue of origin based on light microscopy examination, and there are many possible histologic types. Tumors are also carefully evaluated for grade, which takes into account cellularity, mitotic activity, nuclear atypia, and necrosis. In general, the *grade, size,* and *depth* are more important factors than the histologic type. Immunohistochemistry studies are sometimes used to subclassify STS, and most tumors are positive for vimentin. The two most common types, malignant fibrous histiocytoma (MFH) and liposarcoma, have no specific positive stains. Rhabdomyosarcoma and leiomyosarcoma stain positively for desmin and actin. Epithelioid and synovial sarcomas are positive for cytokeratin. Malignant schwannomas are positive for S-100.

Histologic Subtypes

Subtype is generally not as important as other features, such as grade and size; however, STS is classified by tissue of origin. The three most common types are MFH, liposarcoma, and leiomyosarcoma.

Malignant Fibrous Histiocytoma
MFH is a tumor with peak incidence in the seventh decade. The most common site is the lower extremity. Superficial MFH is generally low grade with a good long-term survival. Deep MFH is high grade and has poor survival.

Liposarcoma

Liposarcoma tumor affects the middle aged and elderly with most cases between 50 and 65 yrs of age. The thigh and retroperitoneum are the most common locations. There are several subtypes with variable degrees of aggressiveness. Survival depends on grade.

Leiomyosarcoma

These may affect any age group and can be present in a diverse range of locations. One-half are retroperitoneal or intraabdominal. In general, these lesions are poorly responsive to chemotherapy and radiotherapy and have poor long-term survival.

Rhabdomyosarcoma

There are four subtypes of rhabdomyosarcoma. All are high grade and may occur in any age group. However, each subtype has a typical age of onset. Pleomorphic rhabdomyosarcoma is most common in those >30 yrs and typically involves the extremity. The alveolar subtype is common in adolescents and young adults and is very aggressive. Embryonal and botryoid variants occur primarily in children and are very sensitive to chemotherapy.

Synovial Sarcoma

Synovial sarcoma occurs mainly from the second to fourth decades. Patients present with hard, painful masses near joints. X-ray shows a typical calcification pattern. All synovial sarcomas are high grade and have high rates of local recurrence and lymph node metastasis.

Angiosarcoma

Hemangiosarcoma affect the elderly and are common in the head and neck, liver, and breast. They are highly aggressive tumors. Liver hemangiosarcoma is associated with thorotrast contrast. Lymphangiosarcoma is also aggressive and affects older adults. It is associated with chronic edema, such as that seen with mastectomy.

Kaposi's Sarcoma

Kaposi's sarcoma classically affects elderly men and is indolent in this subset of patients. Kaposi's sarcoma is also associated with AIDS and human herpes virus (HHV)-8 infection and, by contrast, is often very aggressive in this setting.

Mesothelioma

Mesothelioma develops in adults >50 yrs and is associated with asbestos exposure. Tumors aggressively encase viscera, and long-term survival is rare.

Neurofibrosarcoma

Neurofibrosarcoma tumors affect young and middle-aged adults and are associated with neurofibromatosis I. The superficial variant is low-grade and had good long-term survival. The deep variant is high grade and is locally aggressive and metastatic. It is associated with a worse prognosis.

Staging and Prognosis

The most important prognostic factors for STS include **size, grade, depth,** and **relationship to fascial planes.** American Joint Committee on Cancer guidelines are based on size, grade, site, and the presence of metastases. Stage IA includes small, low-grade sarcomas, and stage IB includes large, low-grade, superficial sarcomas. Stage IIA includes large, deep, low-grade lesions, and IIB includes small, high-grade lesions. Stage IIC includes large, superficial, high-grade lesions. Stage III includes large, deep, high-grade lesions, and stage IV includes metastatic sarcoma. Stage I carries a survival of 99%. Stage II has a survival of 82%. Stage III has a survival of 52%, and metastatic disease carries a survival of 20%.

Treatment

Surgical resection is the most effective therapeutic approach for STS, along with adjuvant radiation in many cases. In general, small, low-grade lesions may be treated by surgery alone. Larger and high-grade lesions require radiation therapy, which may be external beam or brachytherapy. Stage IV disease is generally treated with chemotherapy, although resection of limited pulmonary metastases has been used in some situations.

Surgery

Sarcomas grow along planes and grossly appear to be well-encapsulated. However, they usually extend into the pseudocapsule, and "shelling-out" of lesions is associated with high local failure rates. In the past, radical excision and amputation were common to avoid this problem.

- **Wide resection,** with a goal of 2–3 cm of normal surrounding tissue, is most commonly used along with radiation treatment in current practice. This type of resection and adjuvant radiation is associated with a 6–13% local failure rate. Large tumors often involve multiple compartments or may lie close to bone or neurovascular structures, and therefore wide excision may not be possible. In these situations, preop radiation is often used with attempted wide resection. Amputation is only required in approximately 5% of patients today. For retroperitoneal sarcomas, wide en bloc excision of tumor and involved organs is the only treatment proven to prolong survival. The ability to obtain free margins is the most important factor, but this may be difficult, as these tumors are often large and involve internal organs.
- **Local recurrence** may occur, typically within 5 yrs of treatment. Treatment in the past generally involved amputation, but today, combined conservative surgery and irradiation provide the best combination of local control and function. After resection of isolated local recurrence, patients may still have significant long-term survival, especially in low-grade tumors.
- **Metastasectomy** is occasionally used in patients with isolated pulmonary metastases. Approximately 20–30% of patients undergoing metastasectomy may have significant disease-free survival.

Radiation Therapy

Adjuvant radiation before or after surgery allows for more limb-sparing surgery with good local control. It is used for high-grade lesions and tumors >5 cm. **Postop radiation** is most routinely used. The dosage for radiation is in the range of 50–65 Gy, and the entire tumor bed with wide margins (5–10 cm) must be included. Complications include muscle and joint stiffness, fracture, and wound breakdown. **Preop radiation** is often used for lesions that are very close to neurovascular bundles or bone to allow for wide excision, which otherwise would not be feasible. It has similar rates of local control; however, it is associated with a higher incidence of wound complications. **Brachytherapy** is another alternative, with catheters placed at the time of surgery. It has similar rates of local control and the advantage of being shorter for the patient. In addition, smaller volumes of tissue are irradiated, which may be useful if important structures, such as joints, are nearby. Radiation therapy has *not* been proved to be of benefit in retroperitoneal sarcomas. Doses are often limited by adjacent organ toxicity, and it is not routinely used.

Chemotherapy

- The benefit of **adjuvant chemotherapy** in sarcoma is **controversial.** Four agents are active in sarcoma, including doxorubicin (Adriamycin, Doxil, Rubex), epirubicin (Ellence), ifosfamide (Ifex), and dacarbazine (DTIC-Dome). These agents have single-agent activity above 15–20%. Metaanalysis of 14 randomized controlled trials of doxorubicin-based chemotherapy showed a slight increase in overall survival for extremity STS. The analysis has several limitations, including inclusion of all types of STS and inclusion of low-grade tumors. It is possible that subgroups of patients, such as those with high-grade lesions, may benefit from treatment, and this is actively being investigated. Trials of combination chemotherapy have shown increased response rates but also increased toxicity without change in overall survival. Further studies are needed before adjuvant chemotherapy can be recommended routinely, with the exception of a few unique tumors, including primitive neuroectodermal tumor and rhabdomyosarcoma.
- **Systemic chemotherapy** is the main treatment for metastatic disease with the goal of palliation of symptoms. The same agents are used, with doxorubicin and ifosfamide being most active. Combination chemotherapy in these patients again results

in higher response rates but not overall survival advantage. Surgery and radiation therapy may also be used for palliation.

BONE SARCOMA

Bone sarcoma may arise from any tissue within the bones. The most common bone sarcomas are osteosarcoma, chondrosarcoma, and Ewing's sarcoma (ES).

Epidemiology

There are 2500 cases annually of bone sarcoma, and they account for 0.2% of malignancies. Bone sarcomas occur between the ages of 10 and 20 or from 40–60. They generally do not show a gender predominance. Benign bone lesions have the potential for malignant transformation.

Pathophysiology

Similar to STS, most bone sarcomas are sporadic. However, radiation is a known risk factor, particularly for osteosarcoma. Paget's disease is also associated with fibrosarcoma and osteosarcoma. Familial retinoblastoma is associated with osteosarcoma. ES is associated with t(11;22) chromosomal translocation.

Clinical Presentation and Diagnosis

Pain and swelling are the typical features on presentation. Patients may also present with pathologic fracture. ES may also be associated with systemic symptoms. Physical exam generally reveals a palpable mass. It is also important to consider that multiple malignancies are metastatic to bone and that history and physical should also be directed to evaluate this possibility. Patients who are suspected to have bone sarcoma should undergo imaging studies, including plain films and MRI and biopsy. On lab evaluation, patients with ES may demonstrate anemia. Elevated alkaline phosphatase may be seen in 60% of patients with bone sarcomas.

Imaging

Plain films may demonstrate characteristic lesions for bone sarcoma. Osteosarcoma is associated with destructive lesions showing a moth-eaten appearance. In addition, a spiculated periosteal reaction and cuff of periosteal new bone may be seen. Plain films in chondrosarcoma show lesions with a lobulated appearance with punctuate or annular calcification of cartilage. ES is associated with an "onion peel" periosteal reaction and soft tissue mass. Metastatic disease may be associated with either osteolytic or osteoblastic lesions, depending on the type of primary malignancy. **MRI** is the imaging modality of choice to evaluate the relationship of the tumor to surrounding structures and determine resectability. CT scan may also be used. Bone scan helps to evaluate for the local extent of the tumor as well as to evaluate for other lesions. CT scan of the chest is used to evaluate for pulmonary metastases.

Biopsy and Pathology

An accurate tissue biopsy is needed for diagnosis. Imaging studies may be suggestive of tumor type; however, it can be difficult to distinguish benign and malignant bone tumors. Biopsy specimens are used to determine the histologic type of tumor as well as the grade. As for STS, **open incisional biopsy is often preferred**. The biopsy should be performed by a surgeon experienced in sarcoma so that it does not compromise the definitive surgical procedure.

Histologic Subtypes

The treatment of bone sarcoma, in contrast to STS, is more dependent on histologic subtype.

Osteosarcoma

Osteosarcomas account for 40–50% of bone sarcomas and present with pain and swelling. They are spindle cell neoplasms that produce bone and are more common in long bones. Approximately 60% occur in adolescents and children. 10% may occur in the third decade. There is a second peak in the fifth and sixth decades, which is frequently due to radiation-associated osteosarcoma or transformation of existing lesions. There is a slight male predominance. The majority are classified as "classic," and this type is more common between 10 and 20 yrs. Most of these lesions are high grade and highly vascular. They are generally biopsied by a core biopsy or open biopsy.

Chondrosarcoma

Chondrosarcoma accounts for 20–25% of bone sarcomas. They generally occur between the fourth and sixth decades. They tend to develop in flat bones, including the shoulder and pelvic girdles. They may arise *de novo* or from preexisting lesions. They are indolent and are generally low grade. Chondrosarcoma may arise peripherally or centrally. Imaging studies may be bland, particularly in central lesions, which may make it difficult to distinguish between benign and malignant lesions. New pain, increasing size, and signs of inflammation point toward malignant lesions. In general, these malignancies are resistant to chemotherapy and radiation. However, they may dedifferentiate into MFH or osteosarcoma, which are more sensitive to chemotherapy.

Ewing's Sarcoma

ES accounts for 10–15% of bone sarcomas, and incidence peaks in the second decade. The femoral diaphysis is the most common location, but they may arise in many bones. They are highly aggressive tumors and are best considered a systemic disease. A characteristic chromosomal translocation, t(11:22), is associated with this sarcoma and with peripheral primitive neuroectodermal tumor.

Staging

Bone sarcomas are staged according to criteria set forth by the Musculoskeletal Tumor Society. This system is based on grade and compartmental localization. Stage I refers to low-grade tumors and stage II refers to high-grade tumors. Stage III is used for metastatic disease. Type A designates an intracompartmental lesion, and B designates an extracompartmental lesion. The American Joint Committee on Cancer staging system is an alternative system and is based on grade, tumor size, and metastatic disease [1].

Treatment and Prognosis

Treatment depends on the histologic type of sarcoma as well as the grade. Lower-grade lesions may be treated by surgery alone, but high-grade lesions require multi-modality therapy. Physical therapy and prosthetics are of great importance in these patients because of the highly invasive nature of the treatment.

Osteosarcoma

These tumors generally have micrometastases at presentation, although <20% have measurable metastases. **Standard treatment** includes preoperative chemotherapy, limb-sparing surgery, and adjuvant chemotherapy. With this type of treatment, long-term survival is possible in 60–80% of patients. The most effective agents in osteosarcoma include doxorubicin, ifosfamide, etoposide (Etopophos, Toposar, VePesid), cisplatin, and high-dose methotrexate. Response to chemotherapy is the most important prognostic factor in this disease. Preop chemotherapy allows for tumor shrinkage, which allows for limb-sparing surgery and prostheses to be used more often. In addition, the response to chemotherapy can be assessed. **Radiation therapy is generally not used** in osteosarcoma, as these tumors are relatively radioresistant. However, tumors of the jaw and face are sometimes treated with radiation, as are tumors that cannot be completely resected. **Prognosis** is dependent on tumor size and location, in addition to response to chemotherapy. Small, distal, appendicular tumors have a better prognosis than larger, axial tumors. In addition, elevated lactate dehydrogenase and alkaline phosphatase are associated with poor prognosis.

Chondrosarcoma

Complete resection of the lesion with limb-sparing procedures is the treatment of choice. The ability to fully resect the tumor is the most important prognostic factor. As these tumors are resistant to radiation and chemotherapy, these modalities are not used in treatment. Long-term survival is approximately 50%. If tumors dedifferentiate into osteosarcoma or MFH, they become more responsive to systemic therapy, and these patients may benefit from chemotherapy. Mesenchymal chondrosarcoma is a subtype that is treated similarly to ES.

Ewing's Sarcoma

Multimodality treatment is used for ES. This disease is highly aggressive and is considered systemic, so chemotherapy is the mainstay of treatment. Local control is achieved by limb-sparing surgery or by radiation therapy. Active agents include vincristine (Oncovin, Vincasar PFS), cyclophosphamide (Cytoxan, Neosar), and doxorubicin. Ifosfamide and etoposide are also useful agents. Combination chemotherapy is used to treat ES and results in a long-term survival of approximately 70%. Response to chemotherapy is an important prognostic factor, as are size and location. For tumors that are below the elbow or mid-calf, long-term survival is approximately 80%. The prognosis for the 20–30% of patients with metastatic disease at presentation remains poor.

Metastatic Bone Sarcoma

The goal for patients with advanced disease is **palliation** of symptoms. Surgery may be used for painful, functionless extremities. In addition, resection of solitary pulmonary metastases may provide survival benefit. Radiation therapy may also be used for palliation, although there is variability in response. Combination chemotherapy is also useful for palliation, particularly in ES and osteosarcoma.

KEY POINTS TO REMEMBER

- STSs are a rare, heterogeneous group of tumors best treated by experts.
- Treatment of STS consists mainly of limb-sparing surgery and radiation, with chemotherapy having a less defined role.
- Bone sarcoma is rare, and treatment depends on histologic subtype more than treatment in STS.

SUGGESTED READING

Bramwell V. Adjuvant chemotherapy for adult soft tissue sarcoma. *J Clin Oncol* 2001;19(5):1235–1237.

DeVita VT, Hellman S, Rosenberg SA, eds. *Cancer: principles and practice of oncology*, 6th ed. Philadelphia: Lippincott Williams & Wilkins, 2001.

Fauci AS, et al. *Harrison's principles of internal medicine*, 14th ed. New York: McGraw-Hill, 1998:744–747.

Ferguson WS, Goorin AM. Current treatment of osteosarcoma. *Cancer Invest* 2001;19(3):292–315.

Pirayesh A, Chee Y, Helliwell TR, et al. The management of retroperitoneal soft tissue sarcomas. *Eur J Surg Oncol* 2001;27:491–497.

Rougraff B. The diagnosis and management of soft tissue sarcomas of the extremities in the adult. *Curr Probl Cancer* 1999;23:7–41.

Sarcoma Meta-Analysis Collaboration. Adjuvant chemotherapy for localized resectable STS of adults. *Lancet* 1997;350:1647–1654.

Wunder JS, et al. A comparison of staging systems for localized extremity soft tissue sarcoma. *Cancer* 2000;88:2721–2730.

REFERENCE

1. Beech DJ, Pollock RE. Surgical management of primary soft tissue sarcoma. *Hematol Oncol Clin North Am* 1995;9(4):707–718.

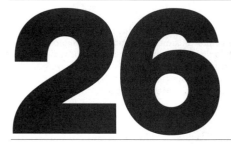

Endocrine Malignancies

Matthew A. Ciorba and
Benjamin B. B. Brennan

INTRODUCTION

Endocrine neoplasms may develop in any of the endocrine organs or in the amine precursor uptake and decarboxylation cells. Overall, this heterogenous group represents only 1.5% of noncutaneous malignancies. However, certain population subsets, such as those who inherit one of the autosomal dominant multiple endocrine neoplasia (MEN) syndromes, are predisposed to developing these relatively rare cancers. Clinical presentations of endocrine tumors vary, but, in general, patients do not uniformly have an associated clinical endocrinopathy. This chapter discusses the MEN syndromes, thyroid carcinoma, carcinoid tumors, and pheochromocytoma.

MULTIPLE ENDOCRINE NEOPLASIA SYNDROMES

MEN syndromes are a group of rare genetic disorders that confer an increased risk of malignancy of endocrine tissues. These disorders are grouped by the major cell types of malignancy that the affected patients are at risk for developing (Table 26-1).

Summaries

MEN I (Wermer's Syndrome)
The mutation is located at the 11q13 interval and codes for a tumor suppressor gene. Inheritance of the mutation is autosomal dominant. Morbidity and mortality are predominately related to duodenopancreatic malignancies.

MEN IIA (Sipple's Syndrome) and MEN IIB
There is autosomal dominant inheritance of an activating mutation of the *ret* oncogene, which is located on chromosome 10. Nearly all patients develop medullary thyroid carcinoma (MTC), which is typically multifocal, bilateral, and occurs at a young age. Other features of these syndromes are expressed variably.

Familial Non-MEN Medullary Thyroid Carcinoma (FMTC)
This disease is also associated with autosomal dominant inheritance of the *ret* oncogene; however, these patients develop MTC without other abnormalities associated with MEN II syndromes. Patients with MEN IIA and FMTC almost invariably develop MTC at an early age, and, therefore, prophylactic thyroidectomy should be considered in patients with a known mutation.

THYROID CARCINOMA

Multiple histologic subtypes of thyroid cancer exist. Together, they account for >90% of all endocrine malignancies. Thyroid cancer is nearly twice as common in women as in men. Previous **radiation exposure** is the main known risk factor in developing well-differentiated thyroid malignancy and has an average lag time of 25 yrs to cancer presentation. The former use of radiation in treatment of benign childhood conditions during the early- to mid-20th century likely, in part, accounts for the increase in follic-

TABLE 26-1. FEATURES OF THE MULTIPLE ENDOCRINE NEOPLASIA (MEN) SYNDROMES

Syndrome	Associated tumors and abnormalities
MEN I	Pituitary adenomas
	Pancreatic islet cell tumors or duodenal (35–75%)
	Parathyroid hyperplasia (90%)
MEN IIA	Medullary carcinoma of thyroid
	Pheochromocytoma (bilateral)
	Parathyroid hyperplasia
MEN IIB	Medullary carcinoma of thyroid
	Pheochromocytoma (bilateral)
	Multiple mucosal ganglioneuromas
	Colonic and skeletal abnormalities with marfanoid body habitus
FMTC	Medullary carcinoma of thyroid

FMTC, familial non-MEN medullary thyroid carcinoma.

ular carcinomas seen since 1970. Cancers of the **parafollicular cells,** termed **MTC,** are not known to be related to radiation exposure and can occur sporadically (2/3) or in individuals who inherit either the MENII or NMTC syndrome (1/3). Although the behavior of thyroid cancer can be variable, the course is usually indolent. Thus, if the cancer is discovered early, cure rates are high (Table 26-2).

TABLE 26-2. THYROID CANCER HISTOLOGIC SUBTYPES AND KEY FEATURES

Histologic subtype	% of all thyroid cancers	Characteristics
Well-differenti-ated		Typically affect younger patients. Course is relatively benign and indolent. Metastases occur late and to bone, lungs, cervical lymph nodes, and skin. Surgery and radioactive iodine are treatments of choice.
Papillary	70	Psammoma bodies present on histology in 50%.
Follicular	12–20	Hürthle cell variety is more aggressive form.
Anaplastic (spindle cell)	2	Typically affect older patients and may arise from differentiated thyroid carcinomas or from a multinodular goiter. Aggressive tumors with local invasion common and always considered stage IV. Metastases to lung common, and advanced disease is uniformly fatal. External beam radiation is marginally effective.
Medullary thyroid carcinoma	5–9	Neoplasia of the parafollicular/C cells for which sporadic and inherited forms exist. Secrete calcitonin and occasionally ACTH. May cause diarrhea in advanced disease. Metastases to inferior surface of liver capsule typical. Treatment is surgical.

Diagnosis and Evaluation

- Evaluation of the **thyroid nodule** is a relatively common medical issue. The majority of thyroid nodules are benign, and the history and exam assist in directing further investigation. For all cases presenting, the chance of a thyroid nodule being malignant is 5–10%. The risk of malignancy is increased in men, individuals younger than 20 or older than 45, those with a positive family history, or those having previous radiation exposure either by medical treatment or from nuclear radiation accidents. A solitary nodule or rapid change in size is also of greater concern, as are symptoms of hoarseness, dyspnea, dysphagia, or a new Horner's syndrome. **Physical exam** should evaluate size, firmness, mobility, and local lymphadenopathy. Symptoms of diarrhea or flushing are occasionally seen in advanced MTC due to hormone secretion. Nodules <1 cm in a patient without other risk factors may be followed with repeat exam in 6–12 mos. However, nodules >1 cm or any size nodule in a patient with one of the previously listed risk factors warrants further evaluation.
- **Histologic evaluation** is essential to diagnosis and is initially obtained by fine-needle aspiration biopsy. This tool, sometimes guided by U/S, is used to obtain a cytologic sample that is subsequently classified on a spectrum from benign to malignant. If malignancy cannot be excluded (in 6–30% of fine-needle aspiration samples) a lobectomy is usually performed to obtain adequate tissue and to determine correct diagnosis.
- Radioactive isotope **scans** and **serologic testing** with TSH and serum thyroglobulin assays are only useful in postop follow-up and not useful in making the diagnosis of thyroid malignancy. Calcitonin levels, however, should be checked at presentation and at follow-up exams for patients with MTC, as it serves as a sensitive tumor marker. In addition, those with MTC need to be evaluated for the *RET* protooncogene mutation and submit a 24-hr urine for vanillylmandelic acid, catecholamines, and metanephrines to evaluate for possible pheochromocytoma.
- Once the diagnosis of malignancy is made, all individuals should have a chest x-ray to evaluate for **metastases** to the lung. An extensive staging workup is necessary only in anaplastic thyroid cancers, as they are often metastatic at presentation. Patients with anaplastic tumors should receive complete imaging of the neck with U/S or MRI and have a contrast CT scan of the chest, and consideration should be given to abdominal imaging with a CT or MRI.

Staging and Survival

- The **staging** of thyroid cancer depends on tumor histology, size, and patient age at presentation. In MTC staging, information comes from evaluation of the total thyroidectomy and ipsilateral cervical lymph node dissection. For patients <45 yrs, well-differentiated papillary or follicular cell carcinomas are never classified higher than stage II, which correlates with metastatic disease. On the other hand, anaplastic tumors are classified as stage IV regardless of anatomic extent due to their aggressive nature and high potential for metastasizing. Staging of MTC is based on tumor size, local or nodal involvement, and the presence of metastases.
- Overall, the **course** for most of these neoplasms is indolent, but some subsets of follicular and papillary tumors may be more aggressive or undergo transformation to an anaplastic carcinoma. Well-differentiated thyroid carcinomas have an excellent prognosis. Cure rates reach nearly 100% at 10 yrs, even with capsular invasion, as long as there is no vascular involvement. However, in individuals >45 yrs with distant metastases, disease is classified as stage IV, and 20-yr disease specific mortality is >75%. Anaplastic tumors carry a grim prognosis, often leading rapidly to death within the first few years after diagnosis regardless of treatment. MTCs have 5-yr survival rates >80% in stages I and II disease but <40% with stage III or IV disease.

Management

Treatment of the three main types of thyroid cancer varies significantly. Radioactive iodine, external beam radiation, surgery, and systemic chemotherapy each have their role in comprehensive therapeutic regimens. The details of specific tumor-directed therapy are addressed below.

- **Surgical resection** is the standard of care in all stages of well-differentiated (follicular and papillary) tumors. Patients younger than 40 have an excellent prognosis with thyroidectomy alone. Factors increasing the chance of recurrence include advanced age and tumor size >1 cm. For these patients, a total thyroidectomy is recommended. Although it is uncommon if performed by an experienced surgeon, recurrent laryngeal nerve damage resulting in hoarseness is a risk of thyroid lobectomy. A total thyroidectomy carries the additional risk of **hypocalcemia** from hypoparathyroidism.
- In more advanced disease, dissection of the central and lateral cervical lymph nodes should be considered. However, the increased morbidity is often not compensated for by a substantial effect on prognosis. Residual disease should be treated with radioactive iodine therapy. Even with spread to bone or lung, a cure may be attained with one or more administrations of iodine-131 (^{131}I), as long as the tumor is of low volume. Chemotherapeutic agents, including platinum, taxane-based regimens, and doxorubicin, have all been attempted but are rarely administered because they are typically less effective and have a worse side-effect profile than radioactive iodine.
- Short-wave beta **radiation** from ^{131}I induces cytotoxicity and is the key **chemotherapeutic agent.** There are two main indications for use of ^{131}I. The first is to ablate residual normal thyroid tissue post–total thyroidectomy to improve the sensitivity of subsequent diagnostic ^{131}I scans in detecting recurrence. Second, it is used to treat metastatic disease and destroy microscopic malignant foci. Radioactive iodine therapy requires withdrawal of thyroid hormone for ≥ 2 wks until TSH levels reach 30 mU/L before administration. Follow-up imaging with ^{131}I determines treatment efficacy by revealing residual normal thyroid tissue as well as carcinoma. Treatment ends when there is no further radioactive iodine uptake present. Recent studies show that, for follow-up diagnostic scans, a two-dose regimen of exogenously administered recombinant TSH effectively mimic hormone withdrawal for imaging purposes, but not for treatment.
- **Adjuvant therapy** with exogenous thyroid hormone is routinely used in well-differentiated thyroid carcinomas to suppress TSH. Both normal and neoplastic thyroid tissue depend on TSH for growth. Thyroid hormone is also necessary to prevent symptoms of hypothyroidism. One should keep in mind, however, the potential side effects of higher rates of bone loss and an increased incidence of atrial fibrillation during this period. **Suppression of TSH** to undetectable levels for the initial 5–10 yrs is reasonable. After this time, if there is no evidence of recurrent disease, exogenous thyroid hormone supplementation may be decreased such that the TSH levels rise to the lower limits of normal.
- **Radiation therapy** rarely has a role in differentiated thyroid carcinomas. Routine patient **follow-up** with physical exam, TSH, thyroglobulin level measurement, and chest x-ray is recommended twice yearly until 4 yrs out, then every year until 10 yrs. Thyroglobulin levels are expected to be <5 ng/mL if complete thyroid ablation has been successful.
- **Anaplastic thyroid carcinoma** is poorly responsive to therapy and is often locally invasive if not metastatic at the time of presentation. These poor prognostic features of anaplastic carcinomas mean that their staging is always assigned as stage IV at diagnosis regardless of size, grade, node involvement, or metastasis. 10-year survival rates are approximately 13% in patients with anaplastic cancers. The invasive nature makes tumor resection difficult or even impossible. At initial presentation, tumor may encompass the carotid arteries, esophagus, and/or trachea. Recurrent or superior laryngeal nerve damage may also occur. The complications of local invasion account for the major morbidity of this cancer, often leading patients to require gastrostomy tubes or a tracheostomy. If the imaging reveals limited disease, resection should be pursued for improved local control and delay of these complications, although survival is not altered. Radiation therapy is a necessary component of treatment, and administration should be undertaken concurrently with systemic radiosensitizing chemotherapy. Doxorubicin is the most commonly used agent, and anaplastic tumors are rarely responsive to radioactive iodine. End-stage care typically includes managing local complications, and approximately 50% of patients die from local airway obstruction.

- Surgical resection is the mainstay of therapy for MTC. Although MTC is somewhat indolent in its progression, no effective systemic chemotherapy regimens exist. For this reason, patients with genetic predisposition to the disease should be highly encouraged to undergo *prophylactic total thyroidectomy* with *central lymph node dissection.* Surgical techniques vary, but many surgeons chose to remotely autograft the parathyroid glands during the operation to avoid hypoparathyroidism. **Complications** of local MCT invasion mirror those of anaplastic tumors, yet progression is less rapid. Doxorubicin (Adriamycin, Doxil) is the most effective cytotoxic chemotherapeutic agent, but any objective response is seen in <40% of patients, with no patients having a complete response.

CARCINOID TUMORS

Carcinoid tumors are the most common neuroendocrine tumors. Benign and malignant tumors occur in approximately equal frequency, and either type may be symptomatic. Although overall relatively rare, they are important, as some secrete various vasoactive substances, including histamine, serotonin, catecholamines, and prostaglandins. The small bowel is the most common location for these tumors, but they may occur in the lung, stomach, or ovary as well. Symptomatic carcinoid tumors usually result from small bowel tumors with metastases to the liver. This is termed the **carcinoid syndrome**, which is due to excessive production of serotonin and other bioactive compounds that then have direct access to the systemic circulation.

Natural History

>95% of GI carcinoids arise from the rectum, appendix, or small intestine. The appendiceal and small (<1 cm) rectal tumors rarely metastasize, cause symptoms, or affect survival. Small bowel tumors are more likely to be problematic. One-third of small intestine tumors are multicentric, and the chance of metastases increases with increased tumor size. In general, the progression of small intestinal carcinoid tumors is indolent. However, once metastasis of tumor cells occurs, prognosis is considerably worse. 5-yr survival with localized disease, only nodal involvement, and finally with liver metastases are approximately 95%, 65%, and 20%, respectively. Urinary 5-hydroxyindoleacetic acid levels inversely correlate with survival.

Diagnosis

Approximately 40% of carcinoid tumors found in living patients are hormonally active, leading to the **carcinoid syndrome.** Symptoms may include facial flushing and edema, abdominal cramping and diarrhea, bronchospasm, hypotension, and cardiac valvular lesions (typically on the tricuspid and/or pulmonic valve if the tumor secretions originate in the bowel.) Alcohol, stress, or exercise may precipitate symptoms. Tumors that are not endocrinologically active can also cause devastating effects such as bowel obstruction, appendicitis, or painful liver metastases. An **elevated 24-hr urinary 5-hydroxyindoleacetic acid test** is the key **lab test** for diagnosis. Levels >25 mg/day are the typical finding, whereas the normal value of excretion is <9 mg/day. Before testing, patients should avoid excessive intake of nuts, bananas, avocados, and pineapples for approximately 2 days, as these may result in erroneously high levels. Other routine tests should be aimed at identifying tumor location. Routine blood tests, with attention to LFTs, hepatic, and upper GI system imaging; a chest x-ray; and eventual tissue acquisition should all be part of the workup. If available, somatostatin receptor scintigraphy is a useful imaging test.

Treatment and Management

As survival with untreated carcinoid tumors can exceed 10 yrs, therapy is usually focused on controlling symptoms. **Dietary** tryptophan restriction along with serotonin antagonists and other symptom-controlling drugs are the initial mainstays of therapy.

The somatostatin analog **octreotide (Sandostatin)** used at doses of 100–600 μg SC/day in 2–4 divided doses is effective at symptom alleviation in nearly 90% of patients. A depot formulation of octreotide available in monthly dosing has become standard. Histamine (H_1 and H_2) blockers, prochlorperazine (Compazine), and cyproheptadine (Periactin) (4–6 mg qid) may decrease flushing. Atropine, diphenoxylate, and cyproheptadine can be used for diarrhea. MAOIs are contraindicated. **Surgery** can be risky, as anesthesia often precipitates attacks. However, resection is indicated and highly successful in localized carcinoid tumors. Preop administration of octreotide is necessary to prevent carcinoid crisis. **Radiation** and various **chemotherapy** regimens are typically reserved for symptomatic control of metastases in advanced disease.

PARATHYROID CARCINOMA

Epidemiology

Although adenomas of the parathyroid glands are a common endocrine abnormality, parathyroid carcinoma is quite rare. Primary hyperparathyroidism is categorized pathologically into three groups: a single parathyroid adenoma (83–85%), multiglandular hyperplasia (15%), and parathyroid carcinoma (0.5–3%). When compared to benign hyperparathyroidism found in the postmenopausal female population, parathyroid carcinoma is found equally in both genders at younger ages. With an incidence of only 0.015/100,000 population, parathyroid cancer is classified as one of the most rare human cancers. Although no etiologic causes are known, parathyroid cancer is documented in the autosomal dominant disease of MEN I.

Clinical Features and Diagnosis

Patients with parathyroid carcinoma often present initially with either hypercalcemia or a neck mass. On physical exam, 30–50% of patients with parathyroid carcinoma have palpable masses in the central neck region. A hyperfunctional parathyroid tumor leads to excessive production of parathyroid hormone, and ultimately the clinical syndrome of primary hyperparathyroidism. Clinical signs and symptoms include fatigue, renal stones, and bone disease. Grossly elevated calcium levels lead to nausea, vomiting, polyuria, and dehydration. Cytologic detail is considered an unreliable criterion for diagnosis of malignancy. Definitive diagnosis of parathyroid carcinoma is made in the operating room where local invasion and metastasis can be assessed.

Staging

Owing to the low incidence of new cases, the American Joint Committee on Cancer has not outlined a staging system for parathyroid carcinoma. Local invasion is determined during surgery, and the technetium-sestamibi scan can be useful preoperatively for localization purposes.

Management

Surgical exploration of the neck with complete resection of the tumor along with the ipsilateral thyroid lobe and central cervical lymph nodes is the mainstay of treatment. There is no effective adjuvant therapy. Likewise, the only effective therapy for recurrent or metastatic disease is complete resection. The value of **radiation therapy** is under scrutiny. The management of severe **hypercalcemia** includes saline hydration, furosemide diuresis, and bisphosphonates. Octreotide as well as calcimimetic agents are occasionally used to lower calcium in patients refractory to other therapeutic interventions.

PHEOCHROMOCYTOMA

Pheochromocytomas arise from chromaffin cells primarily in the adrenal medulla (90%), although they can also arise along the aorta, within the carotid body, intracardiac, and even within the urinary bladder. This widespread distribution reflects the location of chromaffin cells associated with the sympathetic ganglia.

Epidemiology

Pheochromocytoma is present in only 0.1% of hypertensive patients who undergo urinary catecholamine quantification. The incidence of malignancy in pheochromocytomas ranges from 5–45% in several series. Extraadrenal tumors may be more commonly malignant. Pheochromocytomas are associated with several inherited disorders. Bilateral adrenal medullary pheochromocytomas are elements of the inherited MEN IIA and MEN IIB neuroendocrine syndromes. Although approximately 25% of patients with von Hippel-Lindau disease develop pheochromocytomas, <1% of patients with neurofibromatosis and Von Recklinghausen's disease are found to have the tumor.

Clinical Features

The most common presenting complaint of patients with pheochromocytomas is severe HTN unrelated to physical or emotional stress. The production of catecholamines result in the clinical symptoms of episodic or sustained HTN and anxiety attacks. Pheochromocytoma have been known to produce other hormones, including ACTH, somatostatin, calcitonin, oxytocin, and vasopressin. Classically, patients describe spells of HTN, palpitations, headaches, and diaphoresis. Other presenting complaints include lactic acidosis, hypovolemia, or unexplained fever. Clinically, the cluster of symptoms can be recalled by remembering the five "Ps": pain, pressure, palpitation, perspiration, and pallor. However, it should be appreciated that many patients do not exhibit these "classic" episodes and may also have persistent HTN, rather than episodic. The "rule of 10" is also useful in recognizing general features of pheochromocytomas: 10% are malignant, 10% are extraadrenal, and 10% are bilateral.

Diagnosis

Diagnosis and localization of pheochromocytomas are critical, as death secondary to hypertensive crisis, cerebrovascular accident, or myocardial infarction is associated with this relatively rare tumor. Pheochromocytomas represent a potentially curable cause of HTN with tumor resection. Traditionally, diagnosis has been based on a 24-hr measurement of **catecholamines** and **metabolites,** including vanillylmandelic acid and metanephrines in the urine. New data suggest that a **random plasma metanephrine** level is extremely sensitive (approximately 99%) in diagnosing pheochromocytoma and is thus an excellent test choice for initial screening. Although rarely used in clinical practice today, the clonidine suppression test has been used in the past. Normally, clonidine suppresses plasma levels of epinephrine and norepinephrine. In the presence of pheochromocytomas, no such suppression is observed.

Management

- After diagnosis, tumor localization and operative preparation is indicated, as **surgical resection** represents the mainstay of curative therapy. Localization of a pheochromocytoma is accomplished by chest and abdominal imaging with CT or MRI. Nuclear scanning after the administration of labeled metaiodobenzylguanidine can be done if the tumor is not localized by either of these other methods. Metaiodobenzylguanidine is structurally similar to norepinephrine and is selectively taken up by adrenergic tissue.
- **Preop alpha-adrenergic blockade** is necessary for patients with pheochromocytomas. Traditionally, phenoxybenzamine has been used to control HTN. Propranolol may be used to control tachycardia but must always follow alpha-adrenergic blockade to avoid hypertensive exacerbation due to unopposed vasoconstriction. Intraop, hypertensive episodes are controlled with alpha-adrenergic blockers or sodium nitroprusside.

- **Malignant pheochromocytomas** are difficult to distinguish from benign pheochromocytomas by pathology alone. Natural history, secondary tumor sites, and recurrence help determine the nature of the pheochromocytoma. Aggressive disease may require combination chemotherapy with cyclophosphamide, vincristine, and dacarbazine. Some authorities recommend routine BP and urinary catecholamine measurements in addition to a regularly scheduled CT, MRI, or metaiodobenzylguanidine scanning to monitor for recurrence.

KEY POINTS TO REMEMBER

- Endocrine malignancies are on a whole uncommon and do not necessarily result in a clinical endocrinopathy.
- Thyroid cancer is certainly the most common endocrine cancer and is divided into subtypes based on original cellular histology as well as level of differentiation.
- Papillary and follicular tumors generally have an excellent prognosis in the young. These individuals can frequently be cured via surgery and radioactive iodine administrations, if necessary. Negative prognostic indicators include age >45 and distant spread.
- Anaplastic tumors are the undifferentiated versions of papillary and follicular tumors. These very aggressive cancers carry a poor prognosis, as treatment options are almost never curative.
- Medullary thyroid cancers derive from the parafollicular cells and produce calcitonin. Both sporadic and inherited forms exist. Individuals in whom genetic testing indicates MEN II or NMTC should be advised to undergo prophylactic thyroidectomy. This is typically done at a very young age, often at younger than 1.
- Carcinoid tumors may secrete vasoactive hormones. The liver can usually process and deactivate these hormones. However, when metastases reach the liver, a collection of symptoms, including flushing, edema, bronchospasm, and diarrhea, may result. This is termed the carcinoid syndrome.
- Pheochromocytoma is a rare neuroendocrine tumor. It may present with a severe hypertensive episode, palpitations, diaphoresis, headaches, and/or skin pallor. Surgery is the primary therapy, although adjuvant chemotherapy is occasionally used.
- Parathyroid carcinoma is extremely rare and typically presents with a neck mass and/or with symptoms of hypercalcemia. Diagnosis and treatment are dependent on surgery.

REFERENCES AND SUGGESTED READINGS

Brandi ML, Gagel RF, Angeli A, et al. Consensus: guidelines for diagnosis and therapy of MEN type 1 and type 2. *J Clin Endocrinol Metab* 2001;86:5658–5671.

Braunwald E, Fauci A, et al., eds. *Harrison's principles of internal medicine*, 15th ed. New York: McGraw-Hill, 2001.

DeVita VT, Hellman S, Rosenberg SA, eds. *Cancer: principles and practice of oncology*, 6th ed. Philadelphia: Lippincott Williams & Wilkins, 2001.

Hundahl SA, Fleming ID, Fremgen AM, et al. Two hundred eighty-six cases of parathyroid carcinoma treated in the US between 1985–1995. A National Cancer Data Report. *Cancer* 1999;86:538.

Kearns A, Thompson G. Medical and surgical management of hyperparathyroidism. *Mayo Clinic Proc* 2002;77:87–91.

Kulke MH, Mayer RJ. Carcinoid tumors. *N Engl J Med* 1999;340:858.

Mann SJ. Severe paroxysmal hypertension (pheochromocytoma): understanding the cause and treatment. *Arch Intern Med* 1999;159:670.

Pacak K, Linehan WM, Eisenhofer G, et al. NIH Conference. Recent advances in genetics, diagnosis, localization, and treatment of pheochromocytoma. *Ann Intern Med* 2001;134:315–329.

Schlumberger MJ. Papillary and follicular thyroid carcinoma *N Engl J Med* 1998;338:297–306.

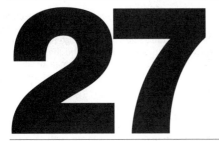

Urologic and Male Genital Malignancies

Matthew A. Ciorba

INTRODUCTION

Prostate cancer is the most common noncutaneous cancer among men. It accounts for approximately 36% of male cancers and 13% of all cancer deaths in men. Although only one-fourth of those with the disease die from it, many more may suffer from its complications. These include but are not limited to bleeding, pain, and urinary obstruction. Urologic cancers, including malignancies of the prostate, urinary bladder, kidney, and testes, affect many individuals and account for a significant portion of health care resources. These topics are discussed in detail throughout this chapter.

PROSTATE CANCER

The lifetime risk of developing cancer of the prostate is approximately 10%, and risk of dying from it is 3%. Despite this sizable risk of having prostate cancer, its course is often indolent, and the average age at presentation is later in life. Thus, in terms of years of life lost per person among all cancers, it ranks comparatively low.

Epidemiology and Risk Factors

Age is the most significant risk factor. Autopsy studies show rates of >10% in men aged 40–49 and up to 80% in men older than 80 yrs. Having a positive family history and being of African-American descent are clearly associated with increased risk. High-fat diets also correlate positively with prostate cancer development. However, symptomatic benign prostatic hypertrophy and history of vasectomy are *not* risk factors.

Screening

Opinions and data surrounding screening for prostate cancer in asymptomatic patients remain controversial. Although treatment outcomes of patients diagnosed with early disease are substantially better than those diagnosed with late-stage disease, high-quality randomized controlled trials have yet to prove that screening decreases the morbidity and/or mortality of prostate cancer. However, much epidemiologic data suggest a benefit to screening. The mortality rate from prostate cancer has declined since the introduction of the prostate-specific antigen (PSA) test. Several randomized studies from Canada and Italy are suggestive that screening may affect long-term outcome. Finally, recent studies have shown that patients with early-stage cancer have a benefit from radical prostatectomy without major compromise in their quality of life. However, physicians should take **age** and **comorbidities** into account when deciding with their patients whether screening should be pursued. The *U.S. Preventive Services Task Force* does not recommend routine screening; however, the *American Cancer Society* recommends patients should discuss screening with their physicians and consider offering yearly digital rectal exams (DREs) starting at age 40 and PSA screening at age 50 yrs in those with no other risk factors.

Clinical Manifestations

- Often, patients with prostate cancer are asymptomatic. However, obstructive **symptoms,** as well as dysuria, back or hip pain, and hematuria, all can be initial presenting symptoms. In some cases, disease may become evident only after investigation of metastatic symptoms such as spinal cord compression, deep venous thrombosis with pulmonary embolus, or bone pain.
- Clues from **physical exam** are dependent on the DRE. Sensation of a hard and irregular nodule(s) is characteristic for the disease. Carcinoma of the prostate sometimes develops within the posterior surfaces of the lateral lobes, which are palpable during the DRE. However, obviously deeper lesions are not detectable on routine DRE. One should recognize that detection sensitivity varies significantly between examiners owing to differences in experience and technique. Trials for detecting early disease suggest that the physical exam, or even an U/S exam, is less sensitive than measurement of the PSA. Locally invasive disease may also be detectable on exam. On occasion, disease disseminates to the lymph nodes, causing evidence of scrotal or lower-extremity lymphedema.

Diagnosis

Because signs and symptoms are often nonspecific or nonexistent, screening or diagnosis by use of lab exams is often performed. The relatively high sensitivity (70–80%) and noninvasive nature of the **total serum PSA assay** have made it the most often-used test. Although PSA levels fall on a continuum, a normal level is considered to be <4 ng/mL. Studies have shown that the sensitivity may increase with lower specificity if a cut-off value of 2.5 ng/mL is used. Of note, levels typically elevate with age and from recent prostatic massage as well as in conditions such as benign prostatic hypertrophy or prostatitis. In the general population, a PSA level of 4–10 ng/mL has a positive predictive value (PPV) of 20–25%, whereas a level >10 ng/mL has a PPV of approximately 50%. Studies show that with both an abnormal DRE and PSA >4 ng/mL, the PPV reaches 60%. Perhaps the most important feature of the PSA testing is the ability to follow its change over time (PSA velocity). An increase of >0.75 ng/mL/yr suggests cancer if the same assay is used.

- Although **transrectal U/S** has been used for screening in some situations, its greatest use is to guide prostatic biopsies. It should then be the next step in diagnosis if screening tests are abnormal or if a nodule is felt on exam.
- **Tissue** is essential for diagnosis and PPVs of a first biopsy attempt range from 75–80% and increase to a 95% cancer detection rate with a second separate biopsy. The sensitivity can also be increased when more needle cores are obtained. A minimum of six cores is standard, although many patients routinely have 8–12 cores/biopsy session. Although uncommon, the procedure does carry the risks of infection and bleeding, along with discomfort during the procedure.

Staging

Histologic **grade** is an important determinant of disease course and patient survival. Adenocarcinomas represent >95% of prostate cancers and are assigned a value using the **Gleason grading scheme.** This system takes the two most predominant histologic patterns in the area of the tumor and assigns each a number from 1–5. These numbers are then added together to give the total score. *Higher scores* correlate with more poorly differentiated tumors and worse prognosis. Squamous and transitional cell tumors make up a majority of the remaining prostate tumors, with another important subset being the high-grade neuroendocrine or small-cell tumors. Table 27-1 describes the current TNM (tumor, node, metastases) staging system and basic treatment guidelines, although each individual's case must be considered separately.

Management Options

Watchful Waiting

Prostate cancer is often indolent in nature, allowing this technique to be viable in some patients. In general, this option is used for patients whose life is expectancy <10

TABLE 27-1. STAGING AND TREATMENT

Stage	Description	Treatment based on life expectancy
T1a	Nonpalpable; ≤5% resected tissue with cancer	<10 yrs: WW >10 yrs: RadP, XRT, WW
T1b	Nonpalpable; >5% resected tissue with cancer	<10 yrs: XRT, HRx >10 yrs: RadP, XRT, HRx
T1c	Nonpalpable; elevated PSA	Same as T1b
T2a	Palpable; <50% of one lobe or less	Same as T1b
T2b	Palpable; >50% of one lobe only	Same as T1b
T2c	Palpable; involves both lobes	Same as T1b
T3a	Palpable; unilateral extracapsular invasion	WW, XRT, or HRx depending on histology
T3b	Palpable; bilateral extracapsular invasion with seminal vesicle involvement	Same as T3a
T3c	Tumor invading seminal vesicle	—
M	Distant metastases	Likely HRx vs supportive care

HRx, hormone therapy; RadP, radical prostatectomy; WW, watchful waiting; XRT, radiation therapy.

yrs and in those who have less advanced disease with a low histologic grade. Older men who may have other significant comorbidities and whose cancer was discovered after surgery for partial prostatectomy for benign hyperplasia are typical patients for whom this method is used. Mortality rates from prostate cancer in this group range from 9–15% in the first 10 yrs, but by 15–20 yrs out, rates rise dramatically. Younger, healthier men rarely qualify for watchful waiting.

Radical Prostatectomy
Younger men in whom life expectancy is >10 yrs and in whom disease is believed to be localized are those commonly considered to benefit from a **surgical** approach. For these patients, surgery offers the best rate of cure or progression-free survival. In addition to the traditional surgical risks after radical prostatectomy, **complications** include urethral strictures, erectile dysfunction, and urinary incontinence. Earlier detection of less advanced disease, partly achieved by screening patients with serum PSA assays, has resulted in a higher number of patients receiving surgery before extracapsular spread of their cancer. In these patients, 15-yr survival reaches 90%. Some of these men are able to benefit from the less extensive, nerve-sparing radical retropubic prostatectomy, which offers preserved erectile function. Some centers are performing laparoscopic radical prostatectomies, but the standard use of this technique awaits more experience.

Radiation Therapy
External beam or implanted radioactive seeds have been used as an alternative to prostatectomy in certain patients with localized (T1 or T2) disease. 15-year disease-free survival rates range from 45–85% in this population. The side effects of erectile dysfunction (40–50%), incontinence (1–2%), and urethral stricture (3–8%) still remain, and radiation proctitis occurs in 5–15% of patients. Older and less healthy men with more aggressive or advanced cancers are frequently those to whom radiation therapy is recommended. Improved 3D imaging techniques combined with increasingly focused radiation delivery systems, termed *conformal radiation therapy*, are improv-

ing outcomes and tolerability of this treatment modality. This is also the treatment of choice in stage III (T3) patients in whom long-term survival can be obtained by radiation therapy in combination with hormones.

Hormonal Therapy

Numerous treatment options are available based on the principle that prostate cancers are testosterone dependent. These hormonal treatment options are typically used for patients who cannot tolerate other interventions but are symptomatic from localized disease or in advanced prostate cancer. An **orchiectomy** is a simple and effective method of decreasing serum testosterone and has the benefit of being free from compliance issues for those who chose this option. Ketoconazole (Nizoral) in very high doses induces a chemical castration in a short period of time, but hepatoxicity limits long-term use. **Estrogen therapy** with diethylstilbestrol is also effective but may increase cardiovascular mortality and cause painful gynecomastia. **Gonadotropin-releasing hormone agonists** used initially with an androgen antagonist are also effective at long-term testosterone suppression and are the most widely used option in the United States. This treatment option is more expensive, but has psychologic advantages over castration or estrogen use. Hormonal therapy comes at a price of subjecting patients to androgen deprivation, which causes hot flashes and decreases in libido and muscle mass. Some data also suggests osteoporosis occurs at a higher rate with long-term androgen deprivation. Maximal androgen ablation by eliminating both gonadal and adrenal androgens can at best offer an improved survival benefit of 6–20 mos, depending on stage of disease. The use of combined androgen deprivation is controversial, because several metaanalyses suggest only minimal benefit to initial blockage of the gonadal secretion of testosterone alone.

Chemotherapy

Most men eventually develop hormone-resistant prostate cancer, and thus they no longer gain benefit from hormonal manipulation. It is now common practice to use systemic chemotherapy in treating this stage of disease. Many different agents have been used in trials, but the optimal regimen has yet to be discovered. The current standard-of-care regimen for hormone-resistant prostate cancers still producing PSA is a combination of mitoxantrone (Novantrone) with a corticosteroid. There may be a role for a combination regimen of estramustine (Emcyt) and a taxane in men with good performance status [1]. Serum PSA levels and quality-of-life measures along with prolonged survival are used to determine regimen success. These regimens have shown quality-of-life benefits for patients and may have survival benefits. Further studies of chemotherapy in conjunction with surgery or radiation therapy are being done in clinical trials.

RENAL CELL CARCINOMA

Less prevalent than prostate cancer, renal cell carcinoma represents 2% of all cancers. However, it rarely produces symptoms or signs until later stages of the disease, at which time the chances of cure have drastically diminished.

Epidemiology and Risk Factors

The overall incidence of renal cell carcinoma is on the rise but remains twice as common in men as women, with equal incidence rates between blacks and whites. The higher incidence in males may change, as smoking rates equalize between men and women. As with most cancers, age is the premier risk factor. Accordingly, disease predominately presents in the seventh and eighth decades of life. Other apparent but not absolute risk factors include cigarette smoking, obesity, HTN, and heavy metal or petroleum product exposure. Although hereditary forms of the disease occur uncommonly, one clear genetic linkage is with von Hippel-Lindau disease. Nearly 40% of these individuals develop multifocal renal cell carcinoma with clear cell histology.

Clinical Features

Hematuria, abdominal pain with a palpable **flank, or abdominal mass** is the classic triad for diagnosis of renal cell carcinoma. Of note, this triad occurs in combination only 10% of the time. Other nonspecific symptoms include fever, night sweats, feeling of malaise, and weight loss. One interesting potential presenting symptom is that of a left-sided varicocele in men, secondary to obstruction of the testicular vein. Although, in general, small tumors rarely produce symptoms. Diagnosis of renal cell carcinoma in modern day medicine has improved predominately because of incidental findings during an abdominal CT or U/S performed for other indications. At diagnosis, 20–30% of tumors are overtly metastatic, often to the lung, bone, liver, and brain. Paraneoplastic syndromes are rare but include erythrocytosis and hypercalcemia from overproduction of erythropoietin or PTH-related protein, respectively.

Diagnosis

Contrast-enhanced CT has a >90% sensitivity in detecting tumors of ≤3 cm. Sensitivity of U/S is approximately 80% for similar tumors. CT scans are also highly useful in determining cancer staging preop. MRI with gadolinium enhancement is superior to CT imaging and appropriate in those who have an IV contrast allergy or in whom inferior vena cava involvement is suspected. Despite the high sensitivity of available imaging techniques, diagnosis still lies with histologic exam of tissue. In addition to renal cell carcinoma, squamous and transitional cell of the renal pelvis, Wilms' tumor, sarcoma, and metastatic disease all remain in the differential diagnosis.

Staging and Survival

The modified Robson staging system or that of the American Joint Committee on Cancer may be used in assigning renal cell carcinoma a pathologic stage. This stage is the most important factor in determining survival. 5-yr survival ranges are included in Table 27-2. It should be noted that significant variance in survival exists for Robson stage III tumors. If there is nodal involvement, survival is <30% but may approach 50% if there is only local vein invasion. Even in localized disease treated by radical nephrectomy, relapse still occurs in 20–30% of patients.

Management

- The mainstay of therapy in localized disease is **surgical resection.** Radical nephrectomy (resection of kidney and perirenal fat) and nephron sparing surgery (partial

TABLE 27-2. STAGING OF RENAL CELL CARCINOMA AND 5-YR SURVIVAL RATES

Description of disease extent	AJCC equivalent	5-yr survival (%)
Confined to renal capsule		65–85
≤ 7 cm	I	
>7 cm	II	
Extends through renal capsule, but not through Gerota's fascia	III	45–80
Renal vein, IVC, or regional nodal involvement	III	15–50
Extends through Gerota's fascia, >1 lymph node, or distant metastases	IV	0–10

AJCC, American Joint Committee on Cancer; IVC, inferior vena cava.
Adapted from American Joint Committee on Cancer. *AJCC cancer staging manual*, 5th ed. Philadelphia: Lippincott–Raven, 1997.

nephrectomy) have both been studied. For patients without large superior-pole tumors or abnormal-appearing adrenal glands on CT scan, overall patient survival data are similar between the two procedures. Laparoscopic nephrectomies have almost become a commonly used technique. Absolute indication for partial nephrectomy exists for patients with bilateral tumors or a functional/anatomic solitary kidney. Nephron-sparing surgery may also be used electively for patients with small unilateral lesions (≤ 4 cm).

- Although numerous regimens have been tried, **chemotherapeutic** and **hormonal therapies** have been largely ineffective at treating metastatic renal cell carcinoma. Recent research, with relatively favorable outcomes, has been focused on use of **immunomodulatory therapies,** including those with interleukin-2 or alpha interferon. Although the number of patients that benefit is often on the order of 20%, a smaller number will have impressive long-term control of their disease with immunotherapy. Some patients, on the order of ≤ 5%, will be cured with immunotherapy. Preliminary reports show that the use of **allogeneic peripheral-blood stem cell transplantation** in select populations with refractory metastatic renal cell carcinoma may be beneficial. Such results are still early, and this technique has high levels of morbidity with chronic graft vs. host disease often required for a response. Two separate randomized trials have also shown a survival benefit to **nephrectomy,** followed by **interferon** for metastatic renal cell cancer. These data also suggest a benefit to the debulking of tumor.
- Postop, follow-up with physical exam, Cr, Hgb/Hct, and chest x-ray. Retroperitoneal imaging may be needed to exclude complications of surgery, metastases, or recurrence.

TESTICULAR CANCER

Although testicular cancer is relatively rare, it is an important cancer to recognize, as it typically affects younger patients. It also is amenable to screening by patient self-exam and is a curable tumor under most circumstances.

Epidemiology

Testicular cancer is the most common cancer among men aged 15–35 yrs. Incidence is much higher in whites than blacks. Cryptorchidism and Klinefelter's syndrome are known predisposing factors. Orchiopexy to the undescended testis does not modify the risk of malignancy in cryptorchidism but does allow easier testicular exam.

Clinical Manifestations

A painless testicular mass is the classic presenting symptom and sign, but diffuse testicular pain or swelling is present in many patients. Physical exam should focus on the testicles, lymphadenopathy (particularly supraclavicular), scrotal edema, and evaluation for gynecomastia. Early metastases to bone are rare but possible, and back pain may result from bulky retroperitoneal lymph nodes. Patients are often treated initially with a course of antibiotics for possible epididymitis or orchitis.

Diagnosis and Evaluation

- The **differential diagnosis** should consist of infectious possibilities as well as the benign epidermoid cyst, spermatoceles, and varicoceles. Lymphoma is the second most common testicular tumor, but metastases to the testicles are rare. If symptoms persist after a course of antibiotics or if a mass is palpated, scrotal U/S is the initial test of choice. Unless U/S results indicate otherwise, an orchiectomy by inguinal approach is necessary for diagnosis.
- Testicular tumors are divided into **seminomas** and **nonseminoma tumors.** The nonseminoma tumors include embryonal carcinomas, teratomas, choriocarcinomas, and mixed germ cell types. Leydig, granulosa, and Sertoli cell tumors occur rarely.

- **Serum tumor markers** beta-hCG, lactate dehydrogenase, and AFP are important in diagnosis and monitoring therapeutic response. All three markers may be present in nonseminomas, with beta-hCG being present in 100% of choriocarcinoma subtype tumors. Seminomas occasionally express beta-hCG but never express AFP.
- **Other preop workup** should include a chest x-ray in addition to routine chemistry and hematology. Abdominal and pelvic CT exams are useful in assessing node status and staging. Stage I disease is localized to the testis, stage II disease has spread to retroperitoneal lymph nodes, and stage III disease is metastatic or has spread to lymph nodes above the diaphragm.

Management

- **Transinguinal orchiectomy** is the preferred surgical approach and is necessary for staging and diagnosis. The transscrotal approach has increased risk of tumor seeding.
- **Seminomas** are extremely sensitive to radiation, and retroperitoneal radiation is the only further therapy for stage I and nonbulky stage II tumors. If nodal involvement is present but not bulky, **radiation therapy** along with orchiectomy is the preferred approach for stage II tumors. **Chemotherapy** is rarely necessary except for stage III disease.
- **Nonseminomatous cancers** are less radiosensitive, and surgery with sympathetic nerve-sparing retroperitoneal lymphadenectomy is the current standard treatment. Adjuvant chemotherapy is often recommended if the surgical resection showed that cancer cells were present on pathology. It is also recommended for bulky retroperitoneal lymphadenopathy or stage III disease. Etoposide and cisplatin ± bleomycin is the chemotherapeutic regimen of choice. Residual disease present after chemotherapy often consists of chemo-insensitive teratomas, and thus it should be removed surgically.
- Patients with testicular cancer should have close **follow-up** over the years after diagnosis and treatment.
- **Relapse** usually becomes evident in the first 8–10 mos. In addition, because many of these patients are cured, long-term toxicities of treatment are important.
- **Surgical side effects** include retrograde ejaculation leading to infertility. Long-term **chemotherapy side effects** are still being collected, as some may not show for decades. However, patients treated with these chemotherapy agents tend to have slightly higher BPs and less favorable lipid profiles, which should be treated the standard way. Many patients also have some high-frequency hearing loss and difficulty with Raynaud's symptoms. Some regimens may also lead to a slightly higher than background risk of acute leukemia.

CANCER OF THE URINARY BLADDER

Bladder cancer is primarily a malignancy of the epithelium, occurring in individuals >60 yrs. It is more common in men than women (2.7:1), and nearly three-fourths of all cases can be linked to cigarette smoking or exposure to industrial dyes and solvents. Occupational exposure to aromatic amines such as benzidone and beta-naphthylamine in the dye industry is a risk factor. Similarly, occupational exposure can also occur in the rubber, leather, textile, paint, printing, and hairdressing industries. Although less common, squamous cell carcinomas also occur and are frequently associated with schistosomiasis.

Clinical Features and Diagnostic Evaluation

Symptoms are not always appreciated by patients, but **hematuria** is present in approximately 90% of individuals with bladder cancer. This may be intermittent or constant, frank or microscopic, and is occasionally associated with symptoms of urinary frequency or urgency. UA reveals or confirms hematuria and, in some, shows pyuria. Cytology can be used, but the gold standard for diagnosis is **cystoscopy with biopsy.** Other imaging modalities, including CT, MRI, U/S, and IV urography, are primarily useful for disease staging.

Staging and Survival

50–80% of bladder cancers are superficial at presentation. These cancers have not yet reached muscular layers of the bladder, lymph nodes, or other distant sites. Proper treatment by transurethral resection and intravesicular chemotherapy leads to survival in >80% of patients.

Management

Local treatment of the bladder via a urethral catheter and intravesicular instillation of drug is effective in eradicating existing disease and at reducing recurrence rates in those who have already undergone resection. Bacillus Calmette-Guérin (BCG) is the most common and effective intravesicular agent used, but others, including mitomycin-C, interferon, and doxorubicin, are also used. If imaging and initial transurethral resection reveal more **advanced cancer,** a partial or radical cystectomy with lymph node dissection may be necessary. Radiotherapy is fairly effective and generally well tolerated. One alternative for patients who hope to preserve their bladder is to combine radiotherapy with systemic chemotherapy. However, with newer surgical techniques to create neobladders, many reasonable options are available for these patients. Chemotherapy may also be used in conjunction with surgical resection in patients found to have metastatic disease at initial presentation (approximately 15%) or in those with high risk of recurrence of their disease. In metastatic disease, cisplatin-based regimens are recommended. More recently, gemcitabine and taxane regimens have shown effective control.

KEY POINTS TO REMEMBER

- Prostate cancer is the most common cancer among men, but many men die with the disease rather than from it.
- The preferred approach to screening for prostate cancer includes the serum PSA test in combination with the DRE. Because no study has unequivocally proven that screening decreases morbidity or mortality, the decision to screen patients may be individualized.
- Histologic grade using the Gleason grading scheme is the most important factor in determining disease course and patient survival.
- Because of prostate cancer's indolent course, treatment options are based on individual patient characteristics and stage of disease.
- Renal cell carcinoma's classic triad is present in only 10% of patients but includes hematuria, abdominal pain, and a palpable flank or abdominal mass.
- Surgery is currently the mainstay of therapy for renal cell carcinoma, but newer therapies are being investigated.
- Testicular cancer is the most common cancer in men aged 15–35 yrs and often presents as a painless testicular mass.
- Treatments for testicular cancer are highly successful with cure rates of >85% for most cases. Orchiectomy is necessary for diagnosis and treatment.
- Seminomas are exquisitely sensitive to radiation therapy if cancer spreads to the retroperitoneal lymph nodes.
- Cigarette smoking or exposure to industrial dyes and solvents can be linked to the majority of bladder cancers.
- Most bladder cancers are superficial at time of diagnosis and can be treated by transurethral excision and intravesicular chemotherapy.

SUGGESTED READING

Bajorin DF, Sarosdy MF, Pfister DG, et al. Randomized trial of etoposide and cisplatin versus etoposide and carboplatin in patients with good-risk germ cell tumors. *J Clin Oncol* 1993;11:598.

Bosl GJ, Motzer RJ. Testicular germ-cell cancer. *N Engl J Med* 1997;337:242–253.

Braunwald E, Fauci A, et al., eds. *Harrison's principles of internal medicine*, 15th ed. New York: McGraw-Hill, 2001.

Catalona WJ. Management of cancer of the prostate. *N Engl J Med* 1994;331(15):996–1004.

Coley C, Barry MJ, Fleming C, et al. Clinical guidelines: early detection of prostate cancer. Parts I & II: prior probability and effectiveness of tests & estimating the risks, benefits and costs. *Ann Intern Med* 1997;126:394–406, 468–479.

DeVita VT, Hellman S, Rosenberg SA, eds. *Cancer: principles and practice of oncology*, 6th ed. Philadelphia: Lippincott Williams & Wilkins, 2001.

Garnick MB, Fair WR. Prostate cancer: emerging concepts. Part I. *Ann Intern Med* 1996;125(2):118–125.

Garnick MB, Fair WR. Prostate cancer: emerging concepts. Part II. *Ann Intern Med* 1996;125(3):205–212.

Holmberg L, Bill-Axelson A, Helgesen F, et al. A randomized trial comparing radical prostatectomy with watchful waiting in early prostate cancer. *N Engl J Med* 2002;347:781–789.

Motzer RJ, Bander NH, Nanus DM. Renal cell carcinoma. *N Engl J Med* 1996;335:865–866.

REFERENCE

1. Gilligan T, Kantoff PW. Estramusine plus taxane is chemotherapy for prostate cancer. *Urology* 2002;60:94–100.

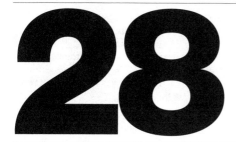

Gynecologic Oncology

Jason D. Wright and
Neil S. Horowitz

INTRODUCTION

Tumors of the female reproductive tract are often diagnosed and managed by the combined efforts of the primary care physician, gynecologist, gynecologic oncologist, and radiation oncologist. This chapter describes the approach to common gynecologic oncology evaluations, as well as briefly discusses selected gynecologic tumors.

VAGINAL BLEEDING

Differential Diagnosis

Vaginal bleeding is caused by either an organic disease or an endocrine imbalance. Organic causes are either related to genital tract pathology or secondary to a systemic disease. Cervical and endometrial cancers are the most common malignancies that result in vaginal bleeding. Dysfunctional uterine bleeding (DUB) is the result of an endocrine imbalance. Table 28-1 displays the most common causes of vaginal bleeding by age group.

Diagnosis

History

A careful menstrual history, including the last menstrual period, as well as the amount and duration of bleeding, should be obtained. Any history of infection, trauma, or systemic diseases should be sought.

Physical Exam

A speculum exam and pelvic exam should be performed. A Papanicolaou (Pap) smear should be obtained. Any suspicious cervical or vulvar lesions should be biopsied. A rectal exam and Guaiac should also be obtained.

Diagnostic Evaluation

Diagnostic evaluation is based on the patient's age and the most likely cause of bleeding. All patients >35 should have an endometrial biopsy performed to rule out endometrial hyperplasia or cancer. Lab assessment includes CBC, hCG, TSH, and ferritin levels.

Management

Patients with a pelvic mass, cervical lesions, and an abnormal Pap smear and postmenopausal patients should be referred to a gynecologist for further evaluation. Acute vaginal bleeding is treated with PO or IV estrogen. Patients with DUB are most often managed with combination oral contraceptive pills, medroxyprogesterone acetate, or endometrial ablation. Hysterectomy provides definitive treatment for patients with vaginal bleeding and no evidence of malignancy.

TABLE 28-1. DIFFERENTIAL DIAGNOSIS OF VAGINAL BLEEDING

Prepubertal	Adolescent	Reproductive	Perimeno-pausal	Postmenopausal
Vulvovaginitis	DUB	Pregnancy	DUB	Endometrial pol-yps
Foreign body	Pregnancy	DUB	Leiomyomas	
Precocious puberty	Exogenous hormones	Leiomyomas	Polyps	Hyperplasia and cancer
		Polyps	Thyroid dys-function	
Neoplasms	Coagulopa-thy disease	Thyroid dis-ease		Atrophic vaginitis
			Exogenous hormones	Other neoplasms

DUB, dysfunctional uterine bleeding.
Adapted from Berek JS, Adashi EY, Hillard PA. *Novak's gynecology*, 12th ed. Philadelphia: Williams & Wilkins, 1996.

PELVIC MASS

Differential Diagnosis

A variety of entities may result in the formation of a pelvic mass. Most common, the pathology arises from the ovary or the uterus. Table 28-2 outlines the most common causes of pelvic masses for each age group.

Ovarian Cysts
Ovarian cysts are the most common cause for a pelvic mass. Follicular cysts are filled with serous fluid, and corpus luteal cysts are often filled with blood.

Benign Ovarian Neoplasms
The most common benign ovarian neoplasm is the cystic teratoma (dermoid cyst). Other benign tumors include mucinous and serous cystadenomas, thecomas, fibromas, and Brenner tumors.

Malignant Ovarian Neoplasms
The incidence of epithelial ovarian tumors increases with age. Germ cell and sex cord stromal malignancies may be found in younger women.

Leiomyomas
Leiomyomas are common in reproductive-aged women. Most leiomyomas (fibroids) regress after menopause.

TABLE 28-2. DIFFERENTIAL DIAGNOSIS OF A PELVIC MASS

Childhood	Adolescence	Reproductive age	Postmenopausal
Ovarian cysts	Ovarian cysts	Leiomyoma	Malignant gyneco-logic neoplasms
Benign neoplasms	Benign neoplasms	Ovarian cysts	
		Benign gynecologic neoplasms	Other malignant neoplasms
		Other malignant neoplasms	

Other Causes
Other less common causes of a pelvic mass include paratubal cysts, ectopic pregnancies, endometriomas, and tuboovarian abscesses.

Diagnosis of a Pelvic Mass

History
History should include any history of urinary or GI symptoms. Any history of pelvic pain or vaginal bleeding should also be elicited.

Physical Exam
The pelvic mass should be evaluated by bimanual exam. An attempt to determine the size and location of the mass should be made. Evidence of ascites or a pleural effusion heightens the suspicion for a malignant ovarian tumor.

Diagnostic Evaluation
A transvaginal U/S is the most sensitive imaging modality to evaluate a pelvic mass. The size, location, and whether the mass is solid or cystic can usually be determined by sonography. CA-125 is a nonspecific tumor marker that may be obtained.

Management

If the pelvic mass appears to be a leiomyoma, observation or surgical management is appropriate. If the pelvic mass arises from the adnexa (ovary or fallopian tube), the patient should be referred to a gynecologist.

Postmenopausal Patients
If the pelvic mass arises from the adnexa, surgery is indicated to rule out an ovarian malignancy.

Premenopausal Patients
Premenopausal patients with a solid adnexal mass should be referred for surgical evaluation. A cystic adnexal mass may be safely observed for 2–3 mos. If the mass persists or enlarges on U/S, surgery is required. Surgery may either be by laparoscopy or laparotomy.

CERVICAL CANCER

In 2001, there were approximately 12,900 new cases of cervical cancer and 4,400 deaths from the disease. Worldwide, 470,000 cases are reported annually. The median age at diagnosis is 51.4.

Epidemiology

Several risk factors are known for cervical cancer. Human papillomavirus is found in >90% of cervical neoplasms. Cervical intraepithelial neoplasia is a precancerous lesion of the cervix. Other risk factors include smoking, multiple sex partners, immunosuppression, and early age at first intercourse. More than 90% of cervical cancers are squamous cell carcinomas. Less common histologies include adenocarcinomas and small cell carcinomas.

Screening

The Pap smear is the standard screening test for cervical cancer. Sexually active women should undergo yearly Pap screening. The role of human papillomavirus testing is uncertain.

Diagnosis

Signs and Symptoms
Many women with cervical cancer are asymptomatic. Symptomatic women most often present with vaginal bleeding, which is often postcoital. Physical exam may reveal a

palpable cervical mass. Palpation of the inguinal and supraclavicular nodes may reveal lymphadenopathy.

Diagnostic Evaluation

If a gross lesion is present, cervical biopsy should be performed. If an abnormal Pap smear yields atypical cytology colposcopy with directed biopsies, a endocervical curettage can be performed. Staging evaluation may include CT, PET, IV pyelogram, cystoscopy, and proctoscopy.

Management

For early-stage disease confined to the cervix, survival is equivalent with either surgery or primary radiotherapy. Patients treated surgically with poor prognostic factors, including positive lymph nodes, lymphovascular space invasion, and large tumor volume, should be treated with adjuvant radiation. Patients with advanced lesions are treated with combination chemoradiation. Radiation is typically delivered with combination intracavitary brachytherapy as well as external beam radiation. Cisplatin with or without fluorouracil administered with radiation improves survival.

Prognosis

Patients with microscopic disease identified by Pap smear have a 5-yr survival of >90%. For patients with spread to the pelvic sidewall at the time of diagnosis, 5-yr survival falls to <40%. Patients treated for cervical cancer require careful follow-up with Pap smears. Pelvic recurrences are most often treated with radiation. Systemic recurrences are most often treated with platinum-based chemotherapy.

OVARIAN CANCER

In 2001, there were approximately 23,400 new cases of ovarian cancer and 13,900 deaths from the disease. The median age at diagnosis is 61 yrs. Epithelial neoplasms account for >85% of ovarian neoplasms. Germ cell tumors and sex cord stromal tumors are less common and typically occur in adolescents and young women.

Epidemiology

Risk factors for ovarian cancer include low parity, infertility, early menarche, late menopause, and anovulatory disorders. 5–10% of ovarian cancers are hereditary. Mutations in BRCA1 and BRCA2, as well as the hereditary nonpolyposis colorectal cancer syndrome, are important risk factors for ovarian cancer. **Serous tumors** are the most common malignant epithelial ovarian tumors. **Less common histologies** include endometrioid tumors, mucinous tumors, clear cell tumors, and transitional cell (Brenner) tumors. Ovarian tumors are often bilateral.

Screening

There is considerable public controversy regarding ovarian cancer screening, given the often dramatic presentation of ovarian cancer and poor prognosis when advanced. However, current methods of screening for ovarian cancer lack acceptable specificity, and thus general population screening is not recommended.

Diagnosis

Signs and Symptoms

Most early ovarian cancers are asymptomatic. **Symptoms** result from abdominal carcinomatosis. Patients often complain of vague GI complaints, including nausea, vomiting, early satiety, bloating, and increased abdominal girth. **Physical exam** may be notable for ascites and an adnexal mass. Pleural effusions are common.

Diagnostic Evaluation

Diagnosis of an ovarian carcinoma requires exploratory surgery. Proper surgical staging is a complex procedure and should be done only by an experienced gynecologic oncologist. If ascites are present, a paracentesis may be performed. Negative cytology does not rule out an ovarian tumor. Staging evaluation may include a CT scan. Colon screening with either colonoscopy or a barium enema should be performed to rule out a colorectal carcinoma. CA-125 is an antigen present on coelomic epithelium. It is elevated in >90% of patients with advanced ovarian cancer. CA-125 is also elevated in a variety of benign abdominopelvic disorders, and thus its value in screening for ovarian cancer is limited. CA-125 is a useful marker to monitor treatment response.

Management

Treatment of ovarian carcinoma **begins with surgical staging** and **cytoreduction.** Cytoreduction (debulking) is the procedure of removing as much gross tumor as is feasible. Optimal cytoreduction is associated with improved survival and responsiveness to chemotherapy. After cytoreductive surgery, adjuvant chemotherapy with paclitaxel (Taxol) and a platinum-containing compound is used unless precluded by toxicity. Recurrences with ovarian carcinoma are common. Treatment of recurrences is with further chemotherapy.

Prognosis

Most patients with ovarian carcinoma present with intraabdominal disease at the time of diagnosis. 5-yr survival for these patients now approaches 40%. After treatment, patients are typically followed with serial CA-125 levels and CT scans to detect recurrences.

ENDOMETRIAL CANCER

In 2001, there were approximately 38,300 new cases of endometrial cancer and 6,600 deaths from the disease. The median age at diagnosis is 61 yrs.

Epidemiology and Risk Factors

The normal endometrium is stimulated by estrogen. Excess estrogen exposure can lead to both endometrial hyperplasia and endometrial cancer. **Risk factors** for endometrial cancer are early menarche, late menopause, obesity, and hormone replacement therapy without estrogen. Tamoxifen (Nolvadex) is also associated with endometrial cancer. The **incidence** of endometrial cancer for patients receiving tamoxifen is 2/1,000. Patients diagnosed with hereditary nonpolyposis colorectal cancer syndrome have a 20–43% lifetime risk of endometrial cancer. Endometrioid adenocarcinoma accounts for >75% of endometrial cancers. Other histologies include uterine papillary serous carcinoma, clear cell carcinoma, and mucinous carcinoma.

Screening

Population-based screening for endometrial cancer is not recommended. Patients with vaginal bleeding should be evaluated as previously described.

Diagnosis

Signs and Symptoms

>90% of patients present with vaginal bleeding. If cervical stenosis is present, pyometra or hematometra may develop. Physical exam is often unremarkable, although slight uterine enlargement may be present.

Diagnostic Evaluation

Diagnosis rests on endometrial sampling. A variety of **endometrial biopsy** devices are available and are >90% sensitive. If cervical stenosis prohibits office-based sampling, fractional dilation and curettage may be performed in the OR. Transvaginal U/S can be used to assess endometrial thickness. If the endometrium is <5 mm, sensitivity is 95% for ruling out endometrial hyperplasia or carcinoma.

Management

All patients who are medically fit should be treated surgically. Surgery should include total abdominal hysterectomy with bilateral salpingo-oophorectomy. Pelvic lymph node dissection should be carried out in all patients except those with low-grade, early-stage, superficially invasive carcinomas. Patients with disease spread beyond the uterus or those with high-grade or deeply invasive tumors should receive adjuvant radiotherapy.

Prognosis

Patients with disease confined to the endometrium have a 5-yr survival of >90%. After treatment, patients should be followed carefully with Pap smears of the vaginal cuff. There is currently no evidence that hormone replacement therapy either increases disease recurrence or decreases survival. The risk and benefits should be discussed with patients who desire hormone replacement therapy. Patients with pelvic recurrences may be salvaged with radiotherapy. Doxorubicin and cisplatin are the most active agents for systemic recurrences.

GESTATIONAL TROPHOBLASTIC DISEASE

Gestational trophoblastic neoplasms (GTNs) are tumors derived from the placental chorion. Tumors may present as either a molar pregnancy or a persistent GTN (PGTN) that develops after a normal or molar pregnancy or after an abortion. GTNs secrete hCG.

Hydatiform Moles

Pathology

Two types of molar pregnancies are known: complete hydatiform moles and partial hydatiform moles. **Complete moles** lack fetal tissue and have chorionic villi with generalized swelling. **Partial moles** have some fetal tissue present and exhibit focal chorionic villi swelling.

Diagnosis

Patients typically present in early pregnancy with an abnormally elevated hCG. Common signs and symptoms include vaginal bleeding (95%), excessive uterine enlargement (50%), preeclampsia (27%), hyperemesis gravidarum (26%), and hyperthyroidism. Incomplete moles often present as incomplete abortions.

Management

Treatment is referral to an obstetrician for suction curettage.

Prognosis

After evacuation, patients should be followed with weekly quantitative hCG levels until normal for 3 mos, then monthly until normal for 6 mos. A rising or plateaued hCG indicates persistent trophoblastic neoplasia.

Persistent Gestational Trophoblastic Neoplasia

PGTN can develop after a molar pregnancy, a normal pregnancy, or an abortion. PGTN may be either locally invasive (in the uterus) or metastatic.

Diagnosis

Patients with locally invasive disease often have vaginal bleeding. 80% of patients with metastatic disease have pulmonary involvement. Other metastatic sites include the vagina (30%), liver (10%), and brain (10%).

Diagnostic Evaluation

Evaluation for patients with a persistently elevated hCG should include CBC; electrolytes; LFTs; and CT scans of the head, chest, abdomen, and pelvis.

Management

GTD is exquisitely sensitive to chemotherapy, and even patients with widespread metastasis can be cured. Patients with locally invasive disease or patients with spread to the pelvis or lungs with low-risk features are treated with single-agent chemotherapy. Methotrexate is most often used, but actinomycin D is also effective. Patients with CNS metastasis or high-risk patients with pulmonary or pelvic spread require combination chemotherapy. Chemotherapy is continued until the hCG has normalized.

Prognosis

After treatment, quantitative hCG is followed weekly until normal for 3 wks, then monthly until normal for 12 mos (24 mos for CNS spread). Contraception is essential during this time. Survival is >97% for patients with nonmetastatic disease. Molar pregnancies recur in 1–1.5% of subsequent gestations.

KEY POINTS TO REMEMBER

- All postmenopausal bleeding should be considered abnormal and investigated for possible malignancy.
- After a history and physical, the first diagnostic step in the evaluation of an adnexal mass is an U/S. Only cystic masses in premenopausal women can be potentially observed.
- Proper surgical staging in ovarian cancer is a complex procedure and must be done only by an experienced gynecologic oncologist.
- Gestational trophoblastic disease is extremely chemosensitive and carries a high cure rate.

REFERENCES AND SUGGESTED READINGS

Berek JS, Adashi EY, Hillard PA. *Novak's gynecology*, 12th ed. Philadelphia: Williams & Wilkins, 1996.

Berek JS, Hacker NF. *Practical gynecologic oncology*, 3rd ed. Philadelphia: Lippincott Williams & Wilkins, 2000.

National Cancer Institute Web site. Available at: http://www.nci.nih.gov. Accessed May 2003.

Stenchever MA, Droegemueller W, Herbst AL, et al. *Comprehensive gynecology*. St. Louis: Mosby, 2001.

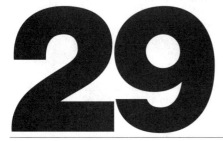

Intracranial Tumors

Stacey K. Knox

INTRODUCTION

Intracranial lesions are fairly rare malignancies—the thirteenth most common in frequency among tumors in adult patients. Primary intracranial tumors have an incidence of 11.5/100,000, whereas approximately 13,000 people die of a primary CNS cancer each year. Metastases to the brain are even more common, with one estimate that >100,000 patients/year die from a systemic cancer that has metastasized to the brain. **Ionizing radiation** is currently the only known unequivocal risk factor for developing a glial or meningeal neoplasm. Irradiation of the cranium, even at low doses, can increase the incidence of meningiomas by a factor of 10 and the incidence of glial tumors by a factor of 3–7. Other potential risks, such as use of cellular phones, exposure to high-tension power wires, head trauma, and exposure to nitrosourea compounds, have provided conflicting and unconvincing data and currently are not considered to be risk factors. It is rare for these neoplasms to run in families unless there is an inherited mutation. There are **four types** of primary intracranial tumors that are considered in this chapter: glial tumors (consisting of oligodendrogliomas and astrocytic tumors), ependymomas, meningiomas, and primary CNS lymphoma. These constitute the majority of primary intracranial tumors. Metastatic tumors from a primary systemic cancer are also discussed. Management of these tumors often involves a multidisciplinary approach involving the neurosurgeon, neuro-oncologist, radiation oncologist, and neurologist, among others. Rehabilitation efforts similarly may be multidisciplinary and involve rehabilitation specialists, physical and occupational therapists, and nurses. The most common parenchymal metastases are associated with primary lung cancer, breast cancer, renal cell cancer, lymphoma, and melanoma. Dural metastases are seen most commonly with breast or prostate cancer.

ASTROCYTIC TUMORS

The epidemiology of these tumors depends on their histologic grade. **Low-grade (grades I and II) astrocytomas** are typically found in children and young adults. The peak incidence in adults occurs in the third to fourth decade of life. **Malignant astrocytomas (grade III)** typically present in the fourth or fifth decade, and **glioblastoma multiforme** (GBM) usually presents in the sixth or seventh decade. Malignant astrocytomas and GBM are the most common glial tumors, with an annual incidence of 3–4/100,000 population. Of these, 80% are GBM. GBM may be either primary or secondary (meaning the GBM has arisen from a tumor that was initially a low-grade astrocytoma). These secondary GBM tend to occur in younger adults, typically ≤45 yrs. The male to female ratio of malignant astrocytic tumors is 3:2.

Clinical Features

Presentation of these tumors depends on their grade. Low-grade astrocytic tumors present with seizure in approximately 90% of cases. Typically, the seizures are focal but may become generalized and cause loss of consciousness. **Headache** is found in 40% of patients. In general, the headache is worse in the morning and improves in a few hours, usually without treatment. On occasion, headache can be unilateral and throbbing, mimicking a migraine or even a cluster headache. Symptoms such as **hemi-**

paresis and **mental status changes** are found in 15% and 10% of patients, respectively. These symptoms reflect the location of the tumor. **Malignant astrocytic tumors,** on the other hand, only present with seizure 15–25% of the time and present with headache 50% of the time. These tumors are much more likely to present with focal neurologic deficits such as hemiparesis, seen in 30–50% of patients, and mental status abnormalities, seen in 40–60% of patients.

Diagnosis

The diagnosis of the tumors is usually established by **MRI. Low-grade** astrocytomas usually are seen as a diffuse, nonenhancing mass that typically has a local mass effect and evidence of cortical infiltration, with abnormal signal reaching the surface of the brain. The radiologic borders of these tumors are usually distinct, with no surrounding edema. **High-grade astrocytomas** have an irregular contrast enhancement, which is often ringlike. These lesions are usually associated with edema, and the mass effect can be severe enough to cause herniation. **Pathologic diagnosis** of these tumors can be done by stereotactic biopsy or surgical excision of the lesion. **Stereotactic biopsy** will provide the diagnosis of an astrocytoma but will not provide enough information to determine the grade of the tumor, because astrocytic tumors are histologically variable from region to region.

Staging

These tumors are graded by the World Health Organization's four-tiered grading system. The criteria used to grade these tumors include the following features: nuclear atypia, mitotic activity, endothelial proliferation, and necrosis.

- Grade I: absence of all features
- Grade II: any one feature
- Grade III: any two features (malignant astrocytoma)
- Grade IV: any three features (glioblastoma multiforme)

Management

- On diagnosis of an astrocytoma, the decision must be made as to whether **treatment is necessary or not.** Some neuro-oncologists argue that **resection** may be delayed safely in patients who are asymptomatic and whose seizures are well controlled. Therapy of these tumors involves **debulking** of the tumor and perhaps excision of the entire tumor surgically if the tumor does not involve critical structures such as the language areas. With low-grade lesions, the next step in treatment is typically low-dose **irradiation.** Irradiation may be done immediately after surgery or may be deferred until there is radiographic evidence of tumor progression. Studies at this time have not shown a difference in survival benefit between immediate and delayed irradiation. Many physicians will wait to start irradiation to provide another treatment option at the time of progression. There is no indication for the routine use of chemotherapy in low-grade astrocytomas at this time.
- Therapy of malignant astrocytoma and GBM is identical. The initial step is to **surgically excise the tumor.** Every effort should be made to remove as much tumor as possible, as this is associated with longer survival and improved neurologic function. Surgery is followed by **high-dose irradiation** of the involved field. Currently, **chemotherapy** is limited to carmustine (BiCNU), which is the agent best studied and has been shown to enhance survival.
- At time of **recurrence,** a second resection should be done, if possible. This should be followed by stereotactic radiosurgery, if it has not been used earlier. Chemotherapy with nitrosourea drugs and procarbazine (Matulane) may also be useful. There may be some role for temozolomide (Temodar) as well.
- **Brainstem** gliomas are inoperable. These tumors are treated with irradiation. If there is increased intracranial pressure, a shunt may be placed.

Prognosis

Prognosis associated with astrocytomas is determined by their grade. The median survival for low-grade astrocytomas is 5 yrs. Most of these patients die from the progression of their disease to a higher grade. The median survival for malignant astrocytomas is typically approximately 3 yrs. The median survival of GBM is typically 1 yr.

OLIGODENDROGLIOMAS

Oligodendrogliomas are usually low-grade neoplasms and account for <5% of intracranial tumors and approximately 20% of glial neoplasms. Mean age at presentation is 38–45 yrs, with a slight male predominance. The **histology** of these tumors shows a uniform population of cells resembling "fried eggs." They arise from oligodendroglial cells, which are responsible for axonal myelination. More than one-third of these tumors have intermixed astrocytic or ependymal elements and are therefore considered "mixed gliomas."

Clinical Presentation

Patients may present with seizure, progressive hemiparesis, or cognitive impairment depending on tumor location. These tumors are known to have delicate vasculature and **hemorrhage** easily, and the patient may present with an acute onset of hemiparesis, headache, and/or lethargy.

Diagnosis

Diagnostic evaluation usually begins with an **MRI.** The radiologic hallmark differentiating this tumor from an astrocytoma is **calcification** of the tumor. Biopsy, as in astrocytoma, is necessary for definitive diagnosis, and **excisional biopsy** is preferred to stereotactic biopsy. Exam by light microscopy shows oligodendroglioma cells that may have regular and rounded nuclei, with some nuclei having a halo-like *appearance* (sometimes termed *fried egg appearance*). There are currently no immunohistochemical stains or markers that definitively establish the diagnosis.

Management

- The median survival for patients with oligodendroglioma is currently 16 yrs. This long survival is attributed to earlier diagnosis of these tumors with MRI and to its chemosensitivity. Most oligodendrogliomas progress by becoming malignant.
- As is seen with astrocytomas, **therapy** may not be necessary at initial presentation if the patient is asymptomatic and seizures are adequately controlled. Therapy of these tumors usually begins with the **excisional biopsy** performed to diagnose these tumors. After surgery and diagnosis, **focal irradiation** and **chemotherapy** are performed. The chemotherapy regimen includes procarbazine, lomustine (CeeNU), and vincristine (Oncovin). Studies have shown that 75% of these tumors respond to therapy, and 50% of tumors will recover completely. Chemotherapy is not curative, but it can induce sustained remissions. Management should be individualized, and there is some evidence that specific molecular genetic changes provide information on the sensitivity of tumors to chemotherapy and prognostic information.

EPENDYMOMAS

- Ependymomas have a bimodal incidence with an early major peak at 5 yrs old and a late minor peak at the median age of 34 yrs. They account for 5% of intracranial tumors in the adult population. There is a 3:2 male predominance.
- **Histologically,** these tumors arise from the ependymal cells, which are normally lining the ventricular chambers and the central canal of the spinal cord. Most are histologically benign. Usually they are classified as either **high or low grade.** These

tumors may metastasize via CSF pathways. Spinal cord metastases that arise from a brain lesion are known as "drop metastases." The overall risk of seeding is approximately 10%, and the greatest risk occurs with high-grade infratentorial lesions.

- **Clinical presentation** depends on the location of the tumor. Most adult tumors occur the spinal canal, especially the lumbosacral region. They are also frequently seen in supra- and infratentorial regions. The supra- and infratentorial lesions usually lead to symptoms of increased intracranial pressure once large enough or focal neurologic deficits and seizures. Ataxia, vertigo, and neck stiffness are common **presenting symptoms** with infratentorial lesions.

- Diagnosis is usually accomplished with an **MRI** of the brain and spinal cord. More than 50% of these tumors will have calcification.

Management

Prognosis for these patients is excellent after treatment. The 5-yr disease-free survival is >80%. 10-yr survival rates range from 40–60%. Age is the most important prognostic factor with younger patients having a worse outcome. **Therapy** is surgical excision followed by irradiation. Gross total resection is the best determinant of outcome. Steroids may be given both before and after surgery to help decrease edema and other complications. Targeting only the local site with methods such as hig-fractionation radiotherapy or stereotactic radiosurgery have shown promise in treating the tumor and limiting some of the complications seen. There is no role for chemotherapy at this time. Evidence of dissemination, as determined by positive CSF cytology or myelographic findings, warrants additional radiation of the spinal axis. The dose and extent of irradiation are also determined by the histologic grade, with anaplastic lesions generally receiving more intensive regimens. Patients should be followed by MRI, as the recurrence rate is significant.

MENINGIOMA

Meningiomas are extraaxial primary brain tumors. They are of leptomeningeal origin, arising from arachnoid cap cells. They account for nearly 20% of intracranial neoplasms. The annual incidence of meningiomas is approximately 7.8/100,000, although most are asymptomatic and discovered incidentally at autopsy. The incidence of symptomatic tumors is approximately 2/100,000 and occurs more frequently in women than men. They are primarily adult tumors with a peak occurrence at age 45 yrs. There is an association with breast cancer, neurofibromatosis, and a history of cranial irradiation.

Classification

They typically are classified as one of four histologic patterns: meningothelial, transitional, fibrous, and angioblastic. The first three subtypes account for the majority of the meningiomas and have benign behavior. The angioblastic subtype is the least common but most aggressive form. **Malignancy** is determined by the amount of brain invasion, increased and atypical mitotic figures, increased cellularity, a papillary histologic pattern, and distant metastases. Malignant meningiomas account for between 1 and 10% of cases. Metastatic disease is seen in <0.1% of cases. Radiation-induced meningiomas are more commonly atypical or malignant. All meningiomas are characterized by the **loss of chromosome 22q.**

Clinical Presentation

Meningiomas can arise virtually anywhere along the leptomeninges. 90% are intracranial, and 90% of those are supratentorial. The three most common sites are adjacent to superior sagittal sinus, over the cerebral convexities, and along the sphenoid ridge. These three sites account for 60% on intracranial meningiomas. Clinical **presentation** of meningiomas varies greatly depending on where they arise. Focal neurologic deficits are common, as are symptoms of increased intracranial pressure. Seizures are particularly common occurring in >50% of patients. Many are found incidentally on CT or MRI.

Diagnosis

Diagnosis of these tumors is usually accomplished using an MRI. They have a characteristic appearance as well as circumscribed, extraaxial, homogenously enhancing, dural-based masses. Peritumoral edema and mass effect are common. 20% have calcification.

Management

- Surgical **resection** of these tumors is considered curative in patients with total resection. Tumors at the base of the skull are usually unresectable, because they are intertwined with vital structures. **Stereotactic radiosurgery** is another option in patients with a tumor that is <3 cm in diameter. At the time of **recurrence,** a second resection should be performed, followed by external beam irradiation.
- Meningiomas have an excellent **prognosis.** Disease-free survival at 10 yrs is 80–90% for all meningiomas. If the tumor is partially resected, the 10-yr progression-free survival is 50–70%. Nearly 65% of malignant meningiomas will recur in 5 yrs, and nearly 80% will recur in 10 yrs. Those patients who are younger, do not have CNS invasion, and those who were able to have more extensive resection do better overall. All patients should be followed closely for recurrence.

PRIMARY CNS LYMPHOMA

These are B cell malignancies of intermediate to high grade, usually diffuse, and large-cell subtype that present within the CNS without any evidence of systemic lymphoma. It represents 1–3% of intracranial tumors. Patients with congenital or acquired immuno-suppression have a markedly increased risk of primary CNS lymphoma. The **incidence** of primary CNS lymphoma peaks in the sixth to seventh decades with a male:female ratio of 2:1. There are no environmental or behavioral risk factors that are associated with the development of this disease. In immunocompromised patients, the risk increases 100- to 1000-fold. This increase is believed to most likely be secondary to infection with Epstein-Barr or other lymphatic viruses, which have been speculated as possible transforming events.

Clinical Presentation

These **lymphomas** are solitary in approximately 40% of patients on presentation, but they typically become multifocal in most patients. They most commonly present with behavioral or cognitive changes, seen in approximately two-thirds of patients. Hemiparesis, aphasia, and visual field deficits are seen in approximately 50% of patients and seizures in 15–20%. Approximately 15% will develop uveitis, sometimes preceding cerebral symptoms by months.

Diagnosis

These tumors are typically diagnosed with the use of MRI. They usually are periventricular in location and have a homogenous pattern of enhancement. Approximately 25% of patients will also have cells identified in the CSF. Stereotactic biopsy is necessary for tissue diagnosis.

Treatment

- **Prognosis** is dependent on treatment regimen. **Radiation** alone usually results in a median survival of 12–18 mos. When **chemotherapy** is used before radiation, the median survival improves to 42 mos, with 25% of patients alive at 5 yrs. Important indicators of poor prognosis include nonambulatory performance status and age (>60 yrs). Additional factors that have been associated with a poor prognosis include the presence of multiple neurologic deficits, elevated CSF protein, and nonhemispheric location.

- Unlike other intracranial tumors, there is **no role for surgery** in primary CNS lymphoma treatment. Treatment usually begins with **high-dose methotrexate** (Folex), which is associated with complete response rates of 50–80%. However, the effectiveness of steroids generally diminishes with disease progression. Typically, patients are treated with systemic steroids and high-dose cytosine arabinoside (Cytosar-U). Addition of radiation after chemotherapy has been beneficial. The radiation ports should include the orbits if retinal or vitreous disease is present and also spinal axis if CSF cytology findings suggest meningeal disease.

METASTATIC TUMORS OF THE CNS

Metastatic lesions to the brain typically occur via hematogenous spread. There typically is a predilection for the gray matter–white matter junction in which cerebral blood flow is greatest. Spinal involvement may be secondary to spread from primary site to the vertebral body, with subsequent compression of the spinal cord, retrograde spread via the vertebral venous plexus, or direct invasion of the epidural space via the intervertebral foramen. 20% of cancer patients will develop brain metastases, and 10% will develop spinal metastases. Refer to Chap. 35, Oncologic Emergencies, for more information regarding spinal cord compression.

Brain Metastases

- Lung is the **most common origin** of brain metastases. Other sources include breast (especially ductal carcinoma), GI malignancies, melanoma, germ cell tumors, and thyroid cancer.
- Metastatic tumors present with the *same clinical features* common to any intracranial mass but occur with a *much more rapid rate of progression*. Focal deficits, seizures, and symptoms of increased intracranial pressure are the usual **presenting symptoms.** The rapid progression is believed to be secondary to the rapid increase in cerebral edema that is usually associated with metastatic lesions.
- **Diagnosis** of these lesions is usually accomplished with CT using contrast. Ring enhancing or diffusely enhancing lesions, typically surrounded by a zone of edema that is out of proportion to the size of the lesion, are most commonly seen. MRI is also useful and is more sensitive in identifying multiple lesions. These cancers are typically considered incurable with few exceptions.
- **Therapy is frequently palliative** in nature. High-dose glucocorticosteroids will frequently provide a rapid improvement in symptoms as the surrounding edema decreases. Improvement occurs within 6–24 hrs, and is sustained with continuous therapy. **Anticonvulsants** are administered empirically, as one-third of patients will develop seizures. **Whole brain radiation** therapy is the primary treatment mode in brain metastases. For those patients who have a single lesion in the brain, surgical excision may be used as a palliative measure. Surgical excision is typically followed by whole brain irradiation. In primary cancers that are chemotherapy responsive, systemic chemotherapy may provide some improvement, although there is typically less of a response than that seen in the primary tumor.
- **Survival** in untreated brain metastases is typically 1 mo. Survival improves to a median of 3–6 mos with the use of steroids and radiation. If the tumor is amenable to surgical excision, the survival may improve to a median of 40 wks.

KEY POINTS TO REMEMBER

- Metastases to the CNS are far more common than primary CNS lesions in adults, and the most common primary CNS lesions are astrocytic tumors.

- There is currently no convincing data that cellular phones or power lines cause CNS tumors.
- CNS lymphoma is the only primary CNS malignancy that does not require surgical excision.
- Metastasis to the CNS is associated with and extremely poor short-term survival.

REFERENCES AND SUGGESTED READINGS

Bigner DD, McLendon RE, Bruner JM, eds. *Russell and Rubinstein's pathology of tumors of the nervous system.* New York: Oxford University Press, 1998.

DeAngelis L. Medical progress: brain tumors. *N Engl J Med* 2001;344(2):114–123.

Galanis E, Buckner J. Chemotherapy of brain tumors. *Curr Opin Neurol* 2000;13(6):619–625.

Landis SH, Murray T, Bolden S, et al. Cancer statistics, 1999. *CA Cancer J Clin* 1999;49:8–31.

Legler JM, Ries LA, Smith MA, et al. Brain and other central nervous system cancers: recent trends in incidence and mortality. *J Natl Cancer Inst* 1999;91:1382–1390.

Murphy G, Lawrence W, Raymond EL, eds. *American Cancer Society textbook of clinical oncology.* Atlanta: American Cancer Society, 1995.

Perry JR, Louis DN, Cairncross MD. Current treatment of oligodendrogliomas. *Arch Neurol* 1999;56:434–436.

Pollack IF, et al. Prognostic factors in the diagnosis and treatment of primary central nervous system lymphoma. *Cancer* 1989;63(5):939–947.

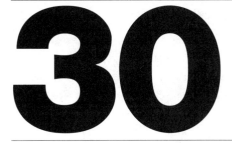

The Leukemias

Judah D. Friedman

INTRODUCTION

The leukemic disorders result from the accumulation of neoplastic WBCs in the bone marrow, peripheral blood, and organs. This may present as bone marrow failure (anemia, thrombocytopenia, and leukopenia), elevated total WBC count, or organ dysfunction. The diagnosis is typically made on a peripheral smear revealing blasts and confirmed on bone marrow biopsy. The prognosis and treatment depend on an accurate determination of the type and staging of the leukemia.

ACUTE LEUKEMIA

The cells of acute leukemia result from the clonal proliferation of an abnormal progenitor stem cell. These cells fail to further differentiate and demonstrate rapid division. These patients are gravely ill from severe bone marrow suppression. The hematopoietic progenitor that loses its ability to differentiate and replicates is usually either a lymphocyte or myelocyte precursor; however, a lesser proportion of cases may have features of both (biphenotypic leukemia). The untreated clinical course is typically very short, and patients can require intense chemotherapeutic regimens or stem cell transplant for treatment.

ACUTE MYELOGENOUS LEUKEMIA

Acute myelogenous leukemia (AML) results from the abnormal proliferation of a myeloid hematopoietic progenitor cell and accounts for 80% of adult leukemias. The median age of diagnosis is 50–60 yrs. In the United States, there is an annual incidence of 2.4/100,000, which increases to 12.6/100,000 in those ≥ 65 yrs. Radiation, previous chemotherapy with alkylating agents or topoisomerase inhibitors, myelodysplasia, myeloproliferative disorders, aplastic anemia, and exposure to benzene are known **risk factors** for the development of AML. People with Down's, Turner's and Klinefelter syndromes are at a higher risk for developing AML. In most cases, very few, if any, risk factors are clearly defined.

Diagnostic Evaluation

Clinical Presentation

Marked cytopenias from leukemic infiltration result in a diverse presentation, including fatigue, pallor, dyspnea on exertion from anemia, hemorrhage from thrombocytopenia, and infection or fever from neutropenia. Leukemic cells may infiltrate many organs, resulting in hepatomegaly, splenomegaly, lymphadenopathy, and, in the case of skin involvement, leukemia cutis. One may see gingival hypertrophy from leukemic infiltrate often with myelomonocytic leukemia. The CNS may also be involved. With leukocyte counts >100,000, leukostasis may occur, resulting in pulmonary infiltrates or cerebrovascular events. Spontaneous tumor lysis syndrome may cause metabolic abnormalities of hyperuricemia, hyperphosphatemia, hypocalcemia, or hyperkalemia. Patients may also present with disseminated intravascular coagulation (with excessive bleeding), more commonly seen in the M3 and M5 subtypes.

TABLE 30-1. ACUTE MYELOGENOUS LEUKEMIA CLASSIFICATION BY FAB

Subtype	Name	Frequency (%)	Peroxidase/ SB/NE[a]
M0	Myeloblastic with minimal differentiation	<5	–/–/–
M1	Myeloblastic without maturation	20	+/+/–
M2	Myeloblastic with maturation	25	+/+/–
M3	Promyelocytic (APML)	10	+/+/–
M4	Myelomonocytic	20	+/+/+
M4Eo	Myelomonocytic with abnormal eosinophils	5–10	+/+/+
M5	Monocytic	20	–/–/+
M6	Erythroleukemia	5	+/+/–
M7	Megakaryoblastic	<5	–/–/+

+, positive; –, negative.
[a]Myeloperoxidase, Sudan black (SB), nonspecific esterase (NE) stains.
Adapted from DeVita VT, Hellman S, Rosenberg S. *Cancer: principles and practice of oncology*, 6th ed. Philadelphia: Lippincott Williams & Wilkins, 2001.

Lab Evaluation

Basic workup should begin with a CBC (pancytopenia may be present), coagulation tests (DIC may be present), electrolytes (check for hyperkalemia, hypocalcemia, hyperphosphatemia, or hyperuricemia as a result of tumor lysis), and possibly an LP (to check for CNS involvement). Leukemic myeloblasts on Wright-Giemsa stain of the peripheral blood and bone marrow aspirate demonstrate large nuclei with scant cytoplasms that may exhibit Auer rods (eosinophilic needle-like inclusions). *Acute leukemia is defined by >30% leukemic blasts in the bone marrow aspirate*. Flow cytometry of peripheral blood or bone marrow may be needed to distinguish acute myeloid leukemias from lymphoid. In addition, morphology, cytogenetics, and histochemical staining may also help make this distinction. These include peroxidase, periodic acid-Schiff, and terminal deoxynucleotidal transferase.

Staging

The **FAB group** identifies nine subtypes of AML that are based on morphology and staining (Table 30-1). They indicate the myeloid lineage and the degree of differentiation. Cytogenetic and molecular subtype should also be obtained and helps to determine prognosis and treatment. For example, the M3 subtype is associated with the translocation 15;17. Recently, the **WHO** developed a classification system of AML based not only on morphologic findings but also on genetic and clinical findings. In the WHO classification (Table 30-2), the blast count necessary for the diagnosis of AML is reduced from 30% to 20%

TABLE 30-2. WHO CLASSIFICATION OF ACUTE MYELOID LEUKEMIA (AML) (SIMPLIFIED)

I	AML with recurrent genetic abnormalities
II	AML with multilineage dysplasia (MDS-related)
III	AML and MDS, therapy related (from alkylator/topoisomerase II inhibitors)
IV	AML, not otherwise categorized

MDS, myelodysplastic syndrome.
Adapted from Vardiman JW, Harris NL, Brunning RD. The World Health Organization (WHO) classification of the myeloid neoplasms. *Blood* 2002;100(7):2292–2302.

TABLE 30-3. POSTINDUCTION THERAPY OPTIONS

	Allogeneic transplant	Autologous transplant	Chemotherapy
Recommended age	<55 yrs	<55 yrs	<60 yrs
Benefits	50–60% cure rate	45–55% cure rate	40% 4-yr survival
Risks	GVHD, transplant-related death	Transplant-related death	Chemotherapy-related morbidity
Comparisons	Theoretical graft vs leukemic effect but highest transplant-related mortality.	Relapse may be higher. Outcomes similar to chemotherapy.	Relapse may be higher.

GVHD, graft-vs-host disease.

blasts in the blood or marrow. Patients with clonal recurrent cytogenetic abnormalities such as t(8;21) inv(16), t(15;17) have AML regardless of the blast percentage. This classification is meant to better highlight biologic behavior and response to therapy.

Management

- Treatment is divided into two phases: **induction** and **postinduction.** The goal is to achieve remission, defined as <5% blasts in the bone marrow and recovery of peripheral blood counts.
  - **Induction** chemotherapy involves 7 days of cytarabine (Ara-C) and 3 days of daunorubicin (DaunoXome) or idarubicin (Idamycin) ("7+3"regimen). Complete remission can be obtained in approximately 70–80% of patients 60 yrs and younger and in approximately 50% of older patients.
  - **Postinduction** therapy is essential to prevent relapse. Three therapeutic options are available: allogeneic bone marrow transplantation, autologous bone marrow transplantation, or further chemotherapy with high-dose cytarabine (Table 30-3).
- For **promyelocytic (M3) leukemia,** all-*trans*-retinoic acid is given twice a day with induction chemotherapy. Maintenance therapy with lower dose all-*trans*-retinoic acid is then necessary.
- In the case of **relapse,** patients should be considered for bone marrow transplantation. Patients who relapse within 6 mos of complete remission should be considered for experimental drugs if they are not bone marrow transplant candidates. For patients >12 mos in remission, their disease may be sensitive to reinduction chemotherapy regimens.

Prognosis

Leukemia can typically be divided into good, poor, and intermediate prognosis groups. These groups often help guide the decision to offer stem cell transplant, as a good-prognosis leukemia often can be cured with standard chemotherapy, whereas poorer-prognosis leukemias are more likely to relapse despite intensive chemotherapy and may benefit from transplant after first remission. "*Good-prognosis*" leukemias are those with favorable cytogenetics: translocation 15;17 (associated with M3 AML), translocation 8;21, and inversion 16 associated with M4 AML with eosinophilia. These patients are typically offered induction therapy followed by consolidation only, as they have a relatively high rate of cure by this strategy (approximately 60–70%). Poor prognostic indicators include age >60 yrs; AML secondary to myelodysplastic syndrome or antecedent hematologic disorder; deletion of 5q, 7q, or trisomy 8; and lack of the favorable cytogenetics [e.g., t(6;9) or t(9;22)] noted earlier. Patients with poor-prognosis leukemia have a high rate of relapse and should be considered for allogeneic bone marrow transplant after induction. Patients with normal cytogenetics fall into an intermediate-risk group, and management should be individualized after remission. Clinical trials are always ongoing, and, whenever appropriate, patients in all groups should be considered for participation. A helpful resource sponsored by the National Cancer Institute can be found at http://cancer.gov/clinicaltrials/. **Survival rates** have improved. Since 1970, the 5-yr survival rate has increased from 15–40% with advances in therapies. Specific subtypes have even better prognoses. For example, in the case of promyelocytic leukemia patients on all-*trans*-retinoic acid, 70% remain disease free at 4 yrs.

ACUTE LYMPHOBLASTIC LEUKEMIA

Acute lymphoblastic leukemia (ALL) results from the abnormal proliferation of a lymphoid hematopoietic progenitor cell. It accounts for 80% of childhood leukemias and 20% of adult leukemias. This section deals only with adult ALL, which has a worse prognosis than childhood ALL.

Diagnostic Evaluation

Clinical Presentation

Patients present with malaise, fatigue, and bone pain. Signs of marrow failure are evident as bleeding, bruising, fever, and infection. 10% of patients present with headache and/or cranial nerve palsies from leukemic infiltration of the CNS; symptoms of a stroke may also be present. In addition, other symptoms may include arthralgias, dyspnea, or hypoxia in part from the leukostasis. Hepatosplenomegaly and lymphadenopathy can be seen. They can be associated with an anterior mediastinal mass (in T-cell subtypes) that can be seen on chest x-ray or large abdominal lymph nodes (in B-cell subtypes).

Lab Evaluation

Basic workup is similar to that of AML (please see Acute Myelogenous Leukemia, Lab Evaluation). A peripheral smear will usually demonstrate the presence of circulating blasts. Bone marrow will be hypercellular with >30% blasts. Cytoplasmic granules and Auer rods should be absent. However, it can be extremely difficult to diagnose ALL on clinical and morphologic grounds alone. Immunophenotyping is often necessary to distinguish ALL from AML. 30% of adult ALL patients exhibit the Philadelphia chromosome t(9;22), as seen in chronic myelogenous leukemia (CML).

Staging

Classification is based on morphologic (FAB system) and immunophenotypic information (Tables 30-4 and 30-5).

Management

- Therapy for ALL consists of three phases of treatment: (a) an initial induction intended to induce a complete remission, (b) CNS prophylaxis to treat the CNS "sanctuary site," and (c) maintenance therapy to maintain remission.

TABLE 30-4. FAB CLASSIFICATION OF ACUTE LYMPHOBLASTIC LEUKEMIAS

Subtype	Morphology
L1	Small lymphoblastic (childhood)
L2	Large lymphoblastic (adult)
L3	Undifferentiated, large vacuolated (Burkitt-like)

Adapted from DeVita VT, Hellman S, Rosenberg S. *Cancer: principles and practice of oncology*, 6th ed. Philadelphia: Lippincott Williams & Wilkins, 2001.

TABLE 30-5. IMMUNOTYPE CLASSIFICATION

Immuno-type	Frequency (%)	FAB subtype	Staining
Pre–B cell	75	L1, L2	+TdT, +CALLA, B-cell markers (CD19, CD20)
T cell	20	L1, L2	+TdT, –CALLA, +acid phosphatase, +T-cell markers (CD2, CD7, CD5)
B cell	5	L3	–TdT, +surface IgG

CALLA, common acute lymphoblastic leukemia antigen; TdT, terminal deoxynucleotidyl transferase.

- **Induction chemotherapy** typically consists of vincristine (Oncovin), prednisone (Deltasone, Orasone), and an anthracycline. Some protocols include L-asparaginase (Elspar) as well. These multiagent protocols carry the burden of profound myelosuppression, and patients must be followed intensely for infectious and cytopenic complications. Complete remissions of 50–70% have been achieved with multiagent therapy. Patients in first remission but with high-risk disease may be offered allogeneic bone marrow transplantation.
- **CNS prophylaxis** is an important component of therapy for ALL, as it has a high incidence of recurrence in the CNS. Regimens typically consist of intrathecal methotrexate (Folex, Rheumatrex, Trexall), usually in combination with either cranial irradiation or high-dose systemic methotrexate.
- **Maintenance therapy** is typically continued for several years, often with mercaptopurine (Purinethol) or methotrexate. However, the optimal regimen for maintenance therapy is not yet clear and is under investigation.
- **Relapse,** unfortunately, is very common in adult ALL. After relapse, patients may be considered for further reinduction chemotherapy, possibly followed by autologous or allogeneic stem cell transplant.

Complications

Leukostasis (especially in patients with AML) may cause symptoms that require emergent leukophoresis. Tumor lysis syndrome, fever, and neutropenia are all concerns as well (see Chap. 36, Oncologic Emergencies). In addition, hematologic abnormalities, such as anemia, thrombocytopenia, and DIC, may be a result of therapies given and should be managed accordingly. If the patient has received a bone marrow transplant, he or she should be followed closely for symptoms of opportunistic infections and graft vs. host disease (see Chap. 32, Introduction to Bone Marrow Transplant).

Prognosis

Although 60–90% of patients can expect to undergo a complete remission with induction chemotherapy, the majority of patients will relapse. Patients who are younger and have good prognostic indicators have a cure rate of 50–70%. Those who are older and have poor prognostic indicators have a cure rate of only 10–30%. Poor indicators include male gender; age >9 yrs and <2 yrs; WBC >15,000–30,000/μL; prolonged time to first remission; L3 Burkitt's morphology; B-cell immunotype; and translocations 8;14, 9;22 (Philadelphia chromosome), and 4;11.

CHRONIC LEUKEMIAS

The chronic leukemias result from the accumulation of differentiated neoplastic WBCs. In comparison to the acute leukemia, they are typically low grade and progress slowly. Some chronic leukemias can be observed for extended periods with no or minimal treatment.

CHRONIC MYELOGENOUS LEUKEMIA

CML, a disorder of hematopoietic stem cells that results in the **overproduction of mature myeloid cells,** accounts for 20% of newly diagnosed leukemias. The median age at presentation is between 50 and 60 yrs. CML patients have the diagnostic t(9;22) translocation. The translocation places the Bcr (breakpoint cluster region) on chromosome 22 next to the Abl gene on chromosome 9. The resulting fusion protein, Bcr-Abl, is a constitutively active tyrosine kinase that drives the cell into uncontrolled proliferation. There are three phases to CML: **chronic** (lasting 3–6 yrs), **accelerated,** and **blast.** Patients are usually diagnosed during the chronic phase and are relatively stable and respond to therapy. Accelerated-phase patients have worsening cytopenias and resistance to therapy. Blast phase is an acute leukemia that is typically rapidly progressive and poorly responsive to therapy. Patients may develop these phases sequentially or progress directly into blast phase from chronic and have an approximately 25%/year chance of doing so.

Diagnostic Evaluation

Clinical Presentation

Most patients are asymptomatic and discovered by routine CBC. However, some may present with generalized fatigue, night sweats, bone pain, fevers, or splenomegaly. Those who present in the blast phase have signs and symptoms of acute leukemia such as fever, weight loss, bleeding, and anemia.

Lab Evaluation

In the *chronic* phase, the CBC is characterized by progressive granulocytosis, often showing a WBC count >50,000/μL with <5% blasts. Basophilia and eosinophilia can be seen as well. Bone marrow shows hypercellularity with <5% blasts. Cytogenetics reveal the Philadelphia chromosome, which is the translocation of chromosomes 9 and 22 (t9;22). This feature is virtually diagnostic for CML but may be seen in other leukemias as well. *Accelerated* phase patients have intermediate numbers of blasts in the bone marrow and blood: >5% but <30% blasts in the blood or marrow. *Blast* phase is myeloblastic in 70–80% of patients and lymphoblastic in 20–30% of patients. It is also an acute leukemia, with marrow or blood blasts >30%.

Management

The treatment strategy for CML is currently in flux. Imatinib mesylate (Gleevec), formally known as *STI571*, is a specific inhibitor of the Bcr-Abl tyrosine kinase that causes CML. In May 2001, imatinib was approved for the treatment of CML refractory to interferon. Imatinib results in a >95% hematologic response and a 76% cytogenetic response in patients who have failed interferon therapy. It may be used in conjunction with standard therapies. Many patients are considered for treatment with imatinib regardless of whether they have failed conventional therapy. Standard treatment for CML includes the following:

- Hydroxyurea (Droxia, Hydrea), an oral agent that reduces leukocytosis, thrombocytosis, shrinks the spleen, and improves quality of life with minimal toxic effects.
- Interferon-alpha, given SC or IM 3×/wk, controls leukocytosis in 75% of patients. Interferon-alpha can delay blast phase and extend survival by approximately 1–2 yrs as compared to hydroxyurea. Side effects include flu-like symptoms.
- Allogeneic bone marrow transplantation for suitable candidates is potentially curative, although carries with it high morbidity. Better results are achieved in young patients (40–50 yrs) with an HLA-identical sibling when transplanted within the first 2 yrs after diagnosis.

In the stable phase, symptoms resulting from leukocytosis, thrombocytosis, and splenomegaly can be managed with oral hydroxyurea. Many patients remain asymptomatic during this phase. Unfortunately, the blast phase is inevitable, and the usual time to transformation ranges from 5–7 yrs. In these patients, the current options are limited to allogeneic bone marrow transplantation, interferon-alpha, or imatinib mesylate. Overall, there is still a poor prognosis for patients who progress to blast phase.

Prognosis

Before the introduction of imatinib, median survival was 5 yrs. Patients who present with an aggressive form of disease survive only months; others have an indolent chemoresponsive CML and live 10 yrs or longer. The cure rate is approximately 60% with allogeneic bone marrow transplantation. There is also a Philadelphia chromosome–negative CML, which carries a poorer prognosis.

CHRONIC LYMPHOCYTIC LEUKEMIA

Chronic lymphocytic leukemia (CLL) results from an accumulation of malignant, immunologically incompetent but mature B-cell lymphocytes. It most commonly presents in men older than 50 yrs. Those with a history of immunodeficiency syndromes are more prone to the development of CLL. The malignant cells of CLL express high levels of the antiapoptotic protein, bcl-2, and express common B-cell antigens CD19, CD20, and CD23. Of note, CD5 antigen, a T-cell antigen, is found in all cases of CLL. A Coombs-positive, warm antibody, hemolytic anemia occurs in 10% of patients, and an immune thrombocytopenia occurs in approximately 5% of patients. In 5% of patients, Richter's syndrome develops, which is a malignant transformation to a diffuse large-cell lymphoma.

Diagnostic Evaluation

Clinical Presentation

Many patients are discovered by routine CBC and are asymptomatic. However, chronic fatigue is one of the more common initial complaints. With bone marrow involvement, patients develop severe fatigue, anemia, bruising, weight loss, and fever. On physical exam, marked splenomegaly, hepatomegaly, and lymphadenopathy can be present. With advancing immunodeficiency, herpes zoster infections, *Pneumocystis carinii* pneumonia, and bacterial infections become more frequent.

Lab Evaluation

- A CBC with differential reveals an absolute lymphocytosis, with >95% small lymphocytes. A blood smear should show **mature lymphocytes.** The classic smudge cell is nonspecific. Anemia and/or thrombocytopenia may be present from bone marrow infiltration or from an autoimmune phenomenon. It is important to assess renal and hepatic function, Coombs antiglobulin, serum protein electrophoresis, chest radiograph, and CT scan of the chest, abdomen, and pelvis. Patients with CLL typically have at least 30% lymphocytes in the bone marrow. A **bone marrow biopsy** should be obtained if the diagnosis is uncertain, or if there is thrombocytopenia or a Coombs-negative anemia.
- It is important to consider *benign* causes of lymphocytosis, including Epstein-Barr virus mononucleosis, chronic infections, autoimmune diseases, drug and allergic reactions, thyrotoxicosis, adrenal insufficiency, and postsplenectomy. The other possible malignancies to consider are hairy cell leukemia (HCL), cutaneous T-cell lymphoma, leukemic non-Hodgkin's lymphoma, prolymphocytic leukemia, and large granular lymphocytic leukemia. Flow cytometry can be helpful in delineating cell markers for diagnosis.

Staging

Classification of CLL is based on the extent of systemic infiltration of lymphocytes. This helps to determine prognosis and the initiation of treatment (Table 30-6).

Management

- It is not necessary to initiate therapy early in the course of CLL. CLL patients are immunocompromised, and fever or any other signs of infection need to be evaluated promptly. **Indications for therapy** include symptoms (fevers, sweats, weight loss), obstructive or advancing lymphadenopathy, spleen or liver enlargement, stages III or IV disease, immune hemolysis or thrombocytopenia, or rapid elevation in lym-

TABLE 30-6. MODIFIED RAI CLASSIFICATION

Stage	Lymphocyte involvement	Prognosis
0	>40% lymphocytes in bone marrow, >5,000/μL blood lymphocytes	Low risk, with >10-yr survival
I	Stage 0 + lymphadenopathy	Intermediate risk, with 7-yr survival
II	Stage 0 or I + hepatosplenomegaly	Intermediate risk, with 7-yr survival
III	Stage 0, I, or II + Hgb <11 g/dL[a]	High risk, with 2-yr survival
IV	Stage 0, I, or II + platelets <100,000/μL[a]	High risk, with 2-yr survival

[a]Anemia and thrombocytopenia resulting from bone marrow infiltration, not from autoimmune destruction.
Adapted from Rozman C, Monserrat E. Current concepts: chronic lymphocytic leukemia. *N Engl J Med* 1995;333:1052–1057.

phocyte count. Conventional treatment is given to control these symptoms, and options include the following:

- Fludarabine (Fludara), a nucleoside, given for 4 wks, is generally chosen as first-line therapy.
- Chlorambucil (Leukeran), an alkylating agent, is given for 3–6 wks. This is an option for resistant disease or for those patients initially treated with fludarabine.
- Combination chemotherapy [e.g., cyclophosphamide (Cytoxan), hydroxydaunorubicin (DaunoXome), vincristine (Oncovin), prednisone] as third-line agents.
- Alemtuzumab (Campath) may also have a role as third-line treatment for CLL.
- Autologous and allogeneic bone marrow transplantations are being explored as options. Young patients with high-risk disease should be considered for this therapy.
- Immune hemolysis or thrombocytopenias should be treated with prednisone or equivalent glucocorticoid at a dose of 1 mg/kg/day, then tapered after control of blood counts. Splenectomy may be needed if the blood counts do not improve on steroids. Local irradiation or splenectomy can control the effects of hypersplenism.

Prognosis

Diffuse marrow involvement, rapidly increasing lymphocyte counts, and initial lymphocytosis of >50,000/μL indicate a poor prognosis for an individual patient with early-stage disease. Anemia and thrombocytopenia correspond with decreased median survival time. Overall, CLL is an indolent disease, and, in the case of stages 0, I, and II, median survivals of >10 yrs are reported. Thus, these patients may die of other comorbid conditions, rather than from CLL. However, if a patient presents with advanced disease, his or her course may be rapid, with a median survival of months to years. It is unclear whether cytotoxic therapy actually improves survival, although it can effectively palliate disease-related symptoms. However, improved supportive care and infection therapy have improved survival and quality of life.

HAIRY CELL LEUKEMIA

HCL is a chronic B-cell leukemia, accounting for only 2–3% of all leukemias, usually affecting men >55 yrs.

Diagnostic Evaluation

Clinial Presentation
Most patients present with malaise and fatigue. On physical exam, splenomegaly or hepatomegaly are evident in 95% and 40%, respectively. With more advanced dis-

TABLE 30-7. THERAPEUTIC OPTIONS FOR HAIRY CELL LEUKEMIA

Therapy	Comment
Cladribine	First-line agent, 7-day IV infusion with >90% response rate.
Interferon-alpha	Given for 1 yr, >90% response rate.
Pentostatin	Given for 3–6 mos, many patients have a complete response. Complicated by neurotoxicity and skin rash.
Splenectomy	Achieves a 75% response rate.

ease, pancytopenia develops, and patients may present with bleeding or recurrent infections (bacterial, viral, fungal, or atypical mycobacterial).

Laboratory Evaluation
A peripheral smear and bone marrow reveal the pathognomonic mononuclear cells. These cells have characteristic irregular hair-like projections around the border of the cytoplasm. CBC frequently shows anemia and thrombocytopenia and, less frequently, granulocytopenia. Although bone marrow aspiration is frequently unsuccessful, the biopsy may show the characteristic hairy cells. Immune studies are CD19, CD20, and typically CD103 positive. Also, hairy cells are TRAP positive (tartrate-resistant acid phosphatase), meaning they have strong acid phosphatase activity that is resistant to tartaric acid inhibition. HCL is differentiated from CLL, lymphomas, and monocytic leukemia based on the characteristic cell morphology, TRAP test, and immune phenotype. There is no formal staging system.

Management

As HCL has a slow course, the decision to treat is based on the development of cytopenias (Hgb <10 g/dL, absolute neutrophil count <1000/μL, platelets <100,000/μL) and recurrent infections. Several treatment options are available (Table 30-7), but are not curative.

Prognosis

Before treatment, median survival was between 5 and 10 yrs. Survival has markedly improved with current therapies.

MULTIPLE MYELOMA

Multiple myeloma is a monoclonal plasma cell disorder that may enter a leukemic phase. Please refer to Chap. 14, Plasma Cell Disorders, for further information.

KEY POINTS TO REMEMBER

- The leukemias are malignant proliferations of WBCs circulating in the blood. An accurate determination of the type and staging of the leukemia is essential for proper treatment and determination of prognosis.
- Acute leukemias are proliferations of immature cells that are rapidly progressive and typically quickly fatal, whereas the chronic leukemias tend to be more indolent and have a longer course, with mature circulating cells.
- It can be extremely difficult to distinguish ALL from AML on clinical and morphologic grounds alone, but AML cells tend to have cytoplasmic granules and Auer rods. The staining characteristics (e.g., Sudan Black, terminal deoxynucleotidyl transferase) are not perfect indicators of type, and subtype and flow cytometry is needed for accurate diagnosis.

- As a **general** rule, ALLs are childhood diseases, and AMLs are adult diseases. ALL in adults typically confers a worse prognosis.
- In promyelocytic (M3) leukemia, all-*trans*-retinoic acid is given with induction chemotherapy to help prevent overt fulminant DIC.
- "Good-prognosis" AMLs include those with cytogenetics of translocation 15;17 (M3 or APML), translocation 8;21, and inversion 16. They can often be managed successfully without stem cell transplant and with relatively high cure rates.
- CNS prophylaxis is an important component of therapy for ALL, as it has a high incidence of recurrence in the CNS.
- CML is often considered a myeloproliferative disorder.
- The Philadelphia chromosome t(9;22) is present in almost every case of CML.

REFERENCES AND SUGGESTED READINGS

Byrd J, Flinn IW, Grever M. Chronic lymphocytic leukemia. *Semin Oncol* 1998;25:4–5.

Casciato DA, Lowitz BB. *Manual of clinical oncology*, 4th ed. Philadelphia: Lippincott Williams & Williams, 2000.

Cassileth PA, Harrington DP. Chemotherapy compared with autologous or allogeneic bone marrow transplantation in the management of acute myeloid leukemia in first remission. *N Engl J Med* 1998;339:1649–1656.

DeVita VT, Hellman S, Rosenberg S. *Cancer: principles and practice of oncology*, 6th ed. Philadelphia: Lippincott Williams & Wilkins, 2001.

Dighiero G, Maloum K. Chlorambucil in indolent chronic lymphocytic leukemia. *N Engl J Med* 1998;338:1506–1514.

Kalidas M, Kantarjian H, Talpaz M. Contempo updates: chronic myelogenous leukemia. *JAMA* 2001;286:895–898.

Kantarjian H, Sawyers C, et al. Hematological and cytogenetic responses to imatinib mesylate in chronic myelogenous leukemia. *N Engl J Med* 2001;346:645–652.

Lowenberg B, Downing JR, Burnett A. Medical progress: acute myeloid leukemia. *N Engl J Med* 1999;341:1051–1062.

Mortimer JE, Brown R. Medical management of malignant disease. Ahya, Flood, Paranjothi, eds. *The Washington manual of medical therapeutics*, 30th ed. Philadelphia: Lippincott Williams & Wilkins, 2001:429–454.

National Cancer Institute Web site. Adult acute myeloid leukemia. Available at: http://cancer.gov/cancerinfo/pdq/treatment/adultAML/healthprofessional/. Accessed August 2003.

Pettitt AR, Zuzell M, Cawley JC. Review: hairy-cell leukemia: biology and management. *Br J Haematol* 1999;106:2–8.

Rozman C, Montserrat E. Current concepts: chronic lymphocytic leukemia. *N Engl J Med* 1995;333:1052–1057.

Vardiman JW, Harris NL, Brunning RD. The World Health Organization (WHO) classification of the myeloid neoplasms. *Blood* 2002;100(7):2292–2302.

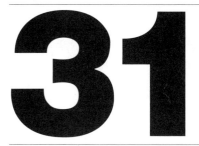

Lymphoma

Ron Bose

INTRODUCTION

The development of lymphadenopathy can be a sign of infection, spread of solid tumor, or indication of the presence of lymphoma. The lymphomas can have a staggering variation in phenotypic expression ranging from slowly growing "indolent" tumors to rapidly progressing disease. This chapter discusses common features of all lymphomas, the evaluation of enlarged lymph nodes, and an overview of the two major types of lymphoma: Hodgkin's and non-Hodgkin's. As a general rule of thumb, Hodgkin's lymphoma tends to affect younger patients and be relatively curable, whereas non-Hodgkin's disease tends to affect older patients and carry a worse long-term prognosis as a group.

LYMPHADENOPATHY AND LYMPHOMA

Clinical Presentation

- The differential diagnosis of **lymphadenopathy** includes many infectious, inflammatory, and neoplastic conditions that may also occur. Other sources of lymphadenopathy should be investigated and ruled out (Table 31-1). Lymphadenopathy, which is painful (due to stretching of the lymph node), is more likely to be related to acute inflammation/infection. Lymphadenopathy in those <40 yrs is typically less concerning than in those >40 yrs. Lymph nodes >2 cm are also more concerning than smaller ones. Location is also important: Generalized adenopathy is more concerning than localized, and supraclavicular nodes are always a concern for malignancy. In general, factors to consider when narrowing the differential diagnosis of lymphadenopathy include age (<40 yrs or >40 yrs), location of lymphadenopathy (generalized or localized), risk factors (e.g., HIV, trauma, exposure to cats), associated symptoms (e.g., fever, chills, weight loss, recent upper respiratory infection), and nodal characteristics (e.g., tenderness, symmetry, consistency, mobility).
- **Workup and management** of lymphadenopathy depends on the cause. The decision to observe and follow lymphadenopathy closely is often made if the cause appears infectious. A trial of antibiotics, further imaging, or lab evaluation may be helpful. If lymphadenopathy does not resolve or improve within 3–4 wks, then further evaluation with either fine-needle aspiration or excisional biopsy (see Diagnostic Evaluation) is appropriate. If the suspicion for malignancy is high and other corresponding symptoms are present, an earlier and more intensive workup is warranted.
- **Lymphoma patients** often present with asymptomatic lymphadenopathy. The involved lymph nodes are commonly rubbery, rather than having the hard texture caused by carcinomas. Extranodal involvement may occur in the spleen or liver, causing enlargement of these organs, or in the bone marrow, causing pancytopenia. Systemic symptoms such as fevers, drenching night sweats, weight loss (these three are known as the **"B" symptoms** of lymphoma), or chronic pruritus may be seen in up to 40% of patients. Pain may occur from mass effect, such as with abdominal pain from splenomegaly or pain related to nerve compression or infiltration. Alcohol-induced pain in areas of involvement is pathognomonic of Hodgkin's lymphomas, but rare. Patients may also present with previously unappreciated lymphadenopathy on radiographic studies.

TABLE 31-1. DIFFERENTIAL DIAGNOSIS OF LYMPHADENOPATHY

Infectious	Inflammatory
Common viral/bacterial pathogens	Rheumatologic: SLE, rheumatoid arthritis, etc.
Less common pathogens	Trauma
Mycobacterium	Allergic, including some drug reactions and serum
Bartonella	sickness
Brucellosis	**Neoplastic**
Tularemia	Lymphoma
HIV	Leukemias and myeloma
Infectious mononucleosis	Solid tumor metastasis
Secondary syphilis	
Toxoplasma	
Fungal	
Others	

Diagnosis

- After a thorough history, a **physical** that includes palpation of all accessible lymph tissue should be undertaken. This includes evaluating all palpable lymph node chains (submental, cervical, supra- and infraclavicular, axillary, epitrochlear, iliac, femoral, and popliteal), liver and spleen for enlargement, and Waldeyer's ring (tonsils and oro- and nasopharyngeal tissue). Additional imaging or procedures, such as a CT scan of the abdomen/pelvis, bone marrow biopsies, or even exploratory laparotomy and lymphangiography, may be necessary depending on the initial physical exam finding and biopsy results.
- A **biopsy** is required for diagnosis, and an **excisional** or incisional biopsy is preferred for initial diagnosis, as lymph node architecture is usually needed to properly diagnose and type lymphoma. Fine-needle aspiration should not be used for initial diagnosis, but may be preferred for staging or evaluation of recurrence. The most easily accessible tissue should be evaluated for diagnosis. Although invasive procedures such as mediastinoscopy, bronchoscopy, or laparoscopy may be needed, identification of superficial tissue by physical exam can significantly reduce the morbidity of invasive biopsy for patients. **Biopsy material** should be sent for both standard pathologic exam and immunostaining to determine subtype. In addition to standard pathologic slides, flow cytometry, cytogenetics, or other studies may be needed.

HODGKIN'S DISEASE

Hodgkin's disease is a malignancy of lymphoid tissue. In contrast to non-Hodgkin's lymphoma (NHL), it tends to spread in an orderly, predictable fashion to adjacent sites of lymph tissue. Hodgkin's disease is comparatively rare, with approximately 7500 new cases diagnosed each year in the United States, but there is a wide geographic range of incidence. Those with higher social class or education, small family size, and early birth order are more at risk. There is a **bimodal age distribution,** with peaks of incidence in the mid-20s age range and a rise in incidence after the age of 50 yrs.

Diagnostic Evaluation

Diagnostic evaluation, described earlier, may be undertaken for tissue diagnosis. **Pathologic specimen** reveals the pathognomonic **Reed-Sternberg** cells in biopsy specimen, which look like "owl's eyes." Histologic subtypes include nodular sclerosing (70–90%), mixed cellular (10–20%), lymphocyte predominant (5%), and lymphocyte depleted (1%).

TABLE 31-2. THE ANN ARBOR STAGING SYSTEM FOR LYMPHOMAS

Stage	
I	Involvement of a single lymph node region or lymphoid structure
II	Involvement of ≥ 2 node regions on the same side of the diaphragm
III	Involvement of lymph node structures on both sides of the diaphragm
IV	Involvement of one or more extranodal sites
Modifiers	
A	No additional symptoms
B	Presence of fever, drenching sweats, or weight loss
X	Bulky disease (nodal mass >10 cm or more than one-third the width of thorax)
E	Involvement of a single extranodal site contiguous or proximal to a known site

Adapted from DeVita VT, Rosenberg SA, Hellman S, eds. *Cancer: principles and practice of oncology*, 6th ed. Philadelphia: Lippincott Williams & Wilkins, 2001.

Workup should also include a CBC; LFTs; lactate dehydrogenase (LDH); creatinine level; uric acid level; ESR; HIV serology; chest x-ray; and CT scan of the chest, abdomen, and pelvis. In addition, gallium scan or bone scan may be undertaken to decide on extent of disease if there is equivocal involvement supradiaphragmatically. Bone scan may be performed if bone pain or elevated alkaline phosphatase is present. **Bilateral bone marrow biopsy** is frequently needed to rule out involvement. Staging laparotomy with splenectomy and staging of multiple lymph nodes are rarely undertaken.

Subtypes and Staging

The Rye classification divides Hodgkin's disease on the basis of pathologic appearance into lymphocyte-predominant, mixed cellularity, lymphocyte-depleted, and nodular sclerosing variants. Hodgkin's disease typically spreads in *contiguous* fashion through lymph node groups, and the **staging system** reflects this tendency. The most common extranodal sites are the spleen, liver, lung, and bone marrow (Table 31-2).

Treatment

- Therapy is based on **stage of disease** at presentation, not on cell subtype.
- **Radiation** can be delivered to local areas of disease or over a wide field (Table 31-3). Radiation is indicated as primary sole treatment of IA or IIA disease and primary combined treatment with chemotherapy in IB and IIB. It is also used as second-line therapy in stage III disease in patients with incomplete chemotherapy response. Radiation also may be part of the preparative regimen for stem cell transplant.

TABLE 31-3. TYPICAL RADIATION SITES AND DEFINITIONS

1. Mantle—cervical, bilateral clavicular, axillary, and mediastinal regions (shielding the lungs, heart apex, and thyroid gland)
2. Paraaortic/splenic
3. Pelvic
- Mantle and paraaortic/splenic—subtotal or extended field
- Paraaortic/splenic and pelvic—inverted Y field
- All three—total lymphoid irradiation

- Indications for **chemotherapy** include primary treatment of stages III and IV disease and as combination therapy in stages I and II disease per what has been previously mentioned (i.e., bulky disease or with "B" symptoms such as a fever >38.5°C, drenching night sweats, and ≥ 10% weight loss over 6 mos). Chemotherapeutic regimens are multiple and include regimens such as MOPP [mechlorethamine (Mustargen), vincristine (Oncovin), procarbazine (Matulane, Natulan), and prednisone (Deltasone)] and ABVD [doxorubicin (Adriamycin), bleomycin (Blenoxane), vinblastine (Velban, Velbe), and dacarbazine (DTIC-Dome)]. Further details regarding specific regimens can be found in other sources. After 3–4 cycles of chemotherapy, repeat imaging of positive areas is needed to assess response to therapy. If the response is complete or partial, chemotherapy is repeated an additional 2–4 cycles, and consolidative radiation may be added.
- **Stem cell transplant** can be performed in an autologous or allogeneic fashion. It is typically indicated for stages III and IV disease that does not respond to chemotherapy or for disease relapse.

Prognosis

Poor prognostic factors include advanced age, presence of "B" symptoms, male gender, age >45 yrs, anemia, leukocytosis, lymphopenia, and hypoalbuminemia. However, all patients should be approached with intent to cure given the high response rates. The majority of Hodgkin's disease patients are cured, with 75–90% of early-stage and 50–70% of stage III and IV patients cured. Patients should be followed closely, as radiation therapy increases the risk of solid tumors in the short term, and chemotherapy increases the risk of acute leukemia in the long term.

Follow-Up

Follow-up in the first 2 yrs involves history and physical, CBC, ESR, LDH, and chemistries q3mos. Chest x-ray, TSH (if neck radiation was given), and additional imaging of the original sites of disease may happen approximately q6mos. Mammography should start in women at age 40 yrs or 8–10 yrs after the initial diagnosis. Labs and history and physical may be spaced out to q6mos in the third year and then annually thereafter. Specific evaluation of symptoms should supersede these general guidelines, which are only appropriate in asymptomatic people.

Recurrence

The management of recurrence first includes a staging evaluation as in an initial diagnosis. Biopsies should be repeated and cell type and architecture reevaluated. If radiation alone was the patient's initial therapy, then typically systemic chemotherapy with or without radiotherapy is offered. If chemotherapy or combined modality treatment was the initial treatment, then bone marrow transplant is offered if the disease-free interval is <1 yr, but combined modality treatment may alternatively be offered if the disease-free interval is >1 yr.

Complications

- **Acute adverse effects** to therapy can include hair loss, mucositis, bone marrow suppression, neuropathy, or GI side effects. Infectious risks typically involve deficient cell-mediated immunity leading to herpes zoster, *Pneumocystis carinii*, CMV, toxoplasma, mycobacterial, or fungal infections. Asplenic patients are susceptible to encapsulated organisms, including streptococcus pneumonia.
- **Other adverse effects** include clinical **hypothyroidism** in 10–20% of patients receiving neck irradiation, and subclinical hypothyroidism occurs in up to 50%. **Infertility** is a frequent complication, particularly with pelvic irradiation, MOPP chemotherapy, and stem cell transplant. **Organ-specific** toxicity from chemotherapy can occur, such as bleomycin lung toxicity or doxorubicin-induced cardiotoxicity

(see Chap. 16, Chemotherapy, for more information). Radiation may also cause pneumonitis, pericarditis, cardiomyopathy, or accelerated atherosclerosis.
- **Secondary malignancies** can occur, and do so, 2–10 yrs after treatment for initial lymphoma. Leukemias that occur are often resistant to treatment and have unfavorable cytogenetics. They may be preceded by a myelodysplastic syndrome. Solid tumors are seen with increased incidence in Hodgkin's disease survivors and typically have a latency of 10 yrs but may be related to less shielding used for patients given radiation in the 1960s and 1970s.

NON-HODGKIN'S LYMPHOMA

There are approximately 60,000 new cases of NHL per year, and the incidence has been increasing over the last few decades. There are associations with pesticides and organic solvents. NHL tends to proceed in a less orderly anatomic fashion than Hodgkin's lymphoma and tends to spread hematogenously sooner.

Diagnostic Evaluation

In addition to the general workup of lymphoma described earlier, CT of the chest, abdomen, and pelvis will delineate extent of disease. CBC, LFTs, alkaline phosphatase, LDH, creatinine level, uric acid level, ESR, HIV serology, and $beta_2$-microglobulin should be drawn. Bilateral bone marrow biopsy should be performed to evaluate for disease presence. Cytogenetics and molecular analysis are needed in many cases to properly subtype the lymphoma. Lumbar puncture and evaluation of the CSF is needed for aggressive or high-grade lymphomas. Additional studies in specific cases include testicular U/S of the contralateral testes to rule out involvement in testicular lymphoma, and upper GI series with small bowel follow-through in patients with involvement of the head, neck, and Waldeyer's ring.

Classification, Grading, and Staging

- The most commonly used classifications are the **Working Formulation and Revised European American Lymphoma/World Health Organization classification** (REAL/WHO). These two classifications are complementary, with the Working Formulation classification emphasizing common lymphomas and clinical behavior, whereas the REAL/WHO system emphasizes correlating the lymphoma cell with a normal stage in lymphocyte development based on cell surface markers. The REAL/WHO classification divides lymphomas into peripheral B-cell, precursor B-cell, peripheral T-cell, and precursor T-cell types. It subsequently divides these major categories into subtypes based on molecular and cell markers. This is meant to more accurately divide the lymphomas into reproducible discrete disease entities. However, the general principle of classification divides the tumors into grades, which have prognostic and therapeutic significance (Table 31-4), as the grade of the tumor determines overall treatment strategy and prognosis.

TABLE 31-4. WORKING FORMULATION CLASSIFICATION OF LYMPHOMAS (REAL/WHO)

Low grade	Intermediate grade	High grade
Small lymphocytic	Follicular large cell	Immunoblastic
Follicular small cleaved cell	Diffuse small cleaved	Lymphoblastic
Follicular mixed cells	Diffuse mixed cells	Small, noncleaved (including Burkitt's)
	Diffuse large cell	

TABLE 31-5. PROGNOSIS OF NON-HODGKIN'S LYMPHOMA

Number of factors present	5-yr overall survival rate (%)
0–1	73
2	51
3	43
4–5	26

- The **Ann Arbor system,** described under Hodgkin's Disease, was specifically designed to stage Hodgkin's lymphoma, but has been applied to non-Hodgkin's as well. However, it should be noted that NHLs do not spread in a contiguous fashion, which is not accounted for in the Ann Arbor system.
- The **International Prognostic Index** was developed as a prognostic model for aggressive NHL. Important factors are (a) age >60 yrs, (b) stage III or IV disease, (c) more than one extranodal site involved, (d) elevated LDH, and (e) decreased functional status (Table 31-5). In addition, tumor size may also be a separate factor in some cases. Using the International Prognostic Index, those patients with 2 or more risk factors have a <50% chance of relapse-free and overall suvival at 5 yrs.

Treatment

Low-Grade Lymphoma
Low-grade lymphomas are typically slow growing and have a long clinical course. Bone marrow involvement is usually present at diagnosis. However, in contrast to their "indolent" course, they typically are poorly responsive to chemotherapy and are not cured by chemotherapy/radiation therapy (XRT) regimens. Stage I–II disease is typically treated by watchful waiting, with XRT to involved areas if they become locally symptomatic. XRT may even induce a complete remission in these stages. Stage III–IV disease is often treated with combination chemotherapy such as CVP (cyclophosphamide, vincristine, and prednisone), FND [fludarabine (Fludara), mitoxantrone (Novantrone), and dexamethasone (Decadron)], or others. After chemotherapy, restaging should be done to assess adequacy of response. Other interventions may include Rituximab, an anti–CD-20 monoclonal antibody. Other options include clinical trials.

Intermediate-Grade Lymphoma (and Some High-Grade Cases)

- Bone marrow involvement is usually not present at diagnosis. Stage I–II nonbulky disease is typically treated with chemoradiation with XRT of the involved field and CHOP [cyclophosphamide, doxorubicin, vincristine (Oncovin), and prednisone]. For bulky stage II and stage III–IV disease, CHOP alone is standard therapy. Although many other regimens have been tested in the last several decades, none have demonstrated clinical superiority.
- **CNS "prophylaxis"** is needed for Burkitt's and lymphoblastic lymphoma due to the high rates of CNS involvement. This typically involves methotrexate or cytarabine, sometimes combined with whole brain irradiation. It also may be indicated for lymphomas involving the testes, sinuses, or with extensive bone marrow involvement.

Relapsed Intermediate-Grade and High-Grade Lymphoma
There are other alternate chemotherapeutic regimens available for relapsed disease (Table 31-6). Autologous or allogenic stem cell transplant is often used after salvage chemotherapy. It may also be used in poor-risk, aggressive cases of lymphoma after first remission.

TABLE 31-6. SAMPLE SALVAGE CHEMOTHERAPY REGIMENS FOR NON-HODGKIN'S LYMPHOMA

ESHAP	Etoposide, methylprednisolone (Solu-Medrol), cytarabine (high-dose ara-C), cisplatin (Platinol)
DHAP	Dexamethasone, cytarabine (high-dose ara-C), cisplatin (Platinol)
CEPP-B	Cyclophosphamide, etoposide, procarbazine, prednisone, bleomycin
MIME	Mesna, ifosfamide, mitoxantrone, etoposide

High-Grade Lymphoma—Special Cases

Lymphoblastic Lymphoma

Lymphoblastic lymphoma is closely related to acute lymphoblastic leukemia and is treated similarly with combined chemotherapy in multiple courses and CNS prophylaxis. The "Stanford regimen" of cyclophosphamide, doxorubicin, vincristine, prednisone, whole brain irradiation, and intrathecal methotrexate followed by maintenance therapy with methotrexate and mercaptopurine is one example. Patients with adverse risk profiles may be considered for stem cell transplant after first remission. CSF cytology should be sent and, if negative, CNS prophylaxis is needed. If there is CSF involvement, additional therapy may also be needed.

Burkitt's Lymphoma

Burkitt's lymphoma has a very rapid growth rate. It is found in an endemic form in Africa, related to EBV infection, and a sporadic form found more typically in the United States. Endemic Burkitt's can often be treated with single-agent chemotherapy (usually cyclophosphamide), whereas sporadic Burkitt's often requires multiagent therapy or stem cell transplant. CNS prophylaxis is needed.

Mantle Cell Lymphoma

Mantle cell lymphoma is another aggressive lymphoma requiring more intensive regimens, such as hyper-CVAD [cyclophosphamide (Cytoxan), vincristine, doxorubicin (Adriamycin), dexamethasone], methotrexate, and cytarabine or CHOP with rituximab followed by stem cell transplant.

Other Lymphomas

AIDS–Associated Lymphoma

See Chap. 32, HIV-Related Malignancy, for more details.

Mucosal-Associated Lymphoid Tissue Lymphoma

Mucosal-associated lymphoid tissue lymphomas are a group of indolent extranodal lymphomas that affect organs such as the stomach, intestines, lung, breast, thyroid, or other sites with lymphoid tissue present. Radiation and surgery are often used in their treatment, but extensive resections are generally not needed. Localized mucosal-associated lymphoid tissue lymphoma of the stomach is associated with *Helicobacter pylori* infection and may regress after treatment with appropriate antibiotic therapy.

Cutaneous T-Cell Lymphoma (Mycosis Fungoides)

Cutaneous T-cell lymphomas invade the cutaneous tissue and typically present as erythematous plaques or exfoliation of skin but may progress to lymph node involvement in advanced stages. They are often treated with local radiation, topical chemotherapy, and PUVA therapy in localized disease.

Complications

Similar complications as described for Hodgkin's lymphoma may occur. In addition, low-grade lymphomas may transform into intermediate- or high-grade lymphoma spontaneously. These transformed lymphomas carry a poorer prognosis. Other complications may occur as well. Immunoglobin production may be either depressed or elevated, and paraproteins are sometimes seen. The result is often increased susceptibility to infection. Patients treated in the past with splenectomy are susceptible to infection by encapsulated organisms. Hypogammaglobulinemic patients may benefit from IV immunoglobulin. Autoimmune hemolytic anemias may occur with lymphomas or chronic lymphocytic leukemia and may be responsive to steroid treatment. Also, like Hodgkin's disease, long-term survivors of NHL are at increased risk for secondary malignancies, with both hematologic malignancies and solid tumors occurring at higher rates in those patients. In the future, molecular profiles of gene expression may be able to target those at higher risk for relapse or adverse effects of NHL treatment.

KEY POINTS TO REMEMBER

- Evaluation of a potential lymphoma includes a broad differential of lymphadenopathy.
- A thorough physical exam assessing all potential lymph tissue involvement may save the patient a more morbid biopsy procedure by identifying a readily accessible biopsy site.
- Most initial lymph node biopsies should be incisional or excisional, with a generous amount of tissue.
- Low-grade NHL is typically incurable but has a long clinical course, whereas high-grade NHL is often more aggressive but potentially curable.
- Hodgkin's lymphoma typically spreads along lymph node groups in an orderly fashion, whereas NHL typically does not.
- Patients treated in the past with splenectomy are susceptible to infection by encapsulated organisms.

REFERENCES AND SUGGESTED READINGS

A predictive model for aggressive non-Hodgkin's lymphoma. The International Non-Hodgkin's Lymphoma Prognostic Factors Project. *N Engl J Med* 1993;329(14):987–994.

Bhatia S, Robison LL, Oberlin O, et al. Breast cancer and other second neoplasms after childhood Hodgkin's disease. *N Engl J Med* 1996;334:745–751.

Coiffier B, Lepage E, Brière J, et al. CHOP chemotherapy plus rituximab compared with CHOP alone in elderly patients with diffuse large-B-cell lymphoma. *N Engl J Med* 2002;346:235–242.

DeVita VT, Rosenberg SA, Hellman S, eds. *Cancer: principles and practice of oncology*, 6th ed. Philadelphia: Lippincott Williams & Wilkins, 2001.

Fauci AS, Hauser SL, Longo DL, et al., eds. *Harrison's principles of internal medicine*, 14th ed. New York: McGraw-Hill, 1998:744–747.

Hansworth JD. Monoclonal antibody therapy in lymphoid malignancies. *Oncologist* 2000;5:376–384.

Hasenclever D, Diehl V. A prognostic score for advanced Hodgkin's disease. *N Engl J Med* 1998;339:1506–1514.

Miller TP, Dahlberg S, Cassady JR, et al. Chemotherapy alone compared with chemotherapy plus radiotherapy for localized intermediate- and high-grade non-Hodgkin's lymphoma. *N Engl J Med* 1998;339:21–26.

Mink SA, Armitage JO. High-dose therapy in lymphomas: a review of the current status of allogeneic and autologous stem cell transplantation in Hodgkin's disease and non-Hodgkin's lymphoma. *Oncologist* 2001;6:247–256.

Mortimer JE, Brown R. Medical management of malignant disease. In: Ahya, Flood, Paranjothi, eds. *The Washington manual of medical therapeutics*, 30th ed. Philadelphia: Lippincott Williams & Wilkins, 2001:429–454.

National Cancer Institute Web site. Adult non-Hodgkin's lymphoma. Available at: http://cancer.gov/cancerinfo/pdq/treatment/adult-non-hodgkins/healthprofessional/. Accessed August 2003.

Socié G, Stone JV, Wingard JR, et al. Long-term survival and late deaths after allogeneic bone marrow transplantation. *N Engl J Med* 1999;341:14–21.

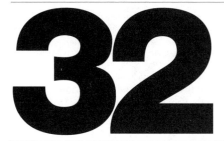

Introduction to Bone Marrow Transplantation

Lisa A. Mahnke

INTRODUCTION

Allogeneic transplant has evolved as a treatment of choice for various hematologic malignancies, including aplastic amenia, chronic myelogenous leukemia, and acute leukemia. It also can be useful for refractory non-Hodgkin's lymphoma, myelodysplastic syndromes and other bone marrow failures, refractory Hodgkin's lymphoma, and multiple myeloma. In addition to these malignant conditions, bone marrow transplantation (or, more accurately, **stem cell transplant**) can effectively treat various hemoglobinopathies and has been used for hereditary immunodeficiencies and metabolic disorders.

CONCEPT OF BONE MARROW TRANSPLANTATION

Stem cell transplant in this chapter is a general term meaning the reconstitution of the patient's hematopoietic cells by the administration of stem cells. Few centers perform actual bone marrow harvesting today. When bone marrow is the source of stem cells, the transplant is referred to as a **bone marrow transplant.** More often, stem cells are collected from a donor's peripheral blood. A transplant using these cells as a donor source is referred to as a **peripheral blood stem cell transplant.**

TYPES OF STEM CELL TRANSPLANTS

Allogeneic stem cell transplants refer to stem cells harvested from a donor and infused into a recipient for the purpose of reconstituting the patient's blood cell lines with those of the donor, resulting in the patient having blood cells of donor origin. In comparison, autologous stem cell transplant is the infusion of a patient's own stem cells to reconstitute all of the hematopoetic lineages (i.e., the monocytes, lymphocytes, and erythrocytes). Autologous stem cell transplant is, therefore, often used to "rescue" a patient's bone marrow after high-dose chemotherapy that would otherwise leave the patient aplastic, whereas in allogeneic transplant, the intention is to give the patient a new set of blood cell lines. When thinking about allogeneic transplants, it is useful to classify them by **donor.** Thus, allogeneic transplants are either **sibling-derived** or are from a **matched unrelated** donor. In general, the sibling transplants suffer fewer problems with rejection, graft failure, or graft-vs-host disease (GVHD) than matched unrelated donor transplants, and, thus, recipients of the latter usually need more intensive immunosuppressive therapy in the posttransplant period (see Complications Related to Transplant).

SOURCES OF STEM CELLS

- The marrow can be harvested **directly,** usually from the iliac crests, with the goal of collecting $> 2.5 \times 10^8$ cells/kg recipient weight.
- More commonly, stem cells are collected from the **peripheral blood of the donor** after "mobilization" or pretreatment with granulocyte colony-stimulating factor (G-CSF) growth factor. Peripheral blood mononuclear cells are then collected by leukapheresis and are selected for the CD34$^+$ (stem cell) population.

- **Placental cord blood** is another potential source of an unrelated donor transplant. This idea first came about because a significant fraction of patients requiring transplant therapy are unable to find a match despite an extensive registry of donors. Placental cord blood contains pluripotent hematopoetic stem cells naturally and in greater concentration than adult marrows. These stem cells have greater proliferative potential as compared to adult precursors and thus may engraft more quickly and robustly. However, they are also more quiescent and thus require stimulation by growth factors. Curiously, such transplants display a lower risk for GVHD (see Transplantation Procedures), which may involve the phenomenon of immunologic tolerance. Such tolerance might mean that cord blood transplants require less strict HLA matching, possibly making the technology more broadly available in the future.

TRANSPLANTATION PROCEDURES

HLA System and Histocompatibility Matching

The major determinants of **histocompatibility,** and thus risk for tissue rejection or GVHD, are encoded by the HLA system on chromosome 6. These proteins normally function in antigen presentation in adaptive immunity. The class I antigens are A, B, C, D, E, F, and G and are found on all nucleated cells. Class II proteins, Dr, Dq, and Dp, are found on a subset of cells, including early hematologic progenitors, mature macrophages, monocytes, B cells and other "antigen-presenting" cells, activated T cells, and endothelial cells. Traditionally, at the time of bone marrow matching of a potential donor, A, B, Dr, and Dq are typed phenotypically by allele. If the donor and the recipient share the same alleles at these loci, then they are considered completely matched. Fortunately, the **HLA locus** can be considered as a haplotype, such that all of the genes on one chromosome are inherited together. This means that the region can effectively be thought of as one gene passed by mendelian inheritance, owing to the low incidence of meiotic recombination between the loci at this site. Thus, for any given patient, the odds are one in four that a sibling will share the same two haplotypes and thus make a complete match. If a sibling donor is not available, then it might be possible for a parent to donate—if the parents happen to share identical alleles at various sites. Barring this, a national or international search is made of unrelated donors to look for a match. As discussed later, such matched unrelated donor transplants are much more prone to GVHD or rejection, likely due to microvariants of histocompatibility, which are as yet poorly defined. The matched unrelated donors may be matched at the serologic level or at the allele level. The allele level may be thought of as a higher "resolution" match. That is, the donor and recipient that are matched at the allele level have a more perfectly matched set of HLA antigens. This leads to a decreased incidence of GVHD.

Preparation for Transplant

Traditionally, the goal of preparation of the recipient has been total hematologic ablation. The intention is complete tumor killing as well as the creation of marrow "space" in which the transplant may engraft. For aplastic anemia, high-dose cyclophosphamide alone may be adequate. However, for all malignancies, total body irradiation is often used in combination with cyclophosphamide or other high-dose agent. All of the preparative regimens and patients subsequently become profoundly pancytopenic (absolute neutrophil count <100, platelet count <10,000 cells/μL) for a period after preparation, until successful engraftment. Time to engraftment depends on source of stem cells, as well as preparative regimen used but often is between 12–24 days.

Preparing the Stem Cells

T-cell depletion of the donor reduces the incidence of GVHD. However, this may also increase the risk of tumor recurrence, likely due to the decreased graft-vs-tumor effect. **Purging** of autologous transplants for tumor cells has been attempted with the hope of decreasing tumor reinfusion; however, the efficacy of this procedure is unclear and is not commonly performed. In patients with **ABO incompatibility,** there is not a barrier to transplantation, but care must be taken to remove erythrocytes from the graft before infusion to prevent against hemolysis and transfusion reaction.

Engraftment

After infusion, the progenitor cells migrate to the marrow. Usually, within 10–14 days, there is evidence for marrow expansion, and by 14–21 days, neutrophils can be detected in the peripheral blood. Factors affecting time to recovery include the use of G-CSF during the mobilization and harvest, degree of pretreatment chemotherapy, and the use of peripheral blood stem cells, which generally have faster recovery than marrow-derived cells. By days 18–21, natural killer cells are expected and will provide antiviral responses. Platelet recovery is more prolonged. Patients will require intense blood and platelet support during this time. Monocytes typically are the first cells to recover, and their presence often heralds initial neutrophil and platelet recovery.

SUPPORTIVE CARE

The posttransplant period is a critical time for stem cell patients. They become profoundly granulocytopenic and thrombocytopenic. During this time, there is significant potential morbidity and mortality from infectious or bleeding complications. Intensive care in a dedicated unit experienced in stem cell transplant is required to support patients and provide optimum outcome.

Blood Products

All CMV-seronegative patients (either during the transplant period or in patients potentially eligible to received a transplant in the future) should receive CMV-negative blood and platelet products. Blood products should also be irradiated or leukodepleted to avoid T-cell responses against host tissue (i.e., graft-vs-host caused by the transfusion). Platelet products are preferably single donor derived to reduce alloantigen exposure.

Hematopoietic Growth Factors

G-CSF and granulocyte-macrophage CSF given to the transplant recipient have been shown to reduce the time to graft recovery and reduce the number of days marked by infectious complications, as well as reduced days of mucositis. They are also used for donor expansion of progenitor cells for harvest. For autotransplants, they should be initiated subsequent to chemotherapy to prevent mobilization of progenitors, which will then be killed, as these may contribute to engraftment after transplant.

COMPLICATIONS RELATED TO TRANSPLANT

Graft Rejection

Graft rejection is usually evident within 1–2 mos of transplant and is defined as either failure to engraft or late loss of engraftment. This process involves residual host cells rejecting the engrafting stem cells. It is more common with matched unrelated allografts or mismatched grafts. Immunosuppression is fundamental to treatment and can usually be successfully tapered months after transplant. Patients can be maintained on cyclosporine (Neoral, Sandimmune) or tacrolimus (Protopic) plus corticosteroids.

Graft-vs-Host Disease

Donor T cells in allogeneic stem cell transplants recognize host HLA antigens causing tissue inflammation and damage. This phenomenon is roughly divided into two fairly distinct clinical entities, acute and chronic GVHD. By convention, acute disease is that occurring within 100 days of transplant. Both forms are more frequent in older patients and in matched unrelated donor transplants and, of course, in any transplant not completely HLA matched. Female donors, older donors, donors previously sensitized by transfusion or pregnancy, or CMV-positive donors are also more likely to cause GVHD. In the acute disease, the skin, mucous membranes, GI tract, and liver are often involved, and the severity is graded 0 (absence of symptoms) to IV (life-threatening disease). Profound immunosuppression can result. Prophylaxis usually includes cyclosporine or methotrexate plus corticosteroids. Treatment consists of high-dose steroids or antithymocyte globulin in addition to cyclosporine. Chronic GVHD can be triggered by infection and is characterized by lichenoid changes of the skin and mucous membranes, vitiligo, nail dysplasia, xerostomia, alopecia, scleroderma-type symptoms, and cholestasis. It also predisposes to infection.

Graft-vs-Leukemia Effect

Much attention has been directed to the study of this phenomenon after it was found that T-cell–depleted grafts often confer a higher rate of relapse of leukemia. It is now recognized that the graft recognition of host malignant cells is very important to the success of treatment. For this reason, T-cell immunodepletion of stem cell grafts has fallen into disfavor.

Venoocclusive Disease

Venoocclusive disease is a feared complication with a high mortality rate, which can occur after either allogeneic or autologous transplant. The major features are jaundice, rising conjugated bilirubin, tender hepatomegaly, and ascites with fluid retention. Risk factors include increased doses of cytotoxic chemotherapy and allografts from matched unrelated donors or mismatched grafts. Therapy is unsatisfactory and has included corticosteroids. Studies of thrombolytics or anticoagulants have not shown efficacy.

Pulmonary Complications

A syndrome resembling ARDS (**a**cute **r**espiratory **d**istress **s**yndrome) occasionally occurs secondary to infection or underlying GVHD, and is referred to as **idiopathic interstitial pneumonia.** CMV is often involved. In patients undergoing autologous bone marrow transplant, a syndrome of diffuse pulmonary alveolar hemorrhage may occur for which the etiology is unclear. It may be related to the cytotoxicity of chemotherapy and may respond to steroids.

Mucositis

Mucositis is extremely common during the neutropenic period, and vigilant attention to oral hygiene with frequent saline flushing with or without antifungals or local anesthetics is required. IV fluids should be used when needed to supplement oral intake. Aspiration precautions and monitoring for potential superinfection with *Candida* or herpes simplex are also needed.

INFECTIOUS COMPLICATIONS
Early Infections

The early period posttransplant is marked by **severe neutropenia.** As such, the patient is at risk for infection with skin and GI organisms due to mucosal breakdown at these sites. Thus, gram-negative bacilli, *Escherichia coli, Pseudomonas, Klebsiella,* and other enterics may cause local infection or sepsis. Enterococci or *viridans* streptococci may also cause bacteremia. Catheter-related bloodstream infection is a problem, and these organisms are usually staphylococci, particularly *Staphylococcus epidermidis.* Fungi are problematic, including *Candida* species and *Aspergillus,* which may cause disseminated disease. Viral reactivation with herpes simplex virus (HSV) is common as is VZV, causing shingles. Human herpesvirus 6 very commonly reactivates and is implicated in graft failure. BK virus is associated with encephalitis, hepatitis, and cystitis. Adenovirus and rotavirus may cause enteritis. Respiratory pathogens include adenovirus, influenza, parainfluenza, and respiratory syncytial virus.

Nosocomial Infection

Special consideration is given to nosocomial transmission of pathogens, including drug-resistant organisms. Thus, vigilance for methicillin-resistant *Staphylococcus aureus* is necessary, and broad coverage with vancomycin (Vancocin) may be appropriate in the setting of neutropenic fevers without a known focus. Vancomycin-resistant enterococcus is commonly isolated from the stool but is often nonpathogenic; however, it may require treatment if isolated from the blood. *Clostridium difficile* causing colitis and diarrhea are problematic, as many patients receive broad antibiotics at some point during transplant. Contact isolation and strict adherence to routine hand washing are necessary to prevent outbreaks of nosocomial pathogens.

Late Infections

The period from 1 mo to approximately 1 yr after transplantation is marked by a **relative cell-mediated immunodeficiency.** CMV reactivation is a major concern and can cause interstitial pneumonitis or pneumonia. CMV reactivation may be stimulated by the transplant process itself, secondary to alloantigen interaction with the host. Patients are at risk for *Pneumocystis carinii* pneumonia. Prolonged immunosuppression with steroids predisposes to *Aspergillus* pneumonia. Graft-related effects can present as interstitial pneumonitis (also known as the **idiopathic pulmonary syndrome** or **idiopathic interstitial infiltrates**) and may contribute to the prevalence of posttransplant pneumonia.

General Principles of Treatment of Infectious Diseases

Workup should be directed at the most likely organisms based on time since bone marrow transplant. Labs and imaging, such as blood and urine cultures, CMV or aspergillus serologies, chest x-ray, and sinus or chest CTs should be considered. (See Chap. 36, Oncologic Emergencies, Neutropenic Fever for further details regarding this complication.) Treatment often requires broad-spectrum antibiotics and antifungals, which can be complicated by serious toxicities, and is only briefly summarized here. Acyclovir is used for HSV and VZV at therapeutic doses. For CMV, ganciclovir (Cytovene) or foscarnet (Foscavir) is required. Human herpesvirus 6 is responsive to ganciclovir or foscarnet as well. *Candida albicans* and *tropicalis* are sensitive to fluconazole but for disseminated infection may require caspofungin (Cancidas), voriconazole (Vfend), or amphotericin (Amphocin, Fungizone). Other *Candida* species, such as *Candida glabrata*, or *Candida krusei*, respond to itraconazole (Sporanox), voriconazole, caspofungin, or amphotericin. For aspergillosis, amphotericin is the standard; however, voriconazole and caspofungin are very effective with fewer side effects. If IV amphotericin is required, lipid formulations may be used to reduce renal toxicity.

Prophylaxis

Strict adherence to hand-washing procedures and isolation precautions (visitor screening, filtered air, no fresh flowers or fruits) is mandatory in the care of the stem cell transplant patient. For CMV-seropositive patients, close surveillance and early treatment of CMV infections is warranted. However, prophylaxis is usually deferred until such infections have been documented and treated, given the toxicities associated with ganciclovir. Routine prophylaxis includes TMP-sulfa against *Pneumocystis*, acyclovir against HSV and VZV, and fluconazole or itraconazole against candidemia. Vaccination with inactivated vaccines can proceed >12 mos posttransplant, and patients will require 23-valent pneumococcal vaccine as well as yearly influenza vaccination (resuming 6 mos posttransplant). Recent data show that a heat-inactivated varicella vaccine may be effective in this population in preventing VZV reactivation. Guidelines for preventing opportunistic infections among hematopoietic stem cell transplant recipients can be found at http://www.guideline.gov.

Prognosis

Despite improving outcomes for a variety of malignancies, complications after bone marrow transplant are still a limiting factor in improving overall survival rates. Many complications are emergent and require admission to an ICU. Respiratory failure is common and may require mechanical ventilation. In addition, GVHD, infections, and medication toxicities may all contribute to multiple organ dysfunction syndrome. The mortality rate is high in these situations, and overall prognosis should be discussed with the patient and family members promptly. Long-term survivors are at risk for secondary malignancies and should be closely followed. Factors such as age, comorbidities, and indication for and type of transplantation all contribute to the overall prognosis in each individual patient.

KEY POINTS TO REMEMBER

- Most "bone marrow transplants" are now typically stem cells collected from peripheral blood.
- Allogeneic stem cell transplant refers to cells from another individual transplanted to give a patient a "new" set of blood cells, while autologous stem cell transplants infuse stem cells from a patient to rescue him or her from treatment-induced bone marrow failure.
- Stem cell transplant is a procedure with a very high morbidity and mortality.
- Neutropenic fever should be treated early and aggressively to avoid mortality.
- Infused blood products must be carefully selected to minimize complications.
- Strict adherence to hand-washing procedures is mandatory in the care of the stem cell patient.
- Posttransplant care includes prophylaxis against organisms such as HSV, VZV, PCP, and CMV.

REFERENCES AND SUGGESTED READINGS

Abeloff MD. *Clinical oncology*, 2nd ed. New York: Churchill Livingstone, 2000.

Antin JH. Long term care after hematopoietic-cell transplantation in adults. *N Engl J Med* 2002;347:1.

Bast RC Jr, ed. *Cancer medicine*, 5th ed. An official publication of the American Cancer Society. New York: B.C. Decker, 2000.

Hata A, Asanuma H, Rinki M, et al. Use of an inactivated varicella vaccine in recipients of hematopoietic-cell transplants. *N Engl J Med* 2002;347:26–34.

Hoffman R, ed. *Hematology: basic principles and practice*, 3rd ed. New York: Churchill Livingstone, 2000.

Janeway CA, Travers P, Walport M, et al., eds. *Immunobiology: the immune system in health and disease*, 5th ed. New York: Garland Pub, 1999.

Mortimer JE, Brown R. Medical management of malignant disease. In: Ahya, Flood, Paranjothi, eds. *The Washington manual of medical therapeutics*, 30th ed. Philadelphia: Lippincott Williams & Wilkins, 2001:429–454.

Tabbara IA, Ghazal CD, Ghazal HH. The role of granulocyte colony-stimulating factor in hematopoietic stem cell transplantation. *Cancer Invest* 1997;15(4):353–357. Review.

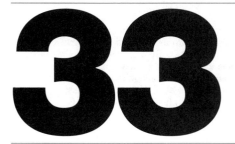

HIV-Related Malignancy

Lisa A. Mahnke

INTRODUCTION

The AIDS-related cancers include Kaposi's sarcoma (KS), primary CNS lymphoma (PCNSL), systemic non-Hodgkin's lymphoma (NHL), and, by AIDS-defining criteria, cervical cancer. Although the mechanisms predisposing HIV patients to such malignancies are not completely known, they are thought to be related to the tumorigenic effects of viruses, poor immune control by the host, release of inflammatory mediators, and, possibly, direct contribution by HIV itself. This is reflected clinically in the profile of AIDS malignancies, which contrasts with other immunocompromised states. The importance of adaptive immunity is paramount. Indeed, in the era of highly active antiretroviral therapy (HAART), many such cancers are now effectively prevented or are seen to regress. Historically, treatment and chemotherapy has been difficult for AIDS patients to tolerate, given poor host immunity, infection risk, and depressed bone marrow reserve, but the advent of HAART and immune reconstitution has significantly improved therapy for many patients. More details regarding some of the malignancies discussed in this chapter can be found in Chap. 28, Gynecologic Oncology, or Chap. 31, Lymphoma.

KAPOSI'S SARCOMA

Epidemiology

KS is the most common HIV-related malignancy. Its incidence is unevenly distributed among AIDS patients, such that in the United States it continues to strongly correlate with homosexual transmission of HIV. This, in turn, correlates with the seroprevalence of the KS viral agent, human herpesvirus 8 (HHV-8). HHV-8 is transmitted sexually and is found in saliva. It is also associated with multicentric Castleman's disease (benign hyperplasia of lymph node groups) and primary effusion lymphoma (discussed later), which, although uncommon, also appear in the AIDS population. With the emergence of effective HAART, the incidence of KS has decreased dramatically.

Pathophysiology

HHV-8 is a gamma-herpesvirus that is uniformly detectable in KS tumors. The virus becomes latent in lymphocytes and encodes a variety of oncogenes that mimic host proteins, including cell cycle analogs and apoptosis inhibitors, as well as cytokines and their receptor homologues. In combination with HIV transcription activators and local release of inflammatory mediators, these viral proteins are thought to transform endothelial cells into the malignant spindle cells seen on histopathology. The tumor is composed of the spindle cells surrounded by collagen bundles with angiogenesis and inflammatory cell infiltration evident.

Clinical Presentation and Diagnosis

KS lesions occur on the skin or mucous membranes and may appear anywhere in the body but rarely involve the CNS. They are plaque-like or macular and are generally violaceous, although they initially appear pink and progress to a deeper color as they grow larger and become indurated. Light-colored perilesional halos may be present. AIDS-related KS is an aggressive cancer, and the majority of patients have multifocal disease with GI involvement at presentation. This may manifest as vague abdominal symptoms or bleeding. Lymphatic obstruction can cause severe lymphedema. Pleuropulmonary disease usually occurs only in the most advanced HIV cases and may cause dyspnea, effusion, or bleeding. **Biopsy** confirms the diagnosis. Thus, colonoscopy, esophagogastroduodenoscopy, or bronchoscopy may be necessary. Serology for anti–HHV-8 antibodies has high sensitivity for previous exposure but is not necessary in the initial workup of KS.

Treatment

The goal of treatment is palliation and control of lesions. Immune reconstitution with HAART should be instituted immediately, because it can effectively contribute to regression of KS lesions. Concurrently, consideration is given to local or systemic therapies. Limited skin or mucosal disease can be treated with radiation, cryotherapy, laser therapy, or intralesional vinblastine. For widespread mucocutaneous disease, visceral disease, or any pulmonary involvement, systemic treatment is required. Interferon-gamma can be efficacious in patients whose CD4 counts are >100. The traditional first-line agent for systemic chemotherapy is liposomal doxorubicin, with paclitaxel as an alternative.

Prognosis

The AIDS Clinical Trials Group guidelines stage cases into "good" and "poor" risk, taking into account tumor characteristics (tumor confined to the skin and/or lymph nodes and/or minimal oral disease vs tumor with associated lymphedema or ulceration; extensive oral, GI, or visceral involvement), CD4 counts (> or <200), and the presence of systemic symptoms (history of opportunistic infection and/or thrush, "B" symptoms of fever, night sweats, weight loss, or diarrhea; performance status). The advent of HAART has markedly improved outcomes.

NON-HODGKIN'S LYMPHOMA

Aggressive B-cell lymphoma is an AIDS-defining disease and includes systemic NHL, PCNSL, and primary effusion lymphoma.

Epidemiology

All HIV patients are at risk for NHL, with the incidence being more marked in patients with lower CD4 counts. The greatest increase in risk over the general population is seen with PCNSL (>3000-fold); however, systemic NHL appears more commonly overall (having a 200-fold risk over the general population). NHL is second only to KS in terms of cancer incidence in patients with with HIV. For AIDS patients with systemic NHL, CNS occurrence is common. Conversely, systemic involvement in the setting of PCNSL is more rare. Risk factors for primary effusion lymphoma correlate with those for KS (and the risks of acquiring HHV-8). Unlike the situation with KS, in which HAART has been shown to have a dramatic impact, the benefits of HAART on lymphoma are as yet undefined but are suspected to be substantial.

Pathophysiology

Systemic Non-Hodgkin's Lymphoma

Systemic non-Hodgkin's lymphomas make up a heterogeneous population of predominately B-cell types. Compared to immunocompetent hosts, they are much more likely to be high grade (40–70% of tumors) and are more often associated with Epstein-Barr virus (EBV) (40–60% of tumors). The etiologies are unclear but are probably a combination of poor host immune surveillance, chronic antigenic stimulation secondary to infections (chronic B-cell stimulation), indirect effects of HIV, release of inflammatory mediators such as cytokines, and transforming properties of EBV itself. Systemic NHL consists of diffuse lymphomas of the (a) large-cell, (b) immunoblastic, and (c) small non-cleaved (or Burkitt-like) subtypes. Burkitt-like NHL presents at relatively higher CD4 counts (>250) compared to either the large-cell or immunoblastic types (<100).

Primary CNS Lymphoma

PCNSL occurs at very advanced stages of HIV, usually when CD4 counts reach 10–50. 100% of tumors are infected with EBV, whose viral gene products are known to be oncogenic. On histology, these B-cell lymphomas are diffuse large cell or immunoblastic.

Primary Effusion Lymphoma (Body Cavity Lymphoma)

Primary effusion lymphoma accounts for only a few percent of all HIV-associated NHL and presents in advanced stages of AIDS. It is an aggressive tumor, high-grade immunoblastic, with a null phenotype (non-B, non–T cell). HHV-8 is universally detectable, and EBV is often found. The strong association with HHV-8 suggests transformation by this virus; several gene products are known to disrupt the cell cycle or are cytokine analogs. The coinfection of the B cells with EBV is probably also important for malignant transformation.

Clinical Presentation

Constitutional symptoms such as fever, weight loss, and night sweats are common with NHL. It is important to remember that *disseminated infection* is part of the differential diagnosis in this situation and must be investigated. However, even after effective treatment for infection in an AIDS host, lymphoma-associated fever may persist. Any prominent lymph node or asymmetric mass suggests tumor and warrants further workup. Common extranodal sites are the CNS, GI tract, lung, and liver. Pleural, peritoneal, or pericardial effusion can be found, especially with primary effusion lymphoma, and fluid aspirates should be examined for cytology.

Diagnosis and Staging

- CT scanning is helpful for **localization of primary lesions.** These will require biopsy. Because imaging alone does not differentiate tumor from infectious focus, **open biopsy** is typically required. The **staging workup** should include CT of the chest, abdomen, and pelvis as well as bone marrow biopsy and lumbar puncture for CSF analysis. Flow cytometry can establish the diagnosis, revealing clonality.
- Special regard to **CNS involvement** is necessary for HIV patients with NHL as follows:
  - After systemic lymphoma is found, MRI scanning of the head is warranted to search for CNS involvement.
  - Also, prophylactic intrathecal chemotherapy may be considered at the time of the initial lumbar puncture.
- Conversely, the **workup of brain mass** in and of itself proceeds somewhat differently. CT or MRI imaging will not distinguish CNS toxoplasmosis from lymphoma, as both lesions can appear ring enhancing. If the lesion is solitary, then it is more likely to be lymphoma. Serology for **toxoplasma** IgG or IgM should be obtained. If both are negative, then the lesion is more likely lymphoma. If the serology is positive, then the patient can be treated with empiric antibiotic therapy followed by repeat imaging in 10 days to look for regression. If the lesions worsen, brain biopsy will be necessary. Also of note, the finding of EBV DNA in the CSF by PCR is very sensitive and specific for the diagnosis of PCNSL.

Treatment

- As with KS, HIV patients often have low bone marrow reserve and suffer intercurrent opportunistic infections that make treatment difficult. **Combination therapies** are preferred, as with HIV-seronegative patients. The addition of **myeloid growth factors** is recommended. Treatment is based on staging, as in non–HIV-infected patients. However, as most HIV-AIDS patients have advanced tumors on presentation, systemic combined chemotherapy is usual. For earlier stages, chemotherapy is followed by consolidation and involved field radiation. Dose reduction has been successfully applied to reduce bone marrow toxicity. For more localized disease (uncommonly encountered), abbreviated chemotherapy [e.g., four cycles with CHOP (cyclophosphamide, doxorubicin, vincristine, and prednisone) with involved field radiotherapy] may be considered.

- Patients having systemic NHL with Burkitt's histology or bone marrow involvement should receive **meningeal prophylaxis,** either with methotrexate (Folex, Rheumatrex, Trexall) or cytosine arabinoside (Cytosar-U). If there is evidence for lymphomatous meningitis, then the patient should also receive whole brain irradiation. As with KS, optimization of HAART is strongly recommended and is predicted to have substantial synergizing treatment benefit.

- For PCNSL, dexamethasone (Decadron) is necessary if there is evidence of brain edema, whole brain radiation is instituted early, and intrathecal chemotherapy should be used, remembering that such treatments are palliative. Patients with advanced HIV disease should be particularly considered for lower-dose combination regimens [e.g., m-BACOD (methotrexate, bleomycin, Adriamycin [doxorubicin], cyclophosphamide, Oncovin [vincristine], and dexamethasone), methotrexate, cyclophosphamide, doxorubicin, vincristine, bleomycin, dexamethasone, and leucovorin]. The standard therapy is CHOP. Restaging evaluation is done after 2 cycles, and therapy is continued for 6–8 cycles beyond complete response.

Prognosis

Poor prognostic factors are low CD4 counts (<100), increased age, elevated lactate dehydrogenase, poor performance status, presence of extranodal disease, prior AIDS-defining illness, or advanced stage or aggressive histology of lymphoma.

CERVICAL CANCER

The Centers for Disease Control and Prevention classifies **cervical cancer** as an AIDS-defining disease. However, current evidence does not strongly reveal an increased incidence in the HIV population, in contrast to NHL or KS. Clearly, cervical cancer is related to the spread of **human papilloma virus** (HPV), and because the risk factors for HPV are similar to those of HIV, incidence studies are often confounded. Given its relation to a virus, it had been predicted that waning host immunity with AIDS would promote cervical cancer and worsen its progression among HPV-positive HIV patients. In terms of severity, some evidence does suggest *more aggressive disease* among AIDS patients and, more clearly, the evidence shows a higher rate of recurrence among treated patients. HPV strains 16, 18, and 31 are the most highly oncogenic, expressing the transforming proteins E6 and E7, which interfere with host tumor suppressor proteins p53 and Rb. It is also possible that HIV-HPV interactions facilitate the development of malignancy. In terms of treatment, therapy is the same for HIV and non-HIV patients, but, again, recurrence is more common among the former. Physicians should be vigilant with preventative measures for cervical cancer in the HIV population. The Centers for Disease Control guidelines promote **Pap smear testing** at the time of diagnosis and 6 mos thereafter. If these are normal, then annual screening is recommended, just as in the general population. If atypical squamous cells of unknown origin or cervical intraepithelial neoplasia are found at any time, then the patient is referred for colposcopy with biopsy. See Chap. 28, Gynecologic Oncology, for further information.

OTHER NEOPLASMS

Hodgkin's Lymphoma

AIDS patients have a significantly increased risk for Hodgkin's disease, and it would be reasonable to classify it among the AIDS-defining illnesses. The mixed-cellularity histologic subtype predominates, in contrast to HIV-seronegative patients, conferring a worse prognosis. The lymphocyte-depleted subtype also occurs more frequently. Patients often present with advanced stages of disease, usually at moderately depleted

CD4 counts (~250–300). Hepatic involvement is not uncommon. Staging is done as with HIV-negative patients and includes CT of the chest, abdomen, and pelvis and bone marrow biopsy. As with treatment of NHL, these patients often have depressed bone marrow reserve and are unable to tolerate myelotoxic agents. The most effective regimen is unclear. ABVD (doxorubicin, bleomycin, vinblastine, and dacarbazine) has been used, and myeloid growth factor should be coadministered. Less myelosuppressive therapies have also been used. For more localized disease, involved field radiotherapy may be considered. See Chap. 31, Lymphoma, for details. All patients should be initiated on HAART, although data for improved outcomes have not been reported.

Anogenital Neoplasia

The incidence of anal cancer correlates with receptive anal intercourse. It is unclear whether the AIDS epidemic has promoted an increase in the rates of anal cancer. As with cervical cancer, HPV is likely etiologic; anal dysplasia correlates with HPV positivity and with oncogenic strains. Treatment is similar to non–AIDS-related anal cancer, which involves a combination of chemotherapy and radiation. See Chap. 21, Colorectal Cancer, for details.

KEY POINTS TO REMEMBER

- Patients with AIDS are at high risk for several malignancies: Kaposi's sarcoma, CNS lymphoma, cervical cancer, and NHL.
- Treatment with HAART helps to effectively prevent the HIV-related malignancies.
- Kaposi's sarcoma is related to a causative viral agent, HHV-8, and is more common in men with HIV.
- HAART can have dramatic benefits in causing regression of Kaposi's sarcoma but is not clearly effective in the case of NHL.
- It can be difficult to distinguish CNS toxoplasmosis from lymphoma by CT or MRI, as both lesions can appear ring enhancing. Checking serologies for toxoplasma or a short trial of appropriate antibiotic therapy to determine response may be useful to distinguish in an attempt to avoid biopsy.
- Cervical cancer is an AIDS-defining disease, related to HPV. Specific serotypes (strains 16, 18, and 31) are most strongly associated with progression to cervical cancer.
- Vigilant cervical cancer screening is required in HIV-positive patients. Guidelines for treatment are similar to non–HIV-positive patients.

REFERENCES AND SUGGESTED READINGS

Abeloff MD. *Clinical oncology*, 2nd ed. New York: Churchill Livingstone, 2000.

Antin JH. Long-term care after hematopoietic-cell transplantation in adults. *N Engl J Med* 2002;347:36–42.

Antman K, Chang Y. Kaposi's sarcoma. *N Engl J Med* 2000;342:1027–1038.

Chang Y, Cesarman E, Pessin MS, et al. Identification of herpesvirus-like DNA sequences in AIDS-associated Kaposi's sarcoma. *Science* 1994;266:1865–1869.

Kaplan LD, Gates AE. AIDS malignancies in the era of highly active antiretroviral therapy. *Oncology (Huntingt)* 2002;16:5.

Krown SE, Testa MA, Huang J. AIDS-related Kaposi's sarcoma: prospective validation of the AIDS Clinical Trials Group staging classification. AIDS Clinical Trials Group Oncology Committee. *J Clin Oncol* 1997;15:3085.

Mandell GL. *Principles and practice of infectious diseases*, 5th ed. New York: Churchill Livingstone, 2000.

Pagano JS. Viruses and lymphomas. *N Engl J Med* 2002;347:78–79.

34

Cancer of Unknown Primary Site

Holly M. Magiera

INTRODUCTION

Cancer of unknown primary site (CUPS) is defined when there is a biopsy-proven malignancy for which the site of origin is not defined by a thorough history and physical, imaging studies, chemistries (including tumor markers), and detailed pathologic evaluation. This is a heterogeneous group of patients, but the majority are >60 yrs, and the median survival is 4–11 mos, with little response to therapy. There are **subgroups,** however, with treatment-responsive disease that may be able to achieve long-term disease-free survival. The workup of the patient with an unknown primary tumor is focused on identifying these patients with treatable disease. An exhaustive search for the primary tumor after these treatable cases have been identified adds little to the overall management of the patient, as the primary tumor site is located in only 15–25% of patients before death, and up to 30% are not found at autopsy.

Epidemiology

CUPS accounts for 2–5% of all initial cancer diagnoses. The median age at diagnosis is 56–60 yrs, with equal numbers of men and women affected. As noted earlier, the **median survival is poor**—4–11 mos—regardless of treatment. A special subgroup is patients who present with poorly differentiated midline tumors and who have a median age at presentation of 39 yrs. Approximately 25% of these tumors as a whole are responsive to treatment.

PRESENTATION
Clinical Features

Patients typically present with symptoms of their metastatic disease and may often have multiple symptoms. Pain is the most common presenting symptom and is present in 60% of patients. Other symptoms include weight loss, fatigue, new mass, lymphadenopathy, CNS abnormalities, and bone pain or fracture. Common **sites of metastasis** include lymph nodes, bone, liver, lung, brain, and skin. Cervical adenopathy can be a manifestation of primary lung, breast, or head and neck cancer, as well as lymphoma. A midline mass in the mediastinum or retroperitoneum is worrisome for an extragonadal tumor.

CLASSIFICATION AND DIAGNOSTIC WORKUP
Classification

- The treatment of CUPS depends to a large extent on the pathology of the specimen. Light microscopy is the first step in the classification of these malignancies. There are **four major classifications,** including poorly differentiated neoplasm, poorly differentiated carcinoma/adenocarcinoma, moderately to well-differentiated adenocarcinoma, and squamous cell carcinoma. In addition, other features may point to a diagnosis.
- **Immunohistochemistry** is widely available and may be useful in classifying these tumors. Common leukocyte antigen can distinguish lymphoma from carcinoma. *Neuroendocrine tumors* often stain for neuron-specific enolase, chromogranin, and synaptophysin. Prostate-specific antigen (PSA) staining is suggestive of *prostate cancer* and estrogen receptor/progesterone receptor (ER/PR) is suggestive of *breast cancer.* hCG

and AFP are markers for *germ cell cancers*. *Melanoma* often stains for vimentin, HMB-45, and S-100. *Sarcoma* may stain for vimentin, desmin, and von Willebrand antigen.

- **Electron microscopy** is not widely available and is expensive but may contribute to the diagnosis in some cases. For example, secretory granules are seen in neuroendocrine tumors, and premelanosomes are seen in melanomas.
- **Cytogenetics** may also be useful. Isochromosome 12p and 12q– are seen in germ cell tumors. The t(11;22) translocation has been seen in Ewing's sarcoma and primitive neuroectodermal tumor. The t(8;14) translocation is seen in some lymphoid malignancies.

Diagnostic Workup

The **workup** of tumor of unknown primary site includes evaluation for the most common malignancies: breast, colon, prostate, and lung. However, lung and pancreatic cancer are the primary tumors most likely to present as an unknown primary metastasis. Evaluation includes adequate **biopsy specimen** of the metastatic tumor with appropriate immunohistochemical pathologic studies, thorough **history and physical** (especially of head, neck, breast, pelvis, rectum), chest **x-ray**, chemistries and blood counts, occult blood testing of stool, and consideration of CT imaging of the abdomen and pelvis. In addition, **mammogram** should be performed in women and PSA screening in men. In some cases, panendoscopy may be an appropriate step. Additional studies depend on the site of the metastasis and features on pathology.

MANAGEMENT

Treatment of Specific Subtypes

Poorly Differentiated Neoplasm

Poorly differentiated neoplasms account for approximately 5% of CUPS. Further pathologic studies are very important in this group, as treatment may radically differ depending on results. 35–65% of these tumors are defined as lymphoma after further studies, and this group is often responsive to multiagent chemotherapy. Most of the remainder of tumors are carcinomas, with melanoma and sarcoma accounting for <15%. If a specific cell type is not identified, patients are treated as for adenocarcinoma.

Poorly Differentiated Carcinoma or Adenocarcinoma

- **Poorly differentiated carcinoma** or **adenocarcinoma** accounts for approximately 30% of CUPS. Two-thirds of these will have poorly differentiated carcinoma, and one-third will have adenocarcinoma. In comparison to patients with moderately or well-differentiated adenocarcinoma, these patients tend to be younger, to have more rapidly progressive symptoms, and to have involvement of lymph nodes—the mediastinum and the retroperitoneum. Certain subsets have good response to chemotherapy as well.
- **Further pathologic evaluation** is needed to confirm the diagnosis of carcinoma, to evaluate for neuroendocrine features, and to identify germ cell neoplasms. If patients cannot be classified into subsets, treatment regimens used include carboplatin or cisplatin and paclitaxel-based regimens. These have been found to prolong survival in some studies. The median survival of patients with carcinoma is 13 mos, and for patients with adenocarcinoma it is 8 mos. Certain clinical features, such as young age, nonsmoking status, single metastatic site, neuroendocrine features, and lymph node location, have been associated with a more favorable prognosis. The decision to treat must be individualized and based on performance status and the patient's desire to proceed.

LOW-GRADE NEUROENDOCRINE TUMOR. These tumors have features typical of carcinoid and islet cell tumors and usually involve liver or bone. They may be associated with syndromes such as Zollinger-Ellison and carcinoid. In some patients, a primary site is found in the small intestine, rectum, pancreas, or bronchus. These tumors are generally indolent and may progress slowly over many years. Patients are treated as they would be for metastatic carcinoid or islet cell malignancies.

EXTRAGONADAL GERM CELL TUMOR. Extragonadal germ cell tumor is defined in patients <50 yrs with midline tumors, short duration of symptoms, good response to chemotherapy or radiation, and elevation of tumor markers (alpha-fetoprotein and beta-HCG). Poorly differentiated carcinoma in young men with mediastinal or retro-peritoneal tumors should be treated as germ cell tumors with platinum-based regimens. Approximately 30–40% of these patients may be cured.

GESTATIONAL CHORIOCARCINOMA. Gestational choriocarcinoma should be suspected in young women with poorly differentiated carcinoma and pulmonary nodules. Recent history of pregnancy, spontaneous abortion, or missed menses may be elicited. hCG is often elevated in these patients. Most patients are curable with chemotherapy.

Well-Differentiated or Moderately Differentiated Adenocarcinoma

- **Well-differentiated** or **moderately differentiated adenocarcinoma** is the most frequent type of CUPS, accounting for 60% of cases. The patients are typically elderly with multiple sites of metastasis. The primary tumor will become apparent in 15–20% of patients. At autopsy, the most common primary malignancies found include lung and pancreas, which account for 40% of cases. The median survival is 3–4 mos with this diagnosis. Immunohistochemistry is of limited value in this group of patients, although identification of **ER/PR status** or **PSA** is valuable for treatment and prognosis. Evaluation of patients should include thorough history and physical, chemistries, urinalysis, and chest x-ray. Women should have a **breast exam and mammogram,** and men should have a **prostate exam and PSA** checked. CT imaging of the abdomen may provide a diagnosis in 10–35% of patients and may identify additional sites of metastasis.
- Approximately 10% of patients fit into subsets with a favorable response to chemotherapy, which is discussed later. The remainder do not fit into these groups and are mainly treated for **palliation** of symptoms. Multiple regimens of chemotherapy have been evaluated in these patients with little evidence of improvement in survival. Features such as lymph node location, female gender, or poor differentiation predict a better response to chemotherapy. Liver and bone involvement predict a poor response. Recent trials have suggested that taxane-based chemotherapy regimens may improve survival, and newer agents, such as gemcitabine and topotecan, are being evaluated. However, randomized controlled trials are lacking. Patients with a good performance status should be considered for regimens such as these and for clinical trials.

WOMEN WITH PERITONEAL CARCINOMATOSIS. Women may present with peritoneal carcinomatosis suggestive of **ovarian cancer,** and histologic features, such as psammoma bodies and papillary structure, may be found. Patients often have elevated CA-125 levels, and metastases outside the peritoneal cavity are rare. These women should be treated as for stage III ovarian cancer with surgical cytoreduction and chemotherapy with paclitaxel and platinum. Approximately 15–25% of patients will have long-term survival with this regimen.

WOMEN WITH AXILLARY LYMPH NODE ADENOCARCINOMA. Breast cancer should be suspected in this group of patients. Breast exam and mammography should be performed, as well as staining for ER/PR. In this group of patients with negative exams and imaging, breast adenocarcinoma is found in 40–80% of mastectomy specimens. Patients should be evaluated for other metastatic disease, and if evaluation is negative, they should be treated for stage IIB breast cancer. Primary therapy consists of modified radical mastectomy vs lymph node dissection and breast irradiation. Patients should receive adjuvant treatment based on their age, lymph node status, ER/PR status, and her-2-neu status. If patients are found to have additional metastatic disease, they should be treated according to guidelines for stage IV breast cancer.

MEN WITH ELEVATED PSA AND/OR OSTEOBLASTIC BONE METASTASES. Patients with these features or with PSA staining of their tumors should undergo hormonal treatment for **prostate cancer** even if the clinical features are atypical, as many will have significant palliation.

PATIENTS WITH A SINGLE METASTATIC LESION. On occasion, only one site of metastasis is found even with complete evaluation. The possibility of a primary cancer of an unusual site, such as apocrine cancer presenting as a skin lesion, should be considered. Treatment should include local therapy with surgical resection or radiation or a combination of the two modalities. Many patients can have prolonged survival with this type of treatment. The role of systemic treatment is not yet defined in these patients but may be considered for patients with good performance status and poor differentiation, especially in the context of clinical trials.

Squamous Cell Carcinoma

Squamous cell carcinoma accounts for 5% of cases of CUPS. Most of the patients are elderly and have a significant history of alcohol and/or tobacco abuse. Most of these tumors arise in the lung or head and neck. Additional sites include the esophagus, cervix, anus, rectum, and bladder. For patients who do not fit into the specific subsets that follow, the prognosis is poor. These patients likely have occult lung cancer and should be evaluated with CT and bronchoscopy. Chemotherapy regimens used for non–small cell lung cancer should be considered. If features are atypical for lung cancer, patients should be carefully evaluated for other sites, as adenocarcinoma may undergo squamous differentiation. Immunohistochemistry may be helpful in these patients.

SQUAMOUS CELL CARCINOMA INVOLVING HIGH CERVICAL LYMPH NODES. Primary head and neck cancer should be suspected in patients with squamous cell carcinoma involving high cervical lymph nodes. CT evaluation of the head and neck may better define the disease and identify a primary site. Careful endoscopic evaluation should also be performed in these patients. These studies usually result in location of the primary cancer, but as many as 15% may not be identified. These patients should be treated for locally advanced head and neck cancer. In patients treated with local therapy alone, long-term survival has been seen in 30–40% of patients. The role of chemotherapy is undefined, but recent trials with concurrent chemotherapy and radiation are promising, and this approach should be considered in appropriate patients.

SQUAMOUS CELL CARCINOMA INVOLVING LOW CERVICAL OR SUPRACLAVICULAR LYMPH NODES. Patients with squamous cell carcinoma involving low cervical or supraclavicular lymph nodes presentation should be evaluated for lung cancer with CT and bronchoscopy. The prognosis is not as favorable for this subgroup as for patients with high cervical lymph nodes, but 10–15% may have long-term survival. These patients do not typically respond well to systemic therapy; therefore, local treatment with radiation therapy should be offered.

SQUAMOUS CELL CARCINOMA INVOLVING INGUINAL LYMPH NODES. In most patients with inguinal lymph node involvement, careful exam of the perineum will reveal a primary site. All patients should undergo sigmoidoscopy, and female patients should undergo pelvic examination. If no primary site is identified with these studies, patients should undergo inguinal lymph node dissection with radiation therapy if extensive disease is identified. The role of systemic chemotherapy is not defined but, given the role of combined-modality therapy in cervical and anal cancers, platinum-based regimens should be considered.

KEY POINTS TO REMEMBER

- CUPS accounts for 2–5% of cancers and includes numerous clinical presentations and histologies.
- There are four main light microscopy classifications for these tumors, and further studies, such as immunohistochemistry, should be used in poorly differentiated tumors.
- A number of patient subsets have been identified with a more favorable prognosis and better response to treatment.
- In most patients, the search for the primary cancer should be brief and based on the site and histology of the metastasis.
- Overall, the median survival is poor regardless of treatment.

REFERENCES AND SUGGESTED READINGS

Chorost MI, McKinley B, Tschoi M, et al. The management of the unknown primary. *J Am Coll Surg* 2001;193:666–677.

DeVita VT, Rosenberg SA, Hellman S, eds. *Cancer: principles and practice of oncology*, 6th ed. Philadelphia: Lippincott Williams & Wilkins, 2001:2537–2560.

Hainsworth JD, Greco FA. Treatment of patients with cancer of unknown primary site. *N Engl J Med* 1993;329:257–263.

Hainsworth JD, Greco FA. Management of patients with cancer of unknown primary site. *Oncology* 2000;14:563–574.

Mortimer JE, Brown R. Medical management of malignant disease. In: Ahya, Flood, Paranjothi, eds. *The Washington manual of medical therapeutics*, 30th ed. Philadelphia: Lippincott Williams & Wilkins, 2001:429–454.

NCCN practice guidelines for occult primary tumors. *Oncology* 1998;12:226–309.

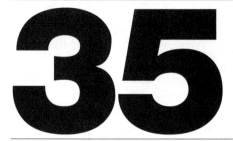

Supportive Care in Oncology

Marcia L. Chantler

INTRODUCTION

Cancer patients have multiple physical symptoms. Symptoms can be related to the cancer itself, side effects of cancer therapy, medications, and comorbid medical conditions. Some cancer symptoms can be alleviated by treatment of the cancer with chemotherapy, radiation therapy, or even surgery. However, these treatments more often than not lead to new or worsening problems, such as fatigue and nausea. In addition to physical symptoms, many patients with cancer suffer psychologic and emotional distress. This chapter focuses on symptom control as an important element of excellent oncology practice, including pain management, nausea and vomiting, mucositis, diarrhea, anorexia, and dyspnea.

PAIN MANAGEMENT

Pain is a prevalent complaint in cancer patients, occurring in 50–70% of all patients with cancer. More than one-half of cancer patients experience moderate to severe pain, with 50–80% of cancer patients not satisfied with their pain relief. The undertreatment of cancer pain can be attributed to multiple barriers, including physician, patient, and societal factors. A convenient and simplified table of analgesics and dosing information may be found in Appendix A.

Definition of Pain

The International Association for the Study of Pain defines pain as "an unpleasant sensory and emotional experience associated with actual or potential tissue damage, or described in terms of such damage. Pain is always subjective. Each individual learns the application of the word through experiences related to injury early in life." Acute pain may be associated with physical signs that are more familiar to the clinician, including tachycardia, HTN, hyperventilation, facial grimacing, or verbalizations. However, patients with chronic pain may not exhibit any of these overt physical signs and may not "appear in pain." It is important to remember that pain is always subjective, and patient self-reporting is a key element to an accurate pain assessment.

Pain Assessment

- The first step in the management of pain depends on a **comprehensive pain assessment** gathered through history, physical exam, and review of lab and radiology studies. Important pain characteristics to elicit from the patient should be descriptions of the pain with regard to onset, duration, intensity, quality, and exacerbating or relieving factors. The physician can use each of these characteristics to aid in the appropriate management plan.
- **Simple tools** can reliably aid in the measurement of pain. The most common clinical assessment tools are verbal rating scales or visual analog scales. A verbal rating scale uses words to describe the pain such as none, mild, moderate, severe, or excruciating. A visual analog scale uses a line with or without verbal clues or numbers and asks the patient to place their pain rating on this scale. The specific scale used to measure pain is less important than the consistent use of a scale over time.

It is important to instruct the patient on how to use the scale. For illiterate or pediatric patients, a visual analog scale can be used with pictures to describe the levels of pain for a better pain assessment tool. Examples of pain scales can be found at http://www.nci.nih.gov/cancerinfo/understanding-cancer-pain/.

- The initial report of pain from the patient, along with the characteristics of the pain obtained through the history, combined with information from the physical exam and review of lab and radiology studies, allows the physician to have a basic foundation of knowledge for the understanding of pain in an individual patient. With this full assessment, the physician should be able to identify potential etiologies and make appropriate clinical decisions for treatment.

Opioid Pharmacotherapy

- **Opioid therapy** can provide effective pain relief to the majority of patients with cancer pain. This success with opioid therapy justifies the use of opioids as the first-line approach for moderate to severe pain in cancer patients. Opioids can be classified as pure agonists or agonist-antagonists, based on their interactions with opioid receptors in the body. The drugs that are included in the agonist-antagonist subclass include butorphanol (Stadol), nalbuphine (Nubain), pentazocine (Talwin), and buprenorphine (Buprenex). Drugs in this subclass have a ceiling effect for analgesia and may reverse the effects of pure agonists. For these reasons, the use of the mixed agonist-antagonist subclass is *not* recommended in the treatment of cancer pain.
- The World Health Organization (WHO) recommends the use of an analgesic ladder in the approach to the selection of opioids to treat cancer pain. Analgesic selection should be guided by the severity of cancer pain. Patients with **mild to moderate** pain are usually started on acetaminophen or NSAIDs. Patients with **moderate to severe** pain or those who had insufficient relief after a trial of acetaminophen or NSAIDs are treated with an opioid used for moderate pain, such as codeine, hydrocodone, dihydrocodeine, and oxycodone (Roxicodone, OxyContin). This opioid may be combined with acetaminophen or an NSAID or an alternative adjuvant drug (tricyclic antidepressant, anticonvulsant, or topical anesthetic). Many of the drugs used for moderate to severe cancer pain are available in the United States as a combination of the opioid and acetaminophen or ASA. The drug can be titrated until the maximum safe dose of acetaminophen (4 g/day) or ASA is reached.
- Patients with **severe** pain, including those who fail to reach adequate pain relief with drugs from the second step on the WHO ladder, should receive an opioid that is useful in the treatment of severe cancer pain. The drugs useful in the treatment of severe cancer pain include morphine (Astramorph), hydromorphone (Dilaudid), fentanyl (Sublimaze), oxycodone, and methadone (Dolophine, Methadose). These opioids may also be combined with acetaminophen or an NSAID or an adjuvant drug when needed. Patients can experience a variation of analgesia and side effects between the different opioids. A clinician may need to rotate among the various opioids to identify the drug that has the correct balance between pain control and side effects. These drugs should be titrated to analgesic effect or intolerable side effects. There is no maximum dose limitation on the opioid medication itself.

Management of Acute and Chronic Pain

- In the treatment of cancer pain, it is important to distinguish between acute and chronic pain, as the goals of treatment are slightly different. **Acute** pain is a linear event; the pain starts, and, with relief of the offending event, the pain stops. Chronic pain is cyclical in nature, repeating itself over time. For acute pain, the goal of treatment is pain relief. To accomplish pain relief, the drugs administered should have rapid onset of action, with the desired duration of action (e.g., 2–4 hrs). The drugs are given prn. Common side effects, such as sedation, are usually acceptable and well tolerated by the patient. An example of an acute pain scenario is the patient who falls and suffers a hip fracture at the site of a previous bone metastasis. The patient is treated with short-acting IV narcotics until surgery can be performed to stabilize the fracture.

- **Chronic** pain management has a different focus. The overall goal is pain prevention and the avoidance of undesirable side effects, such as sedation. The analgesic regimen should include long-acting narcotics administered on a regular schedule and should be individualized for the patient based on side effects. Patients with chronic pain also need to have the understanding of how to manage acute exacerbations with short-acting, rapid-onset analgesics, most commonly referred to as **breakthrough pain relief.** Many cancer patients fall into this category of chronic pain patients. Chronic pain is ineffectively managed when the clinician focuses on acute control of the pain in this setting.
- When **managing chronic pain,** it is important to remember that there are wide variations in dose requirements. This variation is not based on the size or age of the patient or amount of disease present. The analgesic dose required to keep a patient out of pain cannot be predicted, but rather, must be determined by educated trial and error. The following are guidelines for opioid use in chronic pain patients:
  - Start with one drug at the lowest effective dose. Titrate the drug to pain relief or intolerable side effects. If the patient is unable to tolerate one narcotic due to undesirable side effects, switch to an alternative agent.
  - Use around-the-clock dosing schedules to avoid peaks and valleys in serum analgesic levels.
  - Sustained or long-acting release preparations of narcotics are very useful in this population. When converting between modes of administration or drugs, calculate the equianalgesic dosages to avoid undermedicating a patient. See Table 35-1.
  - Breakthrough pain medications should be the same or a similar drug used for long-acting pain relief. The minimum effective breakthrough pain medication dose should be equivalent to 10% of the patient's total daily narcotic requirements.
  - Keep the regimen as simple as possible. Avoid mixing a variety of analgesic regimens.
  - Always start a bowel regimen when placing a patient on narcotics. See Constipation for more tips.
  - Educate the patient and family about dosing and side effects. Discuss and reassure the patient and family about addiction, tolerance, and physical dependence.
- **Morphine** is the drug of choice for moderate to severe cancer pain. It has a wide range of doses available and flexible methods of delivery. Morphine is available as sustained-release, immediate-release, liquid, and parenteral preparations. The sustained-release tablets may be given per rectum in patients unable to swallow. Oxycodone is available orally as immediate- and sustained-release preparations. Fentanyl is available in the parenteral route, as well as the fentanyl (Duragesic) patch for patients unable to swallow or who cannot tolerate morphine or oxycodone. The patches are applied to the chest wall or back and changed q48–72h. The onset of action in these long-acting preparations is 12 hrs. When starting a patient on long-acting agents, the clinician needs to provide the patient with immediate-relief preparations to use in the interim until the long-acting narcotic can achieve adequate serum levels for analgesia.
- **Meperidine** (Demerol) should be avoided in the chronic pain patient population. Meperidine has a very short half-life of 2–3 hrs. This is ineffective in the management of

TABLE 35-1. EQUIVALENT OPIOID DOSES

	PO (mg)	Parenteral (mg)
Morphine	30–60	10
Hydromorphone	7.5	1.5
Meperidine	300	75
Methadone	20	10
Codeine	180	NA
Oxycodone	20	NA
Fentanyl	NA	0.67

NA, not available.

chronic pain. Meperidine has a toxic metabolite, normeperidine, which is a weaker analgesic but a potent CNS stimulant. Normeperidine has a half-life of 25–30 hrs or longer in the setting of renal failure. This can rapidly lead to the accumulation of the drug when used for more than 48–72 hrs. CNS toxicity can include irritability, tremors, myoclonus, agitation, and seizures. When CNS toxicity occurs, it is important to stop the drug. Naloxone (Narcan) should not be administered. The effects of normeperidine are not reversed with naloxone and can precipitate worsening CNS toxicity.

- **Propoxyphene** (Darvon-N) is another narcotic agent that is ineffective in the chronic pain patient. Despite its widespread use, the drug has no more analgesic properties than ASA (650 mg). Propoxyphene has a long half-life of 6–12 hrs. It also has a toxic metabolite, norpropoxyphene, with a half-life of 30–36 hrs. Norpropoxyphene has been associated with pulmonary edema, cardiotoxicity, and cardiac arrest.

- **IM injections** should be avoided for the management of cancer pain. The use of IM injections is painful, and absorption is unreliable. The onset of action can be 30–60 mins, and this is not acceptable in the acute pain setting. IV or transmucosal routes are much more efficacious at getting rapid onset of action in the acute pain setting. The chronic use of IM injections is associated with abscess formation and soft tissue fibrosis.

- The perception that the administration of opioid analgesics for chronic pain management causes **addiction** is prevalent and is a barrier to adequate pain control. Confusion about the differences between addiction, tolerance, and physical dependence is in part responsible. Addiction is a pattern of drug abuse characterized by drug craving and overwhelming behaviors to obtain the drug. Tolerance is a state in which escalating doses of opioids are needed to achieve pain control as the drug effectiveness reduces over time. Tolerance occurs with all of the side effects of narcotics, with the exception of constipation. It is important to educate patients and family members that tolerance to many of the common side effects, such as itching or sedation, will develop, and the *drug should not be abruptly discontinued*. Physical dependence is the onset of signs and symptoms of withdrawal with abrupt discontinuation of the opioid. Abrupt withdrawal may result in tachycardia, HTN, diaphoresis, nausea, vomiting, abdominal pain, psychosis, and hallucinations. This is not the same as addiction. Physical dependence and addiction are not synonymous. When stopping chronic opioid medications, the dose should be reduced in increments of 50% or more q2–3days to avoid the risk of withdrawal symptoms. Finally, it should be remembered that patients experiencing inadequately controlled pain may engage in what appears to be drug-seeking behavior, which is easy to confuse with addiction.

- **Adjuvant analgesics** can be important in the treatment of cancer pain. Adjuvant analgesics include antidepressants, anticonvulsants, corticosteroids, and local anesthetics. Within the antidepressants, the tricyclics are the most effective as an adjunctive therapy for neuropathic pain. Common side effects from the tricyclics include orthostatic hypotension, sedation, urinary retention, confusion, and sexual dysfunction. Doses of the tricyclic antidepressants should be started low and titrated for analgesia. Anticonvulsants are also helpful adjunctive therapies in the treatment of neuropathic pain syndromes. These drugs include carbamazepine (Tegretol), phenytoin (Dilantin), and gabapentin (Neurontin). A wide variation in dose ranges has been used to obtain a clinical benefit. Side effects of these drugs can be self-limiting, including sedation, confusion, and dizziness. Corticosteroids can be useful in the management of bone metastases, nerve compression, elevated intracranial pressure, and obstruction of a hollow viscus. Local anesthetics, such as nerve blocks, lidocaine patches, and eutectic mixture of local anesthetics (EULA) cream, can aid in the treatment of cancer pain. In extreme cases, IV administration of anesthetics can be used in conjunction with IV or intraspinal narcotics to allow the clinician to administer lower doses of narcotics and spare the patient the complications of sedation seen with high doses of narcotics.

CONSTIPATION

- Constipation should be expected during opioid treatment, and **prophylactic measures** should always be initiated with the start of opioid therapy. Constipation occurs with all opioids, and pharmacologic tolerance rarely develops. Symptoms from constipation may become so severe that patients may decide to discontinue pain medications. This is preventable with the use of an aggressive laxative regimen. Dietary interventions are almost never sufficient to prevent constipation. *Combinations of agents* are often necessary. Clinicians should also avoid the use of bulk-forming agents in the absence of a motility agent, especially in debilitated or anorectic patients. When using these agents, it should be remembered that stool softeners and bulking agents do little to relieve constipation but may make stools more comfortable to pass. Their sole use will only lead to constipation with soft stools, and another agent is necessary for adequate treatment. Also, it should be remembered that the onset of abdominal pain or nausea in a patient taking opioids may be due to unrecognized constipation.

- **Laxatives** can be classified into three categories: stimulant, osmotic, and detergent agents. Clinicians frequently fail to dose-escalate a particular agent, and this can lead to the sense that nothing works. Laxatives can be titrated to a maximal therapeutic dose, but this often leads to taking multiple pills. Clinicians should try to simplify the bowel regimen for improvement in patient compliance.
  - **Stimulant** laxatives irritate the bowel, leading to increased peristaltic activity. These laxatives include
    - Senna, start with 2 tablets qhs, titrated to effect (up to ≥ 9/day, can divide bid)
    - Casanthranol (Black-Draught), start with 2 tablets qhs, titrated to effect (up to ≥ 9/day, can divide bid)
    - Bisacodyl (Dulcolax), 5 mg PO or PR qhs, titrated to effect
  - **Osmotic** laxatives draw water into the bowel lumen and increase the moisture content of the stool. In addition, they add to overall stool volume. These agents include
    - Lactulose, 30 mL PO q4–6h, titrated to effect
    - Sorbitol, 30 mL PO q4–6h, titrated to effect
    - Milk of magnesia, 1–2 tbsps 1–2 times/day
    - Magnesium citrate, 1–2 bottles prn
  - **Detergent** laxatives facilitate the dissolution of fat in water and increase the water content of stool. Theses agents include
    - Docusate sodium or calcium, 1–2 PO qd to bid, titrated to effect
    - Phosphosoda enema, prn
- **Prokinetic agents** such as metoclopramide (Reglan) can increase peristaltic activity and facilitate stool movement. This agent can be used in combination with other laxative agents. Lubricant stimulants and large-volume enemas can also be used but are not recommended for the daily use and prophylaxis from opioid-related constipation. The use of these agents is effective while titrating other laxatives to ensure that the patient is having regular bowel movements.

DIARRHEA

- **Diarrhea** can be defined as stools that are looser than normal and may be increased in numbers over baseline. In cancer patients, getting up to go to the bathroom multiple times day and night can be exhausting. If persistent, diarrhea can lead to dehydration and electrolyte abnormalities that can lead to the need for a hospital admission. Potential causes of diarrhea in the cancer patient can include infections, malabsorption, GI bleeding, medications, chemotherapy, radiation to the abdomen or pelvis, and overflow incontinence.
- Patients should be instructed on the establishment of normal bowel habits. Any change from the normal baseline should be reported to the physician to avoid severe dehydration or electrolyte imbalances. Patients should be counseled on the avoidance of foods containing lactose or other gas-forming foods that can increase abdominal cramping and pain. Another general approach to diarrhea is to increase the bulk of the stools with the addition of psyllium, bran, or pectin. However, sometimes bulk-forming agents can worsen abdominal cramping and bloating.
- For the **medical management** of transient or mild diarrhea, the use of attapulgite (Kaopectate) or bismuth salts (Pepto-Bismol) can be useful. Care should be taken to rule out infectious by checking *Clostridium difficile* toxin before using antiperistal-

tic medications in the setting of recent antibiotic use. Potential infectious workup may include checking for fecal leukocytes, ova and parasites, stool culture, and sensitivity. For more persistent and severe diarrhea, agents that slow down peristalsis are more useful, including

- Loperamide (Imodium), 2–4 mg PO q6h (maximum 8 tablets/day).
- Diphenoxylate/atropine (Lomotil), 2.5–5 mg PO q6h (maximum 8 tablets/day).
- Tincture of opium, 0.7 mL PO q4h and titrated. Belladonna can be added as an antispasmodic agent.
- For **persistent, severe diarrhea**, the patient should be admitted for parenteral fluid support and the initiation of octreotide as shown below:
  - Octreotide (Sandostatin), 50 μg SC q8–12h, then titrated to 500 μg q8h SC or higher. May also be given as a continuous IV infusion, 10–80 μg qh.

NAUSEA AND VOMITING

- Nausea and vomiting are commonly associated with advanced malignancies as a direct result of the disease or as known side effects of chemotherapy and other medications. There are multiple potential causes of nausea and vomiting in the cancer patient. Different etiologies for nausea and vomiting may require different interventions for control of the symptoms.
- **Nausea** is the unpleasant subjective sensation that results from the stimulation of the gastric lining, the chemoreceptor trigger zone in the base of the fourth ventricle, the vestibular apparatus, or the cerebral cortex. The neurochemical stimulation of these areas is mediated through the neurotransmitters serotonin, dopamine, acetylcholine, and histamine. All four neurotransmitters can be found in the chemoreceptor trigger zone. Serotonin plays an important role in nausea caused by stimulation of the lining of the GI tract. Acetylcholine and histamine play an important role in nausea related to the vestibular apparatus. Nausea and vomiting that is mediated by the cerebral cortex is not associated with specific neurotransmitters but is related to learned responses and behaviors, such as anticipatory nausea related to chemotherapy.
- A thorough assessment of nausea and vomiting is important to gain an understanding of potential etiologies and allow for an appropriate choice of antiemetics. A common pneumonic for potential **etiologies** is the "11 M's of emesis": metastases, meningeal irritation, movement, mental anxiety, medications, mucosal irritation, mechanical obstruction, motility, metabolic, microbes, and myocardial. See Table 35-2 for a list of etiologies and effective antiemetic agents.
- **Dopamine antagonists** are one of the most frequently used antiemetics. These medications have the potential to cause sedation and extrapyramidal symptoms. Medication dosing options include
  - Haloperidol (Haldol), PO, IV, SC
  - Prochlorperizine (Compazine), PO, PR, IV
  - Droperidol (Inapsine), IV
  - Promethazine (Phenergan), PO
  - Perphenazine (Trilafon), PO, IV
  - Trimethobenzamide (Tigan), PO, PR
  - Metoclopramide (Reglan), PO, IV
- **Histamine antagonists** may also cause sedation and can have a beneficial effect in some patients. The antihistamines also have the added benefit of anticholinergic properties, which can also be beneficial in patients with dual etiologies of nausea. These drugs include
  - Diphenhydramine (Benadryl), PO, IV
  - Meclizine (Antivert), PO
  - Hydroxyzine (Atarax), PO, IV
- **Scopolamine** (Isopto Hyoscine, Scopace, Transderm Scop) is an anticholinergic agent that is useful to treat nausea induced by the vestibular apparatus. It can also be used adjunctively with other antiemetics in empiric therapy. Scopolamine can be given as a SC or IV scheduled or continuous infusion but is also conveniently available in a transdermal patch.

TABLE 35-2. ETIOLOGY AND MANAGEMENT OF NAUSEA AND VOMITING

Etiology	Therapy
Metastases	
Cerebral (increased ICP)	Steroids, mannitol, anti-DA/Hist
Liver	Anti-DA/Hist
Meningeal irritation	Steroids
Movement	Anti-ACH
Mental anxiety	Anxiolytics
Medications	
Opioids	Anti-DA/Hist, anti-ACH, prokinetic agents, stimulant, laxatives
Chemotherapy	Anti-5HT/DA, steroids
Others	Anti-DA/Hist
Mucosal irritation	
NSAIDs	Cytoprotective agents
Gastroesophageal reflux	Antacids
Mechanical obstruction	
Constipation	Manage constipation
Extraluminal	*Reversible:* surgery
	Irreversible: steroids, scopolamine, inhibit secretions with octreotide
Motility	
Opioids, ileus, others	Prokinetic agents, stimulant laxatives
Metabolic	
Hypercalcemia, hyponatremia, hepatic/renal failure	Anti-DA/Hist, hydration, steroids
Microbes	
Esophagitis (e.g., *Candida*, herpes, CMV)	Antibacterials, antifungals, antivirals
Systemic sepsis	Anti-DA/Hist, other systemic support
Myocardial	Oxygen, opioids, anti-DA/Hist, anxiolytics

Anti-ACH, acetylcholine antagonist; Anti-DA, dopamine antagonist; Anti-Hist, histamine antagonist; Anti-5HT, serotonin antagonist.

- **Serotonin antagonists** have been effective in the treatment of chemotherapy-associated nausea and vomiting. They are also useful for refractory nausea but are typically tried when other medications have failed. The medications available are as follows:
  - Ondansetron (Zofran), PO, IV
  - Granisetron (Kytril), PO, IV
  - Dolasetron (Anzemet), PO, IV
- The use of **dexamethasone** (Decadron), **dronabinol** (Marinol), and **benzodiazepines** is beneficial in some patients, but the mechanism of action remains unclear. Benzodiazepines [i.e., lorazepam (Ativan) in a 1-mg dose] are often useful in conjunction with other classes of antiemetics and may have a synergistic effect.
- Nausea and vomiting from a bowel obstruction can be a challenge to treat, especially when surgery is not an option. **Octreotide** has been shown to effectively inhibit the secretion of fluid into the intestinal lumen and decrease the bloating and abdominal

pain, as well as nausea and vomiting. It may be started by continuous infusion or intermittent SC injection at a dose of 100 μg q8–12h and titrated q24–48h for effect.
- Often, **several classes** of antiemetics may be combined to control nausea and vomiting. For highly emetogenic chemotherapy, such as cisplatin, patients are premedicated with dexamethasone and a serotonin antagonist. Many highly emetogenic chemotherapy agents are also associated with *delayed emesis*, occurring up to 72 hrs after chemotherapy. These patients should be given dexamethasone and a dopamine antagonist to take around the clock for 72 hrs after the infusion.

MUCOSITIS

- **Mucositis** refers to painful inflammation and ulceration of the oral mucosa. Mucositis can result from chemotherapy or radiation therapy. Chemotherapeutic agents that are associated commonly with mucositis include melphalan, methotrexate, etoposide, and vinblastine. Patient factors that can contribute to worsening symptoms include poor-fitting oral prostheses, periodontal disease, and overall poor oral hygiene. Patients should undergo repair of ill-fitting prostheses, tooth extraction, and repair of periodontal disease before the initiation of chemotherapy. In the event that repair cannot be done before chemotherapy, the physician should refer to an oral surgeon once the patient's peripheral blood counts have returned to baseline.
- A **mucositis grading system** allows the physician to assess mucositis severity in terms of both pain and the patient's ability to continue to eat or drink. The grading system established by the National Cancer Institute uses a numbering scale from 0–4, as described.

0	No evidence of mucositis.
1	Nonpainful erythema or ulcers. Able to eat and drink without difficulty.
2	Mildly to moderately painful erythema or ulcers. Still able to eat or drink without difficulty. May require intermittent analgesia.
3	Severe erythema, painful ulcers. Interference with eating and drinking. Requires constant analgesia.
4	Severity of symptoms requires parenteral analgesia and/or nutritional support.

- A **standardized approach** to the prevention and treatment of mucositis is essential to quality care in the oncology patient. The prophylactic measures usually used include mouth rinses with sodium chloride, sodium bicarbonate, or chlorhexidine (Peridex). Regimens commonly used for the treatment of mucositis and the associated pain include a local anesthetic such as lidocaine, magnesium-based antacids (Maalox, Mylanta), diphenhydramine (Benadryl), and an antifungal such as nystatin (Mycostatin) or Mycelex. These agents are used either alone or in equal concentrations in a mouthwash. The patient can use the mouthwash up to 5 times/day for relief. Sucralfate (Carafate) is a cytoprotectant that can also be useful in the treatment of mucositis. In the treatment of severe mucositis, narcotics may need to be used in addition to the agents mentioned earlier.

ANOREXIA AND CACHEXIA

- **Anorexia and cachexia** frequently occur with many malignancies, especially when the disease is advanced. The specific etiologies of these symptoms are not well understood. Anorexia and cachexia are significant causes of distress to the patient and family members. These symptoms typically represent progression of disease and are not reversible with parenteral or enteral nutrition. The clinician should assess for other potential etiologies for the loss of appetite and weight such as dysphagia, odynophagia, infections, or side effects of medications. Some medications may improve appetite and allow the patient to gain weight, although none of these therapies improves survival.

- There are several approaches to the **general management** of anorexia and cachexia. Patients should be offered their favorite foods and nutritional supplements if the patient enjoys them. Any dietary restrictions should be eliminated. Portion sizes can be reduced, and food should be made to look appetizing. Foods that have potent odors should be avoided.
- There are a wide variety of **pharmacologic approaches** to improve appetite. Corticosteroids have an appetite-stimulating effect, as well as effects on the patient's mood and energy level. Dexamethasone (Decadron) in doses of 2–20 mg/day is recommended. Dexamethasone is preferred because of the relative lack of mineralocorticoid effects, but any steroid will be efficacious. Megestrol acetate (Megace) has also been shown to improve appetite in cancer patients. There is a large variation in the effective dose of megestrol acetate between individual patients. One should begin with 200 mg PO q6–8h and titrate up or down to the desired effect. The cannabinoids, such as dronabinol (Marinol), also have been shown to promote weight gain in cancer patients. Clinicians can begin with a small dose and titrate up to the desired effect. Androgens are currently under investigation for their effects on appetite and weight and may be a useful choice in the future.

DYSPNEA

- Dyspnea can be one of the most frightening symptoms to patients and family members. For the majority of patients, relief of dyspnea can be achieved with simple interventions. Measurement of respiratory rate, O_2 saturation, and blood gas levels do not correlate with the patient's subjective report. The clinician must accept the patient's self-report and try to identify and/or correct the underlying etiology of the symptom. In patients with known advanced disease, the burden of investigating the etiology of the dyspnea must be weighed with the limited potential benefit from therapeutic interventions. There are three widely used medical approaches for the symptomatic breathlessness: **O_2, opioids,** and **anxiolytics.**
- A therapeutic trial of **supplemental O_2** may be beneficial, although it has been suggested that there is a placebo effect in nonhypoxemic patients. In addition, the cool air moving across the patient's face from the supplemental O_2 can also have a calming effect and help in relieving the feeling of air hunger. A fan in the room can also help achieve this effect.
- **Opioids** have demonstrated relief in dyspnea without any measurable effect on respiratory rate or blood gas measurements. The precise mechanism by which opioids exert this effect is not known. In an opioid-naïve patient, doses lower than those used to achieve analgesia may be effective. Doses of hydrocodone, 5 mg PO q4h, or codeine, 30 mg PO q2h, can be beneficial in these patients. Other opioids can be useful and administered IV for urgent situations or when the PO route is not available. Patients can be maintained on a fixed schedule of opioid IV q4–6h. An additional dose of a short-acting opioid, equivalent to 30–50% of the amount of baseline opioid taken q4h can be used qh for intermittent periods of worsening dyspnea. Nebulized morphine can also be helpful in the terminal dyspneic patient.
- **Dyspnea** may cause severe anxiety. Some patients with dyspnea may need more effective treatment for their anxiety associated with the symptom. The benzodiazepines are highly effective anxiolytic medications. The benzodiazepines can be used in addition to opioids and other nondrug therapies to reduce dyspnea. Suggested benzodiazepines include lorazepam, diazepam (Valium), clonazepam (Klonopin), and midazolam (Versed). The clinician should begin with low doses and titrate for desired effects.

OTHER ISSUES

- **Depression** occurs in a significant number of cancer patients. Specific problems facing these patients include pain, medication side effects, and changes in functional status. Typical features of major depression may also be present, such as depressed mood for at least 2 wks, feelings of guilt or worthlessness, inability to concentrate, decreased energy, preoccupation with death or suicide, anhedonia, and changes in eating or sleeping habits. Pharmacotherapy and psychotherapy are effective treatments. Psychostimulants (e.g., methylphenidate, 5 mg PO 9 a.m. and noon qd) begin to work within a short period of time. Antidepressants may require up to 2–4 wks before symptoms are alleviated. The selective serotonin reuptake inhibitors (e.g., citalopram, usual dosage range 20–80 mg PO qd), bupropion SR (usual dosage range 200–400 mg PO qd), and mirtazapine (usual dosage range 30–45 mg PO qd; has sedating effects, but may aid those with insomnia) are all reasonable first-line agents. Depression should be screened for and treated in all cancer patients.

- **Anemia** in cancer patients may be due to the effects of their underlying malignancy (particularly when there is bone marrow involvement) and/or treatment. The basic mechanisms involved are decreased erythropoiesis, decreased iron metabolism, and decreased survival time for RBCs. In addition, erythropoietin production may be impaired. Current treatment approaches are targeted at treating the underlying malignancy and boosting red cell mass. Recombinant erythropoietin has been shown to reduce transfusion requirements and improve outcomes in terms of quality of life and response to treatment.

- **Fatigue** and **weakness** are often multifactorial and involve the underlying malignancy and the effects of treatment. Therapy for these symptoms is limited and often unsatisfying. Use of sedating medications should be minimized as much as possible and nutritional, fluid, and electrolyte status closely followed and optimized. Steroids (e.g., Prednisone, 20 mg PO q a.m.) may be a helpful adjunct in the short term, but long-term use is limited by side effects.

- **Insomnia** is often a result of pain, medications, anxiety, or a mood disorder. Proper sleep hygiene and adequate management of pain and other symptoms are beneficial. In addition, the use of benzodiazepines (e.g., lorazepam, 0.5–2 mg PO qhs) or antidepressants with sedating effects (e.g., trazodone, 50 mg PO qhs, or amitriptyline, 25–50 mg PO qhs) may be used in conjunction with the nonpharmacologic measures.

- **Hospice** and **palliative care** are essential considerations for any patient with a limited life expectancy of approximately 6 mos or less. Please see Chap. 15, Introduction and Approach to Oncology or the National Hospice and Palliative Care Organization (http://www.nhpco.org/) for more information.

KEY POINTS TO REMEMBER

- Pain is a common complaint in cancer patients, occurring in 50–70% of patients. More than one-half of these patients do not get adequate pain relief.
- The WHO recommends the use of an analgesic ladder based on pain severity in the approach to the selection of opioids to treat cancer pain.
- When starting off with narcotics to manage chronic pain, start with one drug at the lowest effective dose and titrate the drug to pain relief. Sustained-release preparations are extremely useful in the management of chronic pain.
- Breakthrough medications should be offered to all patients on chronic analgesics for acute situations. The minimum effective dose should be equivalent to 10% of the total daily narcotic intake.
- Educating the patient and family members about addiction, tolerance, and physical dependence can lead to more effective pain management and avoid situations in which patients may discontinue the medications and precipitate withdrawal symptoms.
- Meperidine and propoxyphene are not effective narcotic analgesics in chronic pain patients owing to toxic metabolites and potential severe adverse side effects.
- Constipation should always be expected during opioid therapy, and prophylactic laxatives and/or stool softeners should be started with the initiation of narcotic medications.
- Nausea and vomiting are commonly associated with advanced malignancies for a variety of reasons. Effective medications are now available to decrease the morbidity associated with these symptoms.
- A standardized approach to the prevention and treatment of mucositis is essential to the quality care of the oncology patient.

- Diarrhea can be debilitating in an oncology patient. Patient education and management with antidiarrheal agents is most often effective to prevent patients from requiring hospitalization for severe dehydration or electrolyte imbalances.
- Anorexia and cachexia are frequent symptoms of advanced malignancies. Some drugs, such as dexamethasone or megestrol acetate, can assist in improving appetite, but, most often, education of the patient and family members is most beneficial.
- O_2, opioids, and anxiolytics can be useful in the relief of dyspnea in the terminal patient.
- Other issues such as depression, anemia, fatigue and weakness, and insomnia should be screened for in cancer patients and appropriately treated to improve symptoms and quality of life.
- Hospice and palliative care options should be discussed with the patient and family when life expectancy is limited.

REFERENCES AND SUGGESTED READINGS

Bonica JJ, Ventafridda V, Twycross RG. Cancer pain. In: Bonica JJ, ed. *The management of pain*, 2nd ed. Philadelphia: Lea & Febiger, 1990:400–460.

Cancer pain. In: National Comprehensive Cancer Network Practice Guidelines in Oncology. 2001:1. Available at: http://www.nccn.org. Accessed May 2003.

Emanuel LL, von Gunten CF, Ferris FD, eds. *The Education for Physicians on End-of-Life Care (EPEC) curriculum: common physical symptoms.* Copyright EPEC Project, The Robert Wood Johnson Foundation, 1999.

Grunberg SM, Hesketh PJ. Control of chemotherapy-induced emesis. *N Engl J Med* 1993;329:1790–1796.

Levy MH. Drug therapy: pharmacologic treatment of cancer pain. *N Engl J Med* 1996;335:1124–1132.

Martin LA, Hagen NA. Neuropathic pain in cancer patients: mechanisms, syndromes, and clinical controversies. *J Pain Symp Manag* 1997;14:99–117.

Rogakos J, Boyer S. Psychiatric disorders. In: Lin, Rypkema, eds. *The Washington manual of ambulatory therapeutics.* Philadelphia: Lippincott Williams & Wilkins, 2002.

Schultz MZ. Oncology and palliative care. In: Lin, Rypkema, eds. *The Washington manual of ambulatory therapeutics.* Philadelphia: Lippincott Williams & Wilkins, 2002:344–358.

Oncologic Emergencies

Judah D. Friedman

INTRODUCTION

Emergencies in the care of the oncology patient are fairly rare but require prompt attention to avoid morbidity and mortality. Patients may need to be followed in an intensive care setting until the acute issue is resolved. They primarily result from pressure or obstruction by space-occupying lesions, metabolic abnormalities, or cytopenic complications.

PERICARDIAL EFFUSION AND TAMPONADE

- Patients typically present with **symptoms** of dyspnea, tachypnea, cough, chest pain, orthopnea, and weakness. Also, often present are jugular venous distention, systemic hypotension, and dulled heart tones. If the effusion rapidly accumulates, there may be profound hypotension along with agitation and confusion. In cases of slow accumulation, fatigue and peripheral edema may be the only symptoms present. Other manifestations include sinus tachycardia, pulsus paradoxus, and hepatomegaly.
- **Pericardial effusion** is frequently caused by malignancy or therapies used to treat it. At autopsy, approximately 5–10% of patients with cancer have malignant pericardial disease. Breast and lung tumors spread locally. Lymphomas involving the mediastinum can involve the pericardium, whereas leukemias can infiltrate the myocardium, resulting in a small pericardial effusion. Most pericardial effusions are asymptomatic. Tumors in the pericardial space can, however, cause bleeding, resulting in much more rapidly accumulating effusions than in exudative or transudative processes. Radiation and drug-induced effusion, hypothyroidism, autoimmune disorders, infection, and idiopathic pericardial disease are part of the differential in a patient presenting with effusion.
- Other pathologic entities may present with similar symptoms in the cancer patient. Cardiotoxicity leading to **congestive heart failure** can result from drugs (anthracyclines such as doxorubicin, trastuzumab, 5-fluorouracil, cyclophosphamide) and radiation-induced heart disease (especially seen in mediastinal radiation for non-Hodgkin's lymphoma and Hodgkin's lymphoma and left breast radiation for breast cancer). Consider other causes of cardiovascular emergencies in the cancer patient, such as coronary artery disease, heart failure, and infective endocarditis.

Diagnosis

On chest x-ray, if >250 cc has accumulated, the cardiac silhouette is enlarged in a globular, symmetric fashion. It may also reveal signs of pulmonary congestion and/or pleural effusions if heart failure is present. ECG can reveal reduced voltage or, with very large effusions, electrical alternans. Echocardiography is the diagnostic test of choice and should be ordered emergently whenever the diagnosis of tamponade is suspected. It will diagnose the effusion and indicate the degree of hemodynamic compromise. Early signs include right atrial collapse and left atrial and/or right ventricular collapse.

Management

With severe hemodynamic compromise, emergent **pericardiocentesis** by a percutaneous, subxiphoid approach should be performed. Giving a **rapid IV fluid bolus and inotropics** can be a temporizing measure to support BP until echocardiographic guidance is available, as this method is much safer than a "blind" approach. Drains or a pericardial window may be necessary. To prevent recurrence, sclerosing agents such as thiotepa are available but are often less effective than a **surgical pericardial window.** However, small asymptomatic effusions may be observed without therapy.

SUPERIOR VENA CAVA SYNDROME

- Superior vena cava syndrome (SVCS) is a result of **compression of the SVC.** Patients typically present with swelling of the neck, face, and upper extremities. Jugular venous distention, cyanosis, and facial plethora may also be observed. Shortness of breath, dizziness, and, rarely, obtundation from cerebral edema are observed if the onset is rapid. Vocal cord paralysis and Horner's syndrome are possible if neural structures are invaded. With slowly progressive obstruction, collateral flow has time to develop, and symptoms related to vascular obstruction may be milder.
- **Bronchogenic carcinoma** and **lymphoma** are the most common causes (95%), although SVCS has been reported in breast cancer as well. Small cell is the most common histologic type of bronchogenic carcinoma, as it arises from the central and perihilar areas of the lung and can enlarge rapidly. **Thrombosis of the SVC** in patients with central venous catheters is an increasingly common cause of an SVC-like syndrome. Other causes of SVCS include granulomatous infections, goiter, aortic aneurysms, and fibrosing mediastinitis.

Diagnosis

CT scan with IV contrast shows reduced or absent opacification of central venous structures with prominent collateral venous circulation. **Chest radiograph** may show widened superior mediastinum and pleural effusions. There is no advantage of MRI over CT. A diagnosis of the mass should be attempted before treatment is begun if the tissue type of tumor is unknown. Sputum cytology, biopsy of lymph nodes, bronchoscopy, thoracentesis, and occasionally mediastinoscopy or thoracotomy can be diagnostic.

Management

Measures including a low-salt diet, head elevation, and oxygen can be temporizing. Diuretics and corticosteroids are often used for treatment at presentation, although corticosteroids are more helpful in SVCS caused by lymphoma. If compression is not life threatening, then diagnosis should be made before beginning treatment. **Radiation therapy** is useful for non–small cell carcinoma and other metastatic solid tumors. Chemotherapy is more useful in small cell lung cancer and lymphoma owing to their exquisite sensitivity. SVCS resulting from catheter-related thrombus is treated by anticoagulation and, in limited cases, fibrinolysis. Other treatment approaches include an interventional radiology procedure, such as PTCA or stent placement.

ACUTE TUMOR LYSIS SYNDROME

The acute tumor lysis syndrome (ATLS) patient presents with rapid development of hyperuricemia, hyperphosphatemia, hyperkalemia, lactic acidosis, and hypocalcemia. Frequently, this results in oliguria from acute renal failure. This usually happens in the setting of therapy of a rapidly growing tumor. It results from the release of intracellular products by rapidly dividing tumor cells or by the **lysis** of radiosensitive or chemosensitive tumor cells **during therapy.** The most common metabolic abnormalities include an acute rise in BUN and serum phosphorus levels in association with hypocalcemia and increases in lactate dehydrogenase. Acute renal failure develops from precipitation of uric acid and calcium phosphate crystals in the renal tubules.

TABLE 36-1. RISK FACTORS FOR TUMOR LYSIS SYNDROME

Patients at risk for acute tumor lysis syndrome

Tumor type

Burkitt's lymphoma

Lymphoblastic lymphoma

Undifferentiated lymphoma

Diffuse large-cell lymphoma

Leukemias

Extent of disease

Bulky retroperitoneal or intraabdominal tumors; mediastinal mass

Elevated lactate dehydrogenase

Elevated WBC count

Patients at risk for renal failure

Preexisting renal failure

Oliguria

Acute renal failure posttransplant

Adapted from Lake DE, Hudis C, eds. *Semin Oncol* 2000;27:243–383.

ATLS may occur spontaneously or during chemotherapy or radiation of hematologic neoplasms. See Table 36-1.

Management

- The best management of ATLS includes the identification of patients at risk for ATLS and taking preventive measures.
- **IV hydration** should occur 24–48 hrs before initiation of chemotherapy (4–5 L/day) and during therapy. Consider using IV furosemide (Lasix) to improve urine flow rate. Electrolytes, uric acid, BUN, creatinine, phosphorus, calcium, and magnesium should be measured twice a day or more often if ATLS develops.
- **Hyperkalemia** should be treated with standard therapy: glucose and insulin (acutely), sodium-potassium exchange resins, and IV calcium if ECG changes are noted.
- Control **hyperuricemia** with allopurinol (Zyloprim) (600–900 mg/day PO). Initiate allopurinol before chemotherapy in patients with preexisting hyperuricemia or in those at high risk for ATLS. If the patient is still hyperuricemic, consider alkalinization of the urine with the addition of 50–100 mEq of $NaHCO_3$ to each L of IV fluid, and if still refractory, add acetazolamide (Diamox), 250–500 mg IV daily.
- **Do not** administer IV calcium for **hypocalcemia** unless evidence for neuromuscular irritability (Chvostek or Trousseau sign is present). With a high serum phosphate level, IV calcium may result in metastatic calcification.
- In the setting of **hyperphosphatemia,** initiate glucose and insulin therapy and PO antacids (phosphate binders). Finally, **consider dialysis** in patients with poor renal function or metabolic abnormalities not corrected by conservative measures.

HYPERCALCEMIA OF MALIGNANCY

Hypercalcemia is the most common paraneoplastic syndrome, seen in 10–20% of patients with cancer. Lung, breast, head and neck, kidney, and multiple myeloma are most often associated with hypercalcemia. Most common, metastases and cytokines activate osteoclasts. Also, ectopically produced parathormone-related protein stimulates osteoclasts bone resorption and renal tubular calcium retention, resulting in hypercalcemia. Hypercalcemia causes a renal parenchymal damage and may cause a nephrogenic diabetes insipidus, resulting in volume depletion. Presentation is nonspecific, with fatigue, anorexia, constipation, polydipsia, and nausea and vomiting, along with lethargy and apathy. Hypercalcemia can produce a brisk diuresis, and patients are often severely volume depleted. In severe cases, mental status alterations, seizures, and coma can be seen.

Management

Management includes obtaining an ionized calcium level or an albumin level to correct for hypoalbuminemia (frequently seen in cancer patients). Serum intact PTH levels are suppressed. The acute treatment of hypercalcemia **begins with IV fluids** (4–8 L). This should be run at 300–500 mL/hr and decreased after the extracellular volume deficit is partially corrected. At least 3–4 L should be given in the first 24 hrs, and a positive fluid balance of at least 2 L should be achieved. Further saline diuresis (100–200 mL/hr) will aid in calcium excretion. Serum electrolytes, including Ca and Mg should be measure q6–12hrs and K and Mg replaced adequately. Lasix should be avoided except in the setting of heart failure. Although toxicity limits their use, **glucocorticoids** (e.g., prednisone, initial dose 20–50 mg PO bid) may be effective in hypercalcemia that is due to some hematologic malignancies and myeloma. Results may take up to 10 days. In addition, oral phosphate may be considered if serum phosphorous level is low and the patient has normal renal function. Dialysis is effective if other treatments fail. Bisphosphonates, which inhibit bone resorption, are standard for treatment of hypercalcemia, but take days for full effect. **Pamidronate** (Aredia), 60 mg for moderate hypercalcemia (12–13.5 mg/dL) and 90 mg for severe hypercalcemia (>13.5 mg/dL), is infused over 4–24 hrs. Pamidronate must be given q2–3wks to avoid recurrence of hypercalcemia. Other drugs rarely used, mostly in hypercalcemia refractory to bisphosphonates, include calcitonin, gallium nitrate, and plicamycin (mithramycin).

SIADH AND HYPONATREMIA

SIADH is seen most commonly in oat cell bronchogenic carcinoma and use of morphine, vincristine sulfate (Oncovin), and cyclophosphamide (Cytoxan). Patients with SIADH and hyponatremia may present with complaints of anorexia and nausea. With rapid and severe decline in serum sodium concentrations, they may also present with confusion, coma, and seizures. Look for decreased serum osmolarity (<280 mOsm/L) and urine that is not maximally dilute (>75–100 mOsm/L). In addition to the previously mentioned, the diagnosis of SIADH requires absence of hypervolemic states (manifest by ascites, edema) and absence of volume contraction, along with normal thyroid, renal, and adrenal functions. Acute management includes IV normal saline or, in more severe cases, 3% sodium chloride (which should typically *only* be given with the assistance of those skilled in its use, such as a nephrologist). Allow only 1–1.5 mEq/L/hr of correction for the first 3–4 hrs and 0.5 mEq/L/hr thereafter to avoid *demyelination* syndromes. Furosemide may aid in free water loss when given with saline. Demeclocycline (Declomycin) is useful in long-term therapy.

EPIDURAL SPINAL CORD COMPRESSION

- **Epidural spinal cord compression,** occurring in 5% of cancer patients, is one of the most common neurologic emergencies. *If caught early when pain is the only symptom, the patient can be spared significant disability.* The thecal sac is compressed by tumor in the epidural space at the level of the spinal cord or cauda equina. Any malignancy can produce epidural compression with prostate, lung, and breast being the most common. The thoracic spine is the most common location, followed by the lumbosacral and then the cervical spine. Compression occurs by either direct extension from metastases in the vertebral bone or by tumor growth through the intervertebral foramina. On occasion, tumor can metastasize directly to the epidural space.
- **Back pain** is the first symptom in 96% of patients. The pain localizes in the back, near the midline, frequently accompanied by referred or radicular pain. The pain, unlike

the pain of a herniated disk, may be exacerbated by recumbency and improved by the upright position. It can be exacerbated by movement, Valsalva, straight leg raise, and neck flexion. Weakness and sensory impairment may follow from hours to months after the onset of pain. Regardless of the spinal compression site, weakness tends to begin in the legs and is more marked proximally than distally early in the course. The weakness can progress to **paraplegia** and can occasionally develop abruptly without prior clinical signs. Sensory complaints range from paresthesias to loss of sensation. Autonomic dysfunction, including impotence or bowel and bladder dysfunction, occurs late and is never the sole presenting symptom. Ataxia has also been reported.

Diagnosis

Diagnosis is made by MRI. **The entire spine should be imaged because of the high incidence of asymptomatic multilevel disease.** Myelography is necessary for those patients with contraindications for MRI. Consider other causes of spinal cord dysfunction, such as myelopathy, intramedullary metastases, hematoma, or abscess. Lumbar puncture to search for additional causes should not be performed until spinal cord compression is excluded.

Management

Immediate neurosurgical consultation and initial treatment involves a high dose of dexamethasone (Decadron), to be given **before** any imaging is obtained. Initially, a dose of 100 mg is followed by 25 mg q4–6hrs. This is usually followed by fractionated external beam radiation therapy (approximately 3,000 cGy over 10–20 fractions over 2–4 wks). The use of laminectomy and vertebral body resection are less common and still undefined.

OTHER NEUROLOGIC EMERGENCIES

- Raised intracerebral pressure and cerebral herniation (from brain metastases, hemorrhage, venous sinus thrombosis, meningitis, head trauma, infarction, abscess). The patient should be stabilized, and maneuvers to lower intracranial pressures such as hyperventilation and IV mannitol or dexamethasone should be attempted. A head CT scan can aid in determining whether surgery is indicated.
- Status epilepticus (from brain metastases, metabolic derangement, neurotoxicity of cancer therapy). Ensuring an airway and proper resuscitation should be first and foremost. Lab studies such as glucose, electrolytes, Ca, Mg, serum and urine toxicology screens, serum alcohol level, CBC, UA, and any pertinent medication levels may be obtained. IV benzodiazepines, phenytoin, and barbiturates are used in the treatment of status epilepticus. If the patient does not have IV access, benzodiazepines are also available in the rectal, IM, or intranasal formulations.
- Intracerebral hemorrhage (from metastatic tumor, thrombocytopenia, and leukostasis). Headache, vomiting, and mental status changes are indicators of significantly increased intracranial pressure and hemorrhage. Workup should include imaging with a stat head CT scan and possibly an LP. Therapy largely focuses on a gradual decrease in blood pressure, supportive care, and surgical consultation when appropriate.

PATHOLOGIC FRACTURES

Pathologic fractures are defined as fractures occurring in diseased bone. Breast, prostate, kidney, and lung are the more common carcinomas to metastasize to bone and potentially cause fracture. A majority of patients have multiple metastatic lesions. Symptoms are of new-onset bone pain in patients with history of a primary carcinoma. In the management of the pathologic fracture, consider life expectancy, as most fractures are best treated surgically with internal fixation. IV narcotics and fracture immobilization control pain and bleeding. Consultation with orthopedics is necessary. Hip and femur fractures will require traction, whereas casts or splints may be used for distal fractures. Radiographs of the region in two planes are needed. A bone scan may be obtained to locate occult lesions. Radiographs of involved bones may identify other areas of impending fracture. Both the pathologic fracture and impending fractures could thus be repaired during one surgery.

INFECTIOUS COMPLICATIONS

Neutropenic Fever

Neutropenic fever is one of the most common complications of chemotherapy. Risk of infection is slightly increased with granulocyte counts <1000/μL, markedly increased with granulocytes <500/μL, and highest <100/μL. 80% of infections in the neutropenic patient originate from the patient's own flora, with 75% of all septicemias caused by gram-negative organisms. However, as many neutropenic patients also have long-term vascular access in place, these are common sources as well. Likely microbes include either gram-positive (*Staphylococcus, Streptococcus*) or gram-negative aerobes (*Escherichia coli, Klebsiella pneumonia, Pseudomonas aeruginosa*).

Neutropenic fever is defined as a **temperature >38°C** in patients with an **absolute neutrophil count <1000/μL.** Indicators of infections, such as exudate, erythema, or warmth, may not be evident because of the reduced numbers of neutrophils. Pneumonias may only be evident by rales, and an infiltrate on chest x-ray may be lacking. Physical exam should focus on the skin, ocular fundus, sinuses, CNS, pelvis, and rectum.

Management

- Management includes searching for a **source of infection** by obtaining two sets of blood cultures, one set from any indwelling intravascular catheter. Sputum, urine, stool cultures, and chest x-ray should also be obtained. Lumbar puncture is not indicated unless clinical signs of meningitis are present, as neutropenia does not predispose to meningitis. In addition, lumbar puncture in the setting of thrombocytopenia can be dangerous.
- Antimicrobial therapy should not await diagnostic tests, as patients can die of gram-negative sepsis in a matter of hours after their first fever, despite appearing well at initial presentation. **Empiric antimicrobial therapy in neutropenic fever:**
  1. Start: antipseudomonal beta-lactam/aminoglycoside. May use single agent such as cefepime (2 g IV q8h in patients with normal renal function) depending on local sensitivities.
  2. If still febrile after 3 days of treatment: add vancomycin (1 g IV q12h in normal renal function or adjust based on trough levels).
  3. If still febrile after 5–7 days: add amphotericin B (starting at 0.5 mg/kg IV qd and can titrate up to 1 mg/kg IV qd as tolerated). Liposomal formulations may also be used and are often better tolerated.
- The above are only general guidelines. If penicillin allergic, consider substituting a fluoroquinolone. If contraindications to aminoglycosides are present, substitute a fluoroquinolone or aztreonam (Azactam). One should consider using vancomycin (Vancocin) as initial therapy in addition to the previously mentioned antibiotics if the patient is hypotensive, has severe mucositis, is colonized with methicillin-resistant *Staphylococcus aureus*, or has signs of obvious catheter infection. Antibacterial choice may vary depending on organisms and resistance patterns at particular hospitals or communities. Always consider other causes of fever in the febrile neutropenic, such as thrombosis. The role of colony-stimulating factors in neutropenic fever is still not clear, but administration should be considered in critically ill patients. Antimicrobials should be continued until neutrophil count rises above 500/mm^3. Changes in empiric therapy should be based on clinical situation but is rarely solely due to persistent fever. Other precautions, such as visitor screening, hand-washing, and proper isolation measures, should be maintained during this period.

KEY POINTS TO REMEMBER

- The amount of disability after treatment of spinal cord compression is directly related to both the pre-event level of function and swiftness of diagnosis. When suspected, liberally use MRI to diagnose, and image the entire spine.
- Give steroids for suspected spinal cord compression before awaiting the results of imaging studies.
- Antimicrobial therapy for neutropenic fever must start immediately with broad-spectrum gram-negative agents before any test results are back.
- The initial treatment of both hypercalcemia and tumor lysis syndrome includes IV fluids.

REFERENCES AND SUGGESTED READINGS

Brigden ML. Hematologic and oncological emergencies: doing the most good in the least time. *Postgrad Med* 2001;109(3):143–163.

Lake DE, Hudis C, eds. *Semin Oncol* 2000;27:243–383.

Mortimer JE, Brown R. Medical management of malignant disease. In: Ahya, Flood, Paranjothi, eds. *The Washington manual of medical therapeutics*, 30th ed. Philadelphia: Lippincott Williams & Wilkins, 2001:429–454.

Murphy GP, Lawrence W Jr, Lenhard RE Jr, eds. *American Cancer Society textbook of clinical oncology*, 2nd ed. Atlanta: American Cancer Society, 1995:597–618.

Singer, GG. Fluid and electrolyte management. In: Ahya, Flood, Paranjothi, eds. *The Washington manual of medical therapeutics*, 30th ed. Philadelphia: Lippincott Williams & Wilkins, 2001:43-78.

Yamada KA, Awadalla S. Neurologic disorders. In: Ahya, Flood, Paranjothi, eds. *The Washington manual of medical therapeutics*, 30th ed. Philadelphia: Lippincott Williams & Wilkins, 2001:516–535.

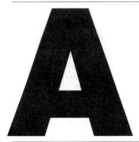

Commonly Used Opioid Analgesics for Chronic Pain

Generic name	Trade name(s) and formulations[a]	Recommended dosing interval
Morphine		
Sustained release	MS Contin, 15, 30, 60, 100, 200 mg	q12h
	Oramorph SR, 15, 30, 60, 100 mg	q12h
	Kadian, 20, 50, 100 mg	q12–24h
	MSIR tablets, 5, 15 mg	q3–4h
Short acting	Roxanol, 20 mg/mL elixir	q2–4h
	Various elixirs, 1, 2, 20 mg/mL	
Oxycodone		
Sustained release	Oxycontin, 10, 20, 40, 80 mg	q12h
Short acting	OxyIR or Roxicodone tablets, 5, 10 mg	q3–4h
	Roxicodone elixir, 5 mg/mL	
	Oxyfast elixir, 20 mg/mL	q2–4h
With APAP	Tablets, mg oxycodone/mg APAP	
	Percocet, 2.5/325	
	Percocet, 5/325	
	Percocet, 7.5/500	
	Percocet, 10/650	
	Roxicet, 5/325 or 5/500	
	Tylox, 5/325	
	Elixir, mg oxycodone/mg APAP	
	Roxicet, 5/325/5 mL	
Codeine	Various	q4–6h
	Tablets, 15, 30, 60 mg	
	Elixir, 15 mg/5 mL	
With APAP	Tablets, mg codeine/mg APAP	q4–6h
	Tylenol #2, 15/325	
	Tylenol #3, 30/325	
	Tylenol #4, 60/325	
Hydrocodone, with APAP	Vicodin, Lortab (5 mg hydrocodone/325 mg APAP)	q4–6h
Hydromorphone	Dilaudid	q3–4h
	Tablets, 1, 2, 3, 4, 8 mg	
	Elixir, 5 mg/mL	
	Suppository, 3 mg	

(continued)

Generic name	Trade name(s) and formulations[a]	Recommended dosing interval
Meperidine	Demerol	Not recommended for chronic pain
Fentanyl		
Transdermal	Duragesic patch, 25, 50, 75, 100 μg/hr	q72h
Transmucosal	Actiq oralet (lollipop), 200, 300, 400 μg	q2h
Methadone	Various	q8h
	Tablets, 5, 10, 40 mg	
	Elixir, 5 mg/5 mL, 10 mg/5 mL, 5 mg/ mL, 10 mg/mL	

APAP, acetaminophen.

[a]The most frequently prescribed brands and formulations are listed. This is not a comprehensive list.

From Schultz MZ. Oncology and palliative care. In: Lin TL, Rypkema SW, eds. *The Washington manual of ambulatory therapeutics*. Philadelphia: Lippincott Williams & Wilkins, 2002:355, with permission.

Index

Page numbers followed by *f* refer to figures; page numbers followed by *t* refer to tables.

Notes

Notes

Notes

Notes